D1233801

Remembering the AIDS Quilt

RHETORIC AND PUBLIC AFFAIRS SERIES

- *Eisenhower's War of Words: Rhetoric and Leadership,* Martin J. Medhurst, editor
- *The Nuclear Freeze Campaign: Rhetoric and Foreign Policy in the Telepolitical Age,* J. Michael Hogan
- *Mansfield and Vietnam: A Study in Rhetorical Adaptation,* Gregory A. Olson
- *Truman and the Hiroshima Cult,* Robert P. Newman
- *Post-Realism: The Rhetorical Turn in International Relations,* Francis A. Beer and Robert Hariman, editors
- *Rhetoric and Political Culture in Nineteenth-Century America,* Thomas W. Benson, editor
- *Frederick Douglass: Freedom's Voice, 1818–1845,* Gregory P. Lampe
- *Angelina Grimké: Rhetoric, Identity, and the Radical Imagination,* Stephen Howard Browne
- *Strategic Deception: Rhetoric, Science, and Politics in Missile Defense Advocacy,* Gordon R. Mitchell
- *Rostow, Kennedy, and the Rhetoric of Foreign Aid,* Kimber Charles Pearce
- *Visions of Poverty: Welfare Policy and Political Imagination,* Robert Asen
- *General Eisenhower: Ideology and Discourse,* Ira Chernus
- *The Reconstruction Desegregation Debate: The Politics of Equality and the Rhetoric of Place, 1870–1875,* Kirt H. Wilson
- *Shared Land/Conflicting Identity: Trajectories of Israeli and Palestinian Symbol Use,* Robert C. Rowland and David A. Frank
- *Darwinism, Design, and Public Education,* John Angus Campbell and Stephen C. Meyer, editors
- *Religious Expression and the American Constitution,* Franklyn S. Haiman
- *Christianity and the Mass Media in America: Toward a Democratic Accommodation,* Quentin J. Schultze

- *Bending Spines: The Propagandas of Nazi Germany and the German Democratic Republic,* Randall L. Bytwerk
- *Malcolm X: Inventing Radical Judgment,* Robert E. Terrill
- *Metaphorical World Politics,* Francis A. Beer and Christ'l De Landtsheer, editors
- *The Lyceum and Public Culture in the Nineteenth-Century United States,* Angela G. Ray
- *The Political Style of Conspiracy: Chase, Sumner, and Lincoln,* Michael William Pfau
- *The Character of Justice: Rhetoric, Law, and Politics in the Supreme Court Confirmation Process,* Trevor Parry-Giles
- *Rhetorical Vectors of Memory in National and International Holocaust Trials,* Marouf A. Hasian Jr.
- *Judging the Supreme Court: Constructions of Motives in Bush v. Gore,* Clarke Rountree
- *Everyday Subversion: From Joking to Revolting in the German Democratic Republic,* Kerry Kathleen Riley
- *In the Wake of Violence: Image and Social Reform,* Cheryl R. Jorgensen-Earp
- *Rhetoric and Democracy: Pedagogical and Political Practices,* Todd F. McDorman and David M. Timmerman, editors
- *Invoking the Invisible Hand: Social Security and the Privatization Debates,* Robert Asen
- *With Faith in the Works of Words: The Beginnings of Reconciliation in South Africa, 1985–1995,* Erik Doxtader
- *Public Address and Moral Judgment: Critical Studies in Ethical Tensions,* Shawn J. Parry-Giles and Trevor Parry-Giles, editors
- *Executing Democracy: Capital Punishment and the Making of America, 1683–1807,* Stephen John Hartnett
- *Enemyship: Democracy and Counter-Revolution in the Early Republic,* Jeremy Engels

Remembering the AIDS Quilt

EDITED BY

Charles E. Morris III

MICHIGAN STATE UNIVERSITY PRESS • *East Lansing*

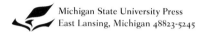
Michigan State University Press
East Lansing, Michigan 48823-5245

Printed and bound in the United States of America.

17 16 15 14 13 12 11   1 2 3 4 5 6 7 8 9 10

LIBRARY OF CONGRESS CATALOGING-IN-PUBLICATION DATA
Remembering the AIDS quilt / edited by Charles E. Morris III.
p. cm. — (Rhetoric and public affairs series)
Includes bibliographical references and index.
ISBN 978-1-61186-007-8 (cloth : alk. paper)
1. AIDS (Disease) and the arts. 2. Social movements. 3. Community arts projects. 4. Persuasion (Rhetoric)
I. Morris, Charles E., 1969–
NX180.A36R46 2011
362.196'979200973–dc22
2010052286

Cover art is "AIDS Quilt—The First Year" © 1991 and is used by permission of the artist, Lola Flash.
Cover design by Erin Kirk New
Book design and typography by Charlie Sharp, Sharp Des!gns, Lansing, Michigan

green press initiative Michigan State University Press is a member of the Green Press Initiative and is committed to developing and encouraging ecologically responsible publishing practices. For more information about the Green Press Initiative and the use of recycled paper in book publishing, please visit *www.greenpressinitiative.org*.

Visit Michigan State University Press on the World Wide Web at *www.msupress.msu.edu*

Contents

Acknowledgments

This project began here in the South End over Sunday morning coffee in November 2005, although the NAMES Project AIDS Quilt has long had a recurrent role in my personal and professional life, from my coming out in 1992 through dozens of seminar conversations in Granville, Nashville, and Boston. It has been a privilege and an honor to edit first the special issue in *Rhetoric and Public Affairs* and then this volume, both of which in some small way I hope will extend engagement with and deepen commitment to those brilliantly embodied—and those strikingly not embodied—in the Quilt, and all those past, present, and future transformed by, lost to, and struggling against AIDS.

That this project came to fruition has everything to do with Martin Medhurst, editor of *Rhetoric and Public Affairs* and the series bearing the same name at Michigan State University Press, and to the talented and dedicated contributors of the essays herein. Marty answered my email and endorsed my pitch in ninety minutes flat, and his support throughout has been enthusiastic and meaningful. As those who know us both can confirm, it would be an understatement to say that Marty and I see and move through the world in different ways. But over more than a decade we have more than discovered common ground, and Marty has taught me much about the meaning of goodwill and generosity of spirit. My friends and colleagues featured in these pages enriched this project—intellectually, emotionally, and politically—with their manifold presence. As you will see, their work graces the Quilt by its moving commemoration and insightful critique.

Many thanks to the staff at Michigan State University Press, especially Kristine Blakeslee and Annette Tanner, whose patience and skill have been much appreciated during the production phase of this project. Martha Bates, in particular, has been a friend to this book, and a delightful fellow traveler. Thanks as well to the staff of the NAMES Project for their assistance and support.

I am grateful to the anonymous reviewers for their thoughtful and helpful feedback. I am grateful, too, for experiencing years of the transformative engagement of Quilt panels and scholarship, Cleve Jones's memoir, and a number of documentaries with so many of my students. I will never forget reading names aloud with them on the campus lawn at Vanderbilt, or the tears in the eyes of the four straight boys who sat with me in Gasson Hall at Boston College watching *Common Threads*—and the many stories of witness that emerged from all those experiences. I strongly believe that the Quilt has induced both mourning and activism among the undergraduates I have taught.

I would never complete any project were it not for the many wonderful people in my world who generously offer ongoing intellectual stimulation and cocktail dish, political comradeship and encouragement, love and friendship, and who abide my ever-increasing idiosyncrasies. Among so many, especially beloved are Rob Asen, Dan Brouwer, Mary Kate Morris, Chuck Morris, Ginny Morris, Jackie Childress, David Morris, Shea Doyle, Tom Nakayama, Andrew Hansen, Jason Black, Dale Herbeck, and Pam Lannutti, who during this book's creation and beyond have constituted my lodestar and laughter, my inspiration and indulgence, my prodding and patience. During the course of this project I lost two from that group who are dearest to me, Virginia Blanck Moore and Alex Hivoltze-Jimenez.

Marvelous muses were they; my work will always bear their inscription. So much, it turns out—and as this book attests—can be measured and forged by profound loss.

Finally, I offer my greatest thanks, accompanied by my deepest love, to Scott Rose, my Gatto, who is my partner, my mainstay, my *sine qua non*. After more than seventeen years, our crazy quilt of a life together continues to amaze and comfort us, a very queer collaboration. I dedicate my labor in this book to my beautiful, darling boy, Augustine, our feline familiar who left us against his and our wills in September 2009. Augustine is now waiting for us with our Ophelia at the limen, apparently a gay bar called the "Rainbow Bridge."

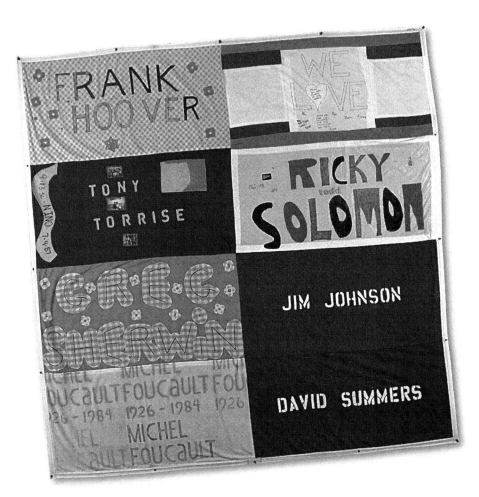

A Vision of the Quilt

Cleve Jones

After eight months on Maui I was back in the Castro. I had no job, no money, and was sleeping on a friend's couch (Jim Foster had taken me in). But I had a plan. I'd written a speech that I hoped would reignite the will to fight. I would give my speech at the candlelight march commemorating the day Harvey Milk and George Moscone had been shot. After that, who knows? I never really worried about career and fortune in those days. I was surviving, and that seemed quite a lot.

It's hard to communicate how awful it was in the fall of 1985. I'd left town out of my own fear and frustration. And somehow that sabbatical had been recuperative. Physically I felt fine. The shingles had left with only lingering tingles. And I'd gotten myself out of the coke and drinking routine, thanks in part to Randy Shilts, an old friend from Haight-Ashbury days. He, alone among my friends, had encouraged me to go to an AA meeting. It was hard as hell to attend those first meetings.

Then, slowly, I broke the pattern and eventually learned to sleep without numbing myself with drink.

But there was something different in the San Francisco I returned to. Everyone seemed exhausted, almost fatalistic about AIDS. I understood that, certainly; but I also detected signs of hope within the despair. For one, the media had caught on to what was happening. Randy, who'd been a staff writer for the *Advocate,* was hired full time by the *Chronicle* to write weekly AIDS columns, and he was extremely dogged in his attempts to puncture all the myths. There was a piece on the fallacy of AIDS being transmitted by mosquito bites, by tainted water, by waiters handling dinner plates. He went into AIDS wards and interviewed the nursing staff and doctors, and the truth was coming out.

Other newspapers followed his lead, and the public began to learn, if not always to accept, that this disease was not divine retribution. And other "points of light" flared up. Bobbi Campbell and his lover sat smiling on the cover of *Newsweek* in an article on the new disease—appearing shockingly alive and productive. There were respected physicians speaking out and against the panic. These were all important achievements, but still it was just so much whistling in the dark. We desperately needed an immediate fix, and it wasn't even on the horizon.

Seven years before, on the night of Harvey Milk's murder, I swore to myself that he would not be forgotten and began organizing a candlelight march to mark the day of his and Mayor Moscone's deaths. It had become a ritual, with thousands attending every year. A few days prior to the 1985 march, my friend Joseph Durant and I were walking the Castro handing out leaflets reminding people of the candlelight memorial. We stopped to get a slice at Marcello's Pizza, and I picked up a *Chronicle*. The front-page headline was chilling: "1,000 San Franciscans Dead of AIDS." I'd known most of them from my work with the KS Foundation. Virtually every single one of them had lived within a ten-block radius of where we were standing at Castro and Market. When I walked up Eighteenth Street from Church to Eureka, I knew the ugly stories behind so many windows. Gregory died behind those blue curtains. Jimmy was diagnosed up that staircase, in that office behind the venetian blinds. There was the house Alex got kicked out of when the landlord found an empty bottle of AZT in his trash can: "I'm sorry, we just can't take any chances." I wasn't losing just friends, but also all the familiar faces of the neighborhood—the bus drivers, clerks, and mailmen, all the people we know in casual yet familiar ways. The entire Castro was populated by ghosts.

And yet, as I looked around the Castro, with its charming hodgepodge of candy-colored Victorians, there were guys walking hand in hand, girls kissing each other hello, being successfully, freely, openly who they were. So much had been accomplished since the closeted days when the community met furtively in a back-alley culture. The Castro was a city within the city, an oasis and harbor for thousands who lived there and millions of gay men and lesbian women around the world for whom it symbolized freedom. And now, in what should have been its prime, it was withering.

Angrily, I turned to Joseph: "I wish we had a bulldozer, and if we could just level these buildings, raze Castro . . . If this was just a graveyard with a thousand corpses lying in the sun, then people would look at it and they would understand, and if they were human beings they'd have to respond." And Joseph, always the acid realist, told me I was the last optimist left standing: "Nobody cares, Cleve. This thing doesn't touch them at all."

November 27, 1985, the night of the memorial march, was cold and gray. As we waited for people to gather, Joseph and I handed out stacks of poster board and Magic Markers, and through the bullhorn I asked everyone to write down the name of a friend who'd been killed by AIDS. People were a little reluctant at first, but by the time the march began we had a few hundred placards. Most of the marchers just wrote first names, Tom or Bill or George; some of the signs said "My brother" or "My lover," and a few had the complete name—first, middle, and last—in bold block letters.

That Thanksgiving night we marched as we had for six years down Market Street to city hall, a sea of candles lighting up the night. One of the marchers asked me who else would be speaking this year, and I said, "No one else. Just me. People are tired of long programs anyway." I was an angry, arrogant son of a bitch. The candles we'd been carrying were stumps by the time we'd gathered at Harvey Milk Memorial Plaza at city hall.

"We are here tonight to commemorate the deaths of Supervisor Harvey Milk and Mayor George Moscone, victims of an assassin's bullets seven years ago this very day." I talked of Harvey and how even back then he was not really our first martyr, that we'd lost many people to murder and suicide and alcohol and AIDS. "Yes, Harvey was our first collective martyr, but now we have many more martyrs and now our numbers are diminished and many of us have been condemned to an early and painful death. But we are the lesbian women and gay men of San Francisco, and although we are again surrounded by uncertainty and despair, we are survivors, and we shall survive again, and the dream that was shared by Harvey Milk and George Moscone will go forward."

Then we moved down Market to the old federal building. At that time it housed the offices of Health and Human Services—not such an effective rallying point as city hall, but perfect for our next demonstration, one that turned out to have more impact than I ever imagined. Earlier in the day, Bill Paul, a professor at San Francisco State University, and I had hidden extension ladders and rolls of tape in the shrubbery around the building's base. As the federal building came into view, I ended the chanting ("Stop AIDS now! Stop AIDS now!") and explained through the bullhorn that we were going to plaster the facade with the posters inscribed with our dead. And that's what happened. The crowd surged forward, the ladders were set in place, and we crawled up three stories, covering the entire wall with a poster-board memorial.

It was a strange image. Just this uneven patchwork of white squares, each with handwritten names, some in script and some in block letters, all individual. We stared and read the names, recognizing too many. Staring upward, people remarked: "I went to school with him" . . . "I didn't know he was dead" . . . "I used to dance with him every Sunday at the I-Beam" . . . "We're from the same hometown" . . . "Is that our Bob?"

There was a deep yearning not only to find a way to grieve individually and together but also to find a voice that could be heard beyond our community, beyond our town. Standing in the drizzle, watching as the posters absorbed the rain and fluttered down to the pavement, I said to myself, *It looks like a quilt.* As I said the word *quilt,* I was flooded with memories of home and family and the warmth of a quilt when it was cold on a winter night.

And as I scanned the patchwork, I saw it—as if a Technicolor slide had fallen into place. Where before there had been a flaking gray wall, now there was a vivid picture, and I could see quite clearly the National

Mall, and the dome of Congress, and a quilt spread out before it—a vision of incredible clarity.

I was gripped by the same terror and excitement that I'd felt standing before other large works commemorating other large issues. Not long ago I'd seen Christo's running fence in Sonoma County. It was a beautiful and moving sight, and I was struck by the grandeur of those vast expanses of shimmering opalescent fabric zigzagging up and down the golden hills. How it billowed in the breeze with the light playing off it, like a string of azure tall ships sailing on a golden sea. And there was the memory of Judy Chicago's *The Dinner Party*. This was a long table, maybe one hundred feet in length, with each place setting designed by a different artist. Both Christo and Judy Chicago had taken commonplace items, sheets drying on a line in his case, plates and utensils in hers, and by enlarging them had made the homely a dramatic, powerfully moving statement. It seemed an apt synthesis: individual quilts, collected together, could have the same immense impact.

When I told my friends what I'd seen, they were silent at first, and as I tried to explain it, they were dubious: "Cleve, don't you realize the logistics of doing something like that? Think of the difficulty of organizing thousands of queers!" But I knew there were plenty of angry queens with sewing machines. I wouldn't be working alone, I told my friends. Everyone understands the idea of a quilt. "But it's gruesome," they said.

That stopped me. Was a memorial morbid? Perhaps it was. And yet there is also a healing element to memorials. I thought of the Vietnam Veterans Memorial wall. I did not expect to be moved by it. I was influenced by the Quakers, who are suspicious of war memorials, which they believe tend to glorify war rather than speak to the horror of it. But I was overwhelmed by the simplicity of it, of that black mirrorlike wall and the power it had to draw people from all across America to find a beloved's name and touch it and see their face reflected in the polished marble and leave mementos.

So I thought about all these things and also about how quilting is viewed as a particularly American folk art. There was the quilting bee with its picture of generations working together, and the idea that quilts recapture history in bits of worn clothing, curtains, jackets—protective cloth. That it was women who did the sewing was an important element. At the time, HIV was seen as the product of aggressive gay male sexuality, and it seemed that the homey image and familial associations of a warm quilt would counter that.

The idea made so much sense on so many different levels. It was clear to me that the only way we could beat this was by acting together as a nation. Though gays and lesbians were winning political recognition in urban centers, without legitimate ties to the larger culture we'd always be marginalized. If we could somehow bridge that gap of age-old prejudice, there was hope that we could beat the disease by using a quilt as a symbol of solidarity, of family and community; there was hope that we could make a movement that would welcome people—men and women, gay or straight, of every age, race, faith, and background.

To this day, critics ignore one of the most powerful aspects of the Quilt. Any Quilt display, no matter how small or large, is filled with evidence of love—the love between gay men and the love we share with our lesbian sisters, as well as love of family, father for son, mother for son, among siblings. Alongside this love, the individual quilts are filled with stories of homophobia and how we have triumphed over it. There's deep and abiding pain in letters attached to the quilts from parents bemoaning the fact that they didn't accept their dead son. And there's implacable anger in the blood-splashed quilts blaming President Reagan for ignoring the killing plague. All these messages are part of a memorial that knows no boundaries. We go to elementary schools, high schools, the Bible Belt of the Deep South, rural America, Catholic churches, synagogues, and wherever we unfold this fabric we tell the story of people who've died of AIDS.

That night, standing with those few men and women in the damp and dark, I saw a way out for all of us, a method of surmounting our fears and coming together in a collective memorial of our experience: all the sadness, rage, and anger; all the hope, all the dreams, the ambitions, the tragedy.

Eleven years later, this picture in my mind's eye became reality. But that night in November 1985 it was just an idea, and on the 8 Market bus up to the Castro, my friends Joseph Durant, Gilbert Baker, and Joseph Canalli were unimpressed. Reagan will never let you do it, they said. Straight families won't join any cause with a bunch of San Francisco queers. It was late, they were tired. An AIDS quilt was a sweet idea, but it was morbid, corny, impossibly complicated. Give it up. But I was on fire with the vision. The idea made so much sense, in so many ways—the irony and truth of it. I couldn't get it out of my head.

The First Displays: D.C. and S.F., 1987

When people ask me today when I knew the Quilt would catch on, I say always. From that first night at the federal building I just knew it would work—that people would be touched and respond. But for all my sureness, it was maddening trying to explain the idea, because I didn't have anything to show. When I told friends I wanted to take ten thousand quilts and lay them out on the Mall in Washington, D.C., on October 11 for the National March for Lesbian and Gay Rights, they really thought I'd lost it.

Finally, after a year and a half of thinking and scribbling on napkins, Joseph Durant and I sat down and made a list of forty men we felt we knew well enough to make quilts for, and in February began cranking them out, each of them three feet by six feet. The panels were that size because of the vision of bulldozing the Castro and leaving only corpses lying in the sun. I wanted to show the space that would be taken up by each of those bodies, about the dimensions of a grave. I told Joseph that we'd sew them into twelve-by-twelve-foot squares, large enough to be efficient and small enough that people could reach out and touch the fabric as they walked around them. Joining them together that way also allowed flexibility, so that some of the panels could be made horizontally and some vertically, like the parquet pattern on the floor of my grandfather's house.

All this was fine with Joseph until he started talking about how we were going to have to build scaffolding to hold it up. I said, no, the power of it comes from laying it flat on the ground. Joseph was adamant that it should be up in the air like a flag, but I knew that that would totally alter the experience. We use both methods of display today, and you can see the difference. If you view the Quilt hanging upright, you have a very different experience from what you have when it's flat on the ground. You're much less conscious of your surroundings when you're looking down and more likely to pause and perhaps kneel and touch it. The argument spiraled out of control, and, unfortunately, Joseph decided he couldn't work with me any longer.

I knew then, as I've always known, that I couldn't do it alone, and I asked Gilbert Baker, who I knew was a good seamstress, to become technical director. But Gilbert, who'd created the rainbow flag, wanted to be called artistic director. And then Ron Cordova came on board also demanding that title. I told them both that there was to be no artistic director. The only artistic director would be the people who made these things. All we do is gather them, uncensored, unedited, and sew them together. Our only job is to display them. Fortunately, Ron decided to put up with me in the end, agreeing to become technical director, and he worked like a dog getting things ready for October.

With the Quilt itself begun, we needed someone with management experience, able to oversee the resources and the money I expected to start coming in. I was living at the time with Atticus Tysen, a sweet young man I'd met at Quaker meeting. He told me about Michael Smith, a fellow Stanford MBA who was looking for work. I couldn't offer a salary, but I had something better, a cause. Mike was the first person I convinced to give me his life. We were a terrible mismatch, and for three years we treated each other with incredible cruelty. But we worked together starting up the Quilt, and it wouldn't have happened without him.

The key to getting any idea off the ground is reaching people, letting them know and see what it is you're pushing, and so sometime in May we called a public meeting. We plastered the Castro with flyers and rented the Women's Building for a couple of hours for our meeting, but as the time drew near, I was stricken with anxiety and became convinced that no one would show up. I was wrong. Two people came: Cindi "Gert" McMullin and Jack Caster. They'd both made quilts much more sophisticated than Joseph's and mine. Gert's was for AIDS activist Roger Lyon: an intricate design containing eighteen notes written to Roger from a class of fifth graders he'd spoken to. The notes were really wonderful, and captured the fierce loyalty and love these kids felt for Roger. They said such wonderfully innocent things, like, "I hope you get out of this tuff spot" and "If you don't get well you owe me 5 dollars." She'd eventually make two more for him.

The quilt Jack made for his lovers Wade and Joe has always been one of my favorites. It's a double panel connected across the top with a ribbon spelling out a line of mystic gibberish. Just before he died, deep in dementia, Wade lifted his head off the pillow and with this joyful look said, "I've got it, the median above to be three!" Jack had no idea what this message meant, but I think it reflected the confusion we all faced—nothing made sense. I love quilts inscribed with something nonsensical, code words and pet names or an evocative sentence like *Remember that night in August. . . .* You're allowed a glimpse of the intimate communication that existed between these people. That's what matters most about the Quilt, that it allows us to lose our cynicism in connection with someone we love and to make private declarations public.

Although Gert and Jack were treasures and quickly became an integral part of our team, the meeting could be looked on only as a failure. The idea was catching on too slowly; we'd never get to D.C. if the Quilt remained an underground effort largely confined to the gay community in San Francisco. In spite of our fears, not one of us gave in to hopelessness. We all had so much riding on it, and so all of us—Gert, Jack, and Mike, the nucleus of the early days—tried to analyze exactly what would make it work. The one thing we'd always had trouble with was explaining the idea in conversation. People needed a visual representation to grasp the idea, something they could see and touch.

Getting the Quilt out there, in front of as many people as possible, became our goal that late spring of 1987. We expected to get a good deal of publicity at the upcoming gay and lesbian pride festival. There'd be upward of 250,000 people attending the event, and we would be able to talk with hundreds of them as they stopped by our booth. Also, I'd been invited to speak at the opening ceremonies and would talk about the Quilt and invite all 250,000 to join us, both in making a quilt and in making the presentation in D.C.

Jack came up with a great idea. I remember him saying, "Cleve, you know Mayor Feinstein. Why don't you get her to hang the Quilt in front of city hall during the week of gay pride?" We were all immediately excited. City hall sits on one of the busiest streets in the city, so no one could miss seeing those panels hanging on the ornate neoclassical facade. It would be a coup. I'd known Mayor Feinstein casually when I worked for Harvey while he was a supervisor, but our relationship had been a little cool since White Night, and I wasn't sure how she'd react. But as always in those early days, we had to make the effort. Also, as Jack quite rightly pointed out, with elections coming up, Dianne's support might help her chances of retaining the mayoralty in ways a refusal would not. "It would be good for her," said Jack. It made sense, so I dredged up the only decent shirt in my closet and went down to make my pitch. It was easy. I remember the mayor twiddling with that ever-present red silk bow at her neck and saying, "I think it would be wonderful." She's got a firm handshake.

Soon after, Warren Caton sent us the stunningly beautiful panels he'd made for Liberace and Rock Hudson. Exquisitely embroidered and dazzling when the light sparkled on the sequins and glitter, these two were like the first in a series of good-luck charms to come. The next break we got came thanks to Scott Lago, who also joined our team. Lloyd Phelps, a coworker of his at Neiman Marcus, had died, and Scott suggested that a quilt would be a wonderful memorial. The company loved the idea, and the entire staff of the visual-display department created a quilt for Lloyd. It was beautiful, a block of golden beige with two kittens on the left side playing with a strand of yarn that curled from their paws into Lloyd's name and then rolled into a ball on the right. Accompanying the quilt was a dedicatory note: "Lloyd Phelps—an Illinois farm boy with a talent for producing the most elegant and sophisticated table settings. He loved his cats and working on his Victorian flat. He was the gentlest of men, with an improbably deep voice. He was kind, giving, and talented, and all of us who worked with him miss him very much."

His panel, along with forty others, was featured in the forty-foot-high front window of the San Francisco Neiman Marcus store in August 1987. The NM display facing Union Square, San Francisco's choicest shopping area, really helped us break through the perception that the Quilt was for and about activist Castro clones. We now had chic! And our new legitimacy translated into a big jump in volunteers, donations, and quilt makers.

Things were really breaking our way in those early months. But as our profile grew, so did the flak. The Quilt was fast becoming "our thing," meaning the property of those who'd lost and continued to lose their gay friends. Feeling ownership of something so explosively emotional was only natural and has propelled the Quilt to its current stature. But in some cases, that proprietary interest fought against the Quilt's overarching goal, which was to connect all people, regardless of age, race, and sexual orientation, in the fight against AIDS.

All this came to a head over the pope's visit to San Francisco in June. He was coming to Mission Dolores, which is right in the middle of the gay and Hispanic neighborhoods. When the pope visits a church, the local congregation decides how to welcome him, and the people at Mission Dolores had asked us to bring some sections of the Quilt to the ceremony.

That set off an uproar. While I saw the pope's acknowledgment as a useful breakthrough, others were outraged. They said the Quilt was made for gays by gays, and it was sacrilege to present it to a homophobe, the man who represents the Catholic patriarchy, two thousand years of oppression. The loudest naysayers were the ACT UP people, a new generation of gay activists for whose identity AIDS was an explosive part. It's not enough to make a quilt, they sneered; the Quilt is a passive thing. The pope's blessing, they felt, would be a mockery of everything they had fought for. I took a few deep breaths and told them then, as I tell them now, that we never said the Quilt is enough. It's one response among thousands, not the final answer. Their faces would harden, and I'd repeat that we would never restrict participation, that we weren't going to exclude anybody. It was no use. I was an Uncle Tom, a sellout, afraid of my own sexuality . . . and on and on. I didn't know it then, but Mission Dolores marked the beginning of a long argument with a small minority of people who hate the Quilt. There's nothing to be done about turning them around.

By mid-July, we had about one hundred panels, all of them stored on Mike Smith's back porch, and we began to look for a workshop to display and assemble them. Though we had absolutely no money, we leased an empty storefront on Market Street, just by the intersection at Castro. This was a huge move for us. Having a space really made us feel as if it were all going to happen. It seemed cavernous—especially when we set up our single sewing machine, a brave little Singer, on a rickety table. We had nothing else back then—no chairs, no tables, nothing but an incredible amount of light fixtures: the previous tenant had been a furniture store, and the ceiling was a maze of track lighting.

I still marvel at our optimism. I just taped a sheet of butcher paper on the front door with the announcement "This is the new home of the NAMES Project and here is our wish list." We needed everything from sequins, beads, fabric, and glue to extension cords, computers, telephones, lights, and furniture. At the end of the list, I added, "back rubs, hugs, and money."

The response was incredible. Within two weeks we were given ten sewing machines (three industrial models!), and volunteers started streaming in. Mike always says it couldn't have happened anywhere else in the country, and he's right. Local merchants paid the first month's rent. Someone left an anonymous gift of five hundred dollars in the donation box, and a hunky chiropractor regularly gave free massages to volunteers who sewed evenings until midnight. Very soon our shelves were overflowing with needles, bobbins, thread, and fabric.

The workshop was magical and at the same time devastating. Every day someone would walk in and recognize a name on the panel, learning for the first time that a friend had died. Guys with AIDS would come in to make their own quilt, then stop coming as they became too sick to work. Sometimes a friend or family member would come by and take the panel to the sick man's house or hospital bed so he could work on it. More often, we just went ahead and finished it for him. There wasn't a day that I didn't cry, but the miracle of it was that over the sound of the sewing machines you'd hear laughter, and it got to be a tradition to sing a rendition of "There's No Business Like Sew Business." Everyone was finally able to train their emotions and energies on something concrete.

Though the majority of volunteers were gay men, there were also lots of straight people coming through our doors to donate time and money: children walked in with their fathers; mothers came by with a quilt they'd made for their husband or son. After a few weeks we realized that the epidemic reached far beyond our little world. And that the Quilt meant something outside the Castro.

In midsummer the *New Yorker* ran an article, and then *People* magazine did a story, as well as the *Dallas Morning News*. After each burst of publicity, we'd get more quilts, including some from people who'd never known the person they were memorializing. When *Newsweek* published a series of photographs profiling 302 people who had died of AIDS, panels began arriving from people who'd been moved by that piece. There was one we received from a man named Michael Lueders to honor Curt Norrup. Curt had broken up with his lover and attempted suicide. The hospital would not release him until he found a place to stay. Michael, who'd never met Curt except through the article, and who had no experience with AIDS, took him into his home and nursed him through the last months, quickly learning how to handle the mundane chores of caring for a bedridden patient, as well as the more difficult tasks, like handling Curt during his seizures.

The quilt he made for Curt is simple: black cloth letters sewn into gray fabric with pink elephants. Attached was a note: "I spent 14 hours sewing with a lot of love and needle pricks but it was well worth it. I knew nothing of his life when I took him in and because of that we became good friends. I pray that our short time together provided him some laughter and hopefully some joy."

During that first summer it felt very much like we were launching a small business on a shoestring budget. Nothing was easy, and most of the day-to-day strains fell on Mike Smith. He was part sergeant, part nanny, dealing with everything from overdue bills to staffing problems. While Mike was putting out fires, I was on the road trying to raise our national profile. Begging plane tickets from rich friends and flight attendants, I'd go to cities around the country, hit every gay bar, and convince the manager to let me into the DJ booth and make an announcement about the Quilt presentation at the National March for Lesbian and Gay Rights in Washington. I learned to keep my speech short or suffer the taunts of queens impatient for a disco fix. But for every jerk there were ten or twenty men and women who listened and promised to come.

Every morning I was at home, I'd go to the post office on Eighteenth Street to see if there were any packages. It was a great day if there was one. Usually there weren't any, and as we went into summer things looked bleak. By mid-July we had less than a hundred quilts, and those were overwhelmingly from the Castro. We'd set the deadline for August 1, just a few weeks away.

One day in late July, having returned from a weeklong swing through Texas, I was standing in line at the post office when one of the clerks looked at me and said, "Oh, it's Mr. Jones!" And his pal raised an eyebrow and chirped, "Does Mr. Jones want his mail?" I was used to a certain amount of ribbing. I knew I'd been a pest and that the Castro post office had a high camp quotient, but I was really puzzled when they opened the door to the back room and asked, "Did you bring a truck?" I went through and saw bins, big canvas postal bins, filled with paper packages, hundreds of them.

I called over to the workshop and told them to bring whatever cars were available and park them on Eighteenth and Collingwood. We set up a relay line, picking bundles up out of the bins and passing them through the post office lobby and over the sidewalk into the cars. As we did this, I read out the postmarks and everybody cheered. Two more from Texas! *Yeah, Texas.* Here's some from New York City! *Yeah, New York City.* Here's one from Delaware. *Yeah, Delaware!* Here's one from Virginia! Montana! . . . *Montana?*

After several minutes, it got very quiet. I think all of us, without saying anything, realized how weird this was, that all across the country people were taking the names of their dead loved ones and pouring all their anger and pain and grief and love into creating works of art and then sending them to a group of strangers at a post office box.

Seeing these panels piled up in the workshop got me thinking about how we'd display them. We all agreed it was very important for people to be able to get close enough to touch the quilts they'd made. We expected they would want to leave mementos like flowers or notes. So we decided to take four of the twelve-foot squares and link them together with grommets and cable ties to form a larger square that was twenty-four feet by twenty-four feet. Canvas walkways would separate each square, so everyone would be able to get within twelve feet of a panel.

The next question was, How do we present it? How do we unfold it? Is there a ceremony, a ritual? Many ideas were advanced, but with all my Quaker mistrust of rituals, I did not want anything fancy or portentous, no music or fanfare or sermons. What we needed was a very simple, dignified, powerful way of revealing the Quilt. Nothing seemed quite right. One morning Jack Caster stumbled in with a terrible hangover and pockets full of wadded-up cocktail napkins, which he excitedly unfolded on my desk. "I've figured it out," he announced. With a rather grand flourish he said, "I call it the lotus fold!" He showed me sketches of a twelve-by-twelve section with eight panels, then began folding them in, corners to the center, corners to the center, until it was a neat bundle. The idea was to position one bundle in the center of each twelve-by-twelve square of the grid. "When it comes time, we'll have a team of eight people do the unfolding. The first four will reach in and pull out the first four corners, the second four will do likewise, and so on until it's flat. Then we'll just pull it out and it will fit into the grid." Sheer genius.

We all agreed it was a simple and elegant solution. But what would the unfolders wear? Should they be dressed alike? If they wore street clothes, wouldn't the colors clash with the Quilt? Black seemed too dark and Druidic; maybe something neutral would work best. White was suggested, then shot down as too nurselike. I thought of the all nurses I'd met in the last few years in AIDS wards across the country and how much love and support they had given. Maybe that wasn't such a bad idea. They were heroes. Many were lesbians who had volunteered to care for the AIDS patients others feared to touch. So we decided that the unfolding ceremony would consist of teams dressed in white, unfolding the lotus-folded panel squares while the names were being read. We went to practice at the Stanford University football field and got it all down.

That final week before the display was exhausting and inspiring. Everything was coming down now to hours and minutes. Though we'd moved the deadline to September 15 and had by then received 720 panels, another 1,200 had just arrived. Each one had to be hemmed to exactly three feet by six feet, then sewn into a twelve-by-twelve square, and then the entire piece again edged in canvas. Grommets were sewn on to hold the fabric in place within the grid of intersecting walkways. The walkways were made of nine-foot-wide white fabric, which in turn had to be measured and cut to the exact size that Ron Cordova, the technical director, had worked out over so many nights pacing up the street from our warehouse to the Café Flore, precisely the right distance.

We had so much help from so many people. Jeff Kuball, an attendant for the air-freight company Flying Tigers, not only had organized a quilt to be made in honor of three coworkers, but had persuaded seventy Tigers employees to donate time and money so that we could fly the Quilt to D.C. and back. It weighed just under seven thousand pounds. Thousands of yards of fabric, thousands of metal grommets, 1,920 names, so much love and loss.

When we got to D.C. for the display, Michael Bento snuck us into some empty dorms at Georgetown University (which had just voted to ban gay and lesbian organizations). We used their computers and phone lines to prepare for our invasion of the District of Columbia.

At about one in the morning on October 11, 1987, ten years after Harvey Milk first called for the National March for Lesbian and Gay Rights, we formed a caravan and made our way through Georgetown up Pennsylvania Avenue to the Mall: the trucks with the Quilt, a thirty-three-foot Winnebago, and a pickup truck with a four-ton scissor lift. It was eerily quiet, and so dark that we used flashlights to layout the walkways and set up the tables and microphone. Plastic sheeting was set down to protect the cloth panels from the damp grass. At 5 A.M. we were only halfway through laying out the grid, but at dawn we were ready, bundles in position. At 7 A.M. the set-up team held hands in a circle. We'd done it! Ron Cordova's calculations had worked out, Steve Abbeyta's grommets held the panels in place—my vision had come true.

And then things went wrong. At the precise moment we began the unfolding, a panicked voice hissed urgently on my earphone, "We fucked up, it doesn't fit." Somehow, we'd set the bundles at wrong angles and when the Quilt was laid out, it extended over the walkways. Thank God for Gert. Very calmly and without the least hesitation, she got on the radio and told the unfolders to lift the Quilt in unison, move it a quarter turn to the left, then set it down. They performed faultlessly. The fabric billowed skyward, catching the first rays of sunlight on the sequins and rhinestones, and then settled gently, perfectly, into place—now a permanent part of every display procedure.

As dawn became day, thousands of people lined the perimeter, and I stepped slowly to the podium in the shadow of the Jefferson Memorial. I have almost no memory of walking to the podium, no words to describe the emotion flooding my heart as I read those twenty-four names, each so precious and containing in a few syllables entire lives. I began with Marvin Feldman. It was extremely difficult to speak slowly and deliberately, pausing between each name, and my voice began breaking down at the end of the list. Other readers were Art Agnos, Whoopi Goldberg, Robert

Blake, Lily Tomlin, Harvey Fierstein, and Congresswoman Nancy Pelosi. Joseph Papp, producer of the New York Shakespeare Festival, ended his list of names with a tribute to "my dear friend and colleague Michael Bennett." Then, in front of photographers, with his wife, Gail, at his side, Papp untied the ribbons around the red fabric roll under his arm and flourished a shimmering panel emblazoned with Michael Bennett's name and a metallic sunburst, the design from Bennett's most famous Broadway production, *A Chorus Line*. He then walked over to the check-in area and turned it in with the other panels that continued to arrive through the day.

And so, a year and a day after Marvin's death, on October 11, 1987, we unfolded nearly two thousand quilts on the National Mall. It looked incredible. Nothing prepared me for its beauty. There were plain panels of stark white with black lettering and extravagant ones with gold lamé encrusted with rhinestones and silver braid. There was every material, from tweed to leather to silk, and of course ribbons and beads and glitter galore. And everything you could imagine was sewn onto the fabric: locks of hair, record albums, souvenir postcards, a Barbie doll, whistles, crystals, a motorcycle jacket, a tuxedo, a shard of glass, foam rubber french fries, toy cars, a thimble, a cowboy hat, teddy bears, a pink Lacoste shirt, a Buddhist's saffron robe, and even a padded jock strap. Notes were scribbled in corners; others were sewn in. Some panels held the ashes of the people they memorialized.

And then there were the letters, hundreds of them, that people had sent along with the panels they'd made. On the back of one of those, decorated with a drawing of twelve candles, three lighted and nine extinguished, Lance Hecox wrote, "To 12 men I expected to grow old with. Nine who have passed on and three who will join them soon."

My friend Gert McMullin wrote of her own grief in one of the most touching letters of them all:

> Roger, The day I met you, my best friend of ten years told me he had fallen madly in love with you and that you would be living together. Oh yes, and that you had AIDS. Oh Roger—please forgive me for the ten minutes that it took me to stop hating you. I didn't know you and all I could feel was anger and then panic that David might become ill. And I had loved him for so long and I didn't know you at all!

Memories of you are not ones most people share. Wheelchairs, hospital waiting rooms, watching you fall, trying to help you up without you being mad that someone had to help you, watching you sleep, and (the most fun!) talking about all of David's faults and nasty habits while lying in bed.

Few memories, true . . . but what I have is all stored very tenderly in my heart.

Roger, I have learned one thing in my life. Don't get to know someone and become friends after they died. I never got the chance to run and play with you or to watch you have the time to be happy.

You have given me one thing—a determination to be the kind of person you would admire. One who touches, wants to be touched and cares. Your respect is my ultimate goal.

Love you so, Gert

Most of the letters came from men mourning their dead lovers. This one, from Paul Hill, talked of the secrecy that was necessary even after his friend's death:

Out of all those people who loved Ric and attended his funeral, only a handful knew that he died of AIDS. Being gay and having lived a lie, it was no problem lying about death as well. My lover who died of pneumocystis quickly became a roommate who died of viral pneumonia. This sham angers me now, but during that period of vulnerability which occurs immediately after a great loss, one can be talked into just about anything. This scenario repeats itself many times a day all over the United States. There are just too many people who don't realize that this awful disease has already touched their lives.

Art Peterson from Atlanta made a quilt for his lover Reggie Hightower and enclosed this note:

Ours was a unique relationship. We had lots of obstacles which we overcame to make our relationship grow: He was deaf, I was hearing; he was black, I was white; we were both gay and proud. We agreed that these were the happiest times of our lives. We lived and shared a totally "married" life.

I don't have many ideas on how he should be memorialized—perhaps a carving on the side of Stone Mountain here in Georgia. I feel it's a shame that I can't convey to others how great a life he lived—for he left no mark to be forever immortalized except deep within those people he loved and those who loved him. How do I fully express his life to those who never met him? The memories are so wonderful and yet they cause so much pain.

His panel is composed of shirts that he wore—some his, some mine. They were hand-sewn (by me) with double thread and double sewn in places for strength and durability. Please display it prominently.

The handsign in the middle is sign language for "I Love You."

Sincerely, Art

There are so many stories from that first display. Years before, Hank Wilson had introduced me to Donald Montwell and Jim Maness. They had organized the protest when Dan White was released from jail and fifty thousand people shut down San Francisco. By 1987 Jim was very ill. At the behest of Donald, who'd managed the Valencia Rose cabaret, where Whoopi Goldberg got her start, Whoopi agreed to come to the first display. On Saturday, before we opened the Quilt to the public, Whoopi and Donald and I took Jim out in his wheelchair for a private viewing. As it was quite chilly, Jim borrowed Whoopi's jacket, a shiny silk road crew jacket emblazoned with "Whoopi." He never gave it back and was buried in it not long after returning to San Francisco. I think he was holding on just to be at display. It meant so much to so many people.

The response to that first display was overwhelming, something I had not imagined or planned for. I'm convinced that every single person who saw the Quilt with their own eyes became an evangelist, telling a few friends who told others, really turning the tide of grassroots support. And certainly the newspaper coverage spread the word. We were on the front page of newspapers around the world, even as far away as New Delhi.

But the thing that put us front and center in millions of Americans' minds was the night I was profiled on television by Peter Jennings as a

"Person of the Week" on the *ABC Evening News*. I first heard about it just two hours before airtime in a phone call from ABC. I thanked the man and hung up, not really believing it. A few friends came over, and we sat around the TV. Nobody bothered to set up a VCR. Jennings started out by saying, "This week the plight of a little girl who fell down a hole has drawn us together," and I thought, *OK, I've been bumped by little Jessica Mc-Clure.* And then he went on, "But tonight we're honoring another person who's brought us together in a different way." And there I was, big as life, walking around the Quilt on television in living rooms all across America. If we thought press coverage had been good, it soon became great. The impact of the Quilt beamed to millions of homes, with mourners walking among two football fields of panels, packed an incredible emotional wallop. It seemed like the whole country was watching television that night, and the calls and letters just poured into the workshop.

When we got home to San Francisco, the mailbox was overflowing. People all over America had been inspired by the panels and had sent us poems and photographs, paintings, screenplays, and play scripts. There were designs for posters, for T-shirts, and caps. And every day brought letters from all over the country and around the world, many accompanied by quilts. I remember one letter from a mother whose two sons had died. She opened by saying she hoped it was acceptable that she has put their names together on a single panel. They were very close friends, she explained, and then she asked to pray for all of us: "I have two more gay sons. I live in fear." Another woman wrote of her ignorance and shame, telling of a time when a dying friend who'd been deserted by his lover and family had reached out for a hug and she's hesitated, afraid of being infected. She hoped he would forgive her.

Some of the letters came from people who'd made quilts for a person they'd never known. "I'm just a housewife," wrote a woman from Nebraska. "I thought there would be no recognition from his family. I felt bad about that. I feel bad about all the people who die of AIDS that nobody knows."

Every letter was different, but they all said that same thing: please bring us the Quilt, let us remember our dead. And that's when I knew that we couldn't close up shop. We had to go on the road and bring the

Quilt to everyone, in whatever town they lived, large or small. The letters and the quilts have never stopped coming.

We had no idea that Quilt would last beyond that day. I was looking for a symbol to focus the nation on the epidemic at a time when many of us had lost hope. I hoped it could be a tool for healing families divided by homophobia and believed it might unite the nation against the plague. But I saw it mainly as evidence, as mediagenic proof of the enormity of the crisis of killing thousands. For all the beauty and tenderness of each panel, the hard fact was that someone of value had died to make it happen. The Quilt was and is an activist symbol—comforting, yes, but mortally troubling. If it raised a single question, it was, What are we going to do about it? That was the challenge we laid at the national doorstep.

On December 17, 1987, we displayed the Quilt in San Francisco. I'd like to say we had a sense of returning victorious to our hometown and that, back with so many familiar faces, we had a feeling of accomplishment, but for me it was a bittersweet time. Even the fact that the display was held at the newly built Moscone Center, named for Mayor George Moscone, contained an element of ambiguity. And I couldn't help wondering, as I walked among the panels, which of my friends would soon have their names stitched with so many others.

I don't mean to suggest that any of my reflections betrayed doubt of our mission. Of that I was rock certain. Neither then nor in the intervening years, over innumerable interviews with reporters and journalists, did I ever flag in telling the story of the Quilt and what we stood for and what we were trying to do. My date book for that month is filled with appointments with ABC, CBS, the *Chronicle,* the *Examiner,* and many smaller local papers. Telling one person who would tell hundreds or thousands of people what we're about has always given me a sense of fulfillment, and in that sense the Moscone display was wonderful.

Certainly, the red-carpet embrace from our fellow San Franciscans was encouraging. All the politicians were there for the opening ceremonies, including Art Agnos, then the newly elected mayor, along with Congresswoman Nancy Pelosi, who'd been one of our earliest supporters and has continued to steer us around bureaucratic tar pits to this day. It was through her good offices that we secured space on the Mall in D.C. just weeks before, and later, in February 1989, she nominated the Quilt for a Nobel Prize. I remember one conversation with her at the San Francisco display when I'd thanked her for the fund-raisers she'd hosted early that summer. She smiled and said with a combination of relief and amazement that she and other politicians had helped raise money out of to loyalty to me, admitting that for all her enthusiasm she'd never imagined that the Quilt would catch on as it had. In this and so many other instances, it was wonderful to be able to return in faith to the people—especially the volunteers and donors—who'd placed their trust in us.

For all the good strokes and sheer relief of being home, I had a sense that we had just begun, that we must hurry. Being HIV-positive may have played a part in my wanting to rush on. I was symptom free, but many others were not. Though we had elevated AIDS to a new level of awareness, mobilized hundreds of thousands of people in the fight against the disease, there had been no accompanying breakthrough in medicine. The fear that dogged my trail that fall was a very simple question: Has our work come in time to make a difference?

One evening after the closing ceremonies I returned to the workshop, exhausted both physically and emotionally, and sat down alone in that quiet, cavernous room, sorting through the stacks of mail at a small table in the back. After a while, I got the feeling I was being watched. We never did lock the doors in those days; never saw the need. I turned and saw an old black woman staring through the front window. She had on a blue dress and matching hat and had a deeply lined, dark face. I went out and said, "We're open, if you want to come in." She just crossed her arms and looked down, wouldn't make eye contact, and came in sideways through the door without saying anything. I went back to my desk, and she walked around. I saw her touch one of the quilts. She picked up a brochure and left without saying a word.

A few days passed. I was again at the workshop. The radio was blaring, the sewing machines were going, there was a couple crying in one corner, there was a group laughing in another corner—just the general chaos and hubbub. And in the middle of this confusion I again got this back-of-the-neck sensation that I was being watched. I turned, and it was the same woman, standing on the sidewalk, scowling through the door, her arms across her chest, wearing the same blue dress.

As she came in the door, I noticed a bundle of fabric in her arms. She walked straight over to me and began her story. She'd come on a Greyhound bus from a small town in Kentucky. A year and a half earlier, her oldest son had returned from Los Angeles, where he'd settled after being discharged from the army. He'd come home to die. Though she was the choir director at her church and had a large, close family, she cared for her son for a year without ever revealing the nature of his disease to anyone.

When it was time for her son to die, she took him to the county hospital. After two days he died. She walked back home and, opening the front door, looked across the living room to her son's bedroom; and through the doorway she could see the hospital bed, the stack of towels, the IV rack, the bedpan. She closed the door to his room and locked it shut.

Several months passed, and she grieved alone, never uttering a word of the truth, never opening the door to her son's room. One day, while she was waiting at the dentist's office, she happened to read a story about the Quilt in a back issue of *People* magazine, went home, and packed a bag. For four days she'd ridden the bus from Kentucky to San Francisco, and now, she said, "I'm at the end." The whole time she'd talked she had been standing ramrod straight. Now she handed me the bundled quilt in her arms and said, "This is my son. I'm going to go home now and clean out his room."

There was nothing to say to this woman that she didn't already know. I stood still and she made her quiet way out the door, pausing only once to give a quick wave—not to me in particular, but to all of us and the quilts and what it all meant. And I felt so proud at that moment, that we in San Francisco, who were mainly young and white and gay, had created a symbol that had traveled across America to this old black woman alone with her grief in the hills of Appalachia and connected her and her son and their struggle with all of us.

I never doubted the Quilt or my place within its mission, but whatever lingering fears I had at the end of that first year about whether I would be up to the task of shepherding a national, even international, project simply vanished after my encounter with that old black woman. Her fortitude gave me the strength and confidence to carry on and brought me to a final acceptance of something I'd struggled with for a long time—my place as a gay man in the world.

The Quilt required me to change. Whether it is the pope or the woman from Kentucky, the Quilt touches something intensely private and personal in everyone who sees it. I had to learn to listen to those feelings, those fears and hopes—not just of my sorrowing brothers, but of everyone who even for a moment had opened up and recognized a common humanity, a link between all of us. For ten years I lived in the gay ghetto, shouted through the bullhorn, marched, and been arrested and jailed. My friends were gay, the music I listened to was gay oriented, the movies I saw had something to do with being gay, and except for a few family holidays it was a closed world. But now our goals demanded a different attitude, a wider reference. Certainly I wanted to startle Middle America and shake them up, but shocking people, hollering, "Look out, America, we're coming!" just didn't work. Times had changed, and the Quilt was part of the way we would survive and possibly prevail.

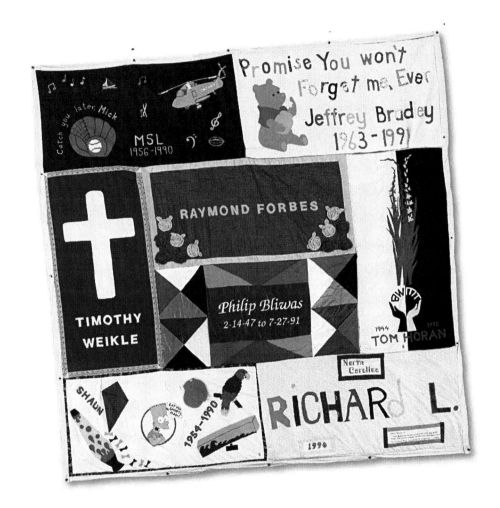

The Mourning After

Charles E. Morris III

Anniversaries, by convention, invite and invent time passages: rhetorical embodiments of retrospective and retroactive experiences; mappings of routes from those pasts through contemporaneous frames into prospective futures; interpellations of us as chronological or epochal or historically contingent and contiguous beings. This project began as a special issue of *Rhetoric and Public Affairs* marking the twentieth anniversary of the NAMES Project AIDS Memorial Quilt, and by the time of this volume's publication we will be approaching its twenty-fifth. Commemorating an anniversary of the AIDS Quilt complicates the familiar epideictic mode because commemoration in this case must always be substantially eulogistic. As such, we must always return to the fundamental questions asked by Eve Sedgwick:

> From a tombstone, from the tiny print in the *New York Times*, from the panels on panels on panels of the NAMES Project Quilt, whose

voice speaks impossibly to whom? From where is this rhetorical power borrowed, and how and to whom is it to be repaid? We miss you. Remember me. She hated to say goodbye. Participating in these speech acts, we hardly know whether to be interpellated as survivors, bereft; as witnesses or even judges; or as the very dead.[1]

With Sedgwick in mind, as well as Paula Treichler's now-idiomatic description of AIDS as an "epidemic of signification," I begin *Remembering the AIDS Quilt* with three time passages that for me exemplify the spirit of commemoration and critique that animates these engaging essays on this epidemic text.[2]

In his posthumously published volume of essays on AIDS, *Queer and Loathing* (1994), author and activist David B. Feinberg opened his tribute to "David P." by lamenting how the epidemic had left him bereft not only of the lost, but also of the rhetorical resources to convey their histories: "In these horrible times we have been forced to abbreviate the mourning process. How many people can you grieve for properly when everyone is dying? I wrote a novel for Jim Bronson, whom I barely knew. I wrote stories about my friends Saul Meissler, Glenn Peter Pumilia, and Glenn Person. Now I am reduced to brief essays in memoriam. Eventually all will be reduced to nothing but a litany of names chanted at the Quilt, panels of cloth the size of a coffin."[3]

The impetus for this book came in a start on a Sunday morning in November 2005 while rereading Christopher Capozzola's essay on the AIDS Quilt for my course on public memory. That I was seized by an awareness of the imminent anniversary is ironic given that Capozzola insightfully places the AIDS Quilt in history within the very specific contexts of gay liberation and AIDS activism in the Reagan era.[4] But I think it was, in fact, such historical precision that precipitated my recognition of the momentous present, what that present might mean, and the ways in which the past might envelop you at the expense of the here and now. When a week later I wrote to ask Cleve Jones for permission to reprint material from his memoir *Stitching a Revolution,* he responded, "I must admit that I was taken aback by the realization that next year marks the 20th anniversary of the first display." What did Jones mean by this? I imagine that, in no small part, and perhaps with lamentation, he had in a start measured the distance between then and now.

On the 2004 DVD edition of Jeffrey Friedman and Rob Epstein's documentary *Common Threads: Stories from the Quilt* (1989), we twice find the beloved activist Vito Russo waxing prophetic about a time after AIDS, about legacies and the archive. In the peroration of his 1988 speech "Why We Fight," memorably delivered at two ACT UP actions that year, Russo observed:

> Don't ever forget . . . remember, that some day, the AIDS crisis is going to be over. And when that day comes, when that day has come and gone, there are going to be people alive on this earth, gay people and straight people, and black people and white people, men and women, who are going to hear the story, that once, a long time ago there was a terrible disease and that a brave group of people stood up and fought and in some cases died so that others might live and be free.

Russo's visionary eloquence also provides in voiceover the peroration of the documentary itself, as we glance one last time at the Quilt displayed at sunset in the sightline of, in juxtaposition against, the White House: "I think what we want to see eventually is an end, a day when we can stop adding panels to this quilt and put it away, as a symbol of a terrible thing that happened and that's now over. You know we forget that some day this is going to be over. Some day there's going to be no such thing as AIDS, and people will just look back and remember that there was a terrible tragedy and we survived."[5]

Yesterday

> In the untimely loss of your noble son, our affliction here, is scarcely less than your own. So much of promised usefulness to one's country, and of bright hopes for one's self and friends, have so rarely been so suddenly dashed, as in his fall. . . . In the hope that it may be no intrusion upon the sacredness of your sorrow, I have ventured to address you

this tribute to the memory of my young friend, and your brave and early fallen child.

> —Abraham Lincoln to the Father and Mother
> of Col. Elmer Ellsworth, May 25, 1861[6]

I meditate on Lincoln, during a period of politicized bicentennial com-memoration, because his funereal voice, his epideictic eloquence, is perhaps without equal in U.S. history, although the AIDS Quilt richly echoes all that made Lincoln's eulogies wise and powerful; because it has often been said that the scope and depth of loss suffered during the first wave of the AIDS epidemic compare only to the toll of war; because of the torturous irony, given the Reagan and Bush regimes, in quoting a U.S. president whose first impulse in the face of tragic human loss was to name and to honor the dead, and to console those intimates left behind—to sincerely mourn. And also because of time: Lincoln's memorial is poignant because it is conjured out of grief for his beloved friend who died, literally, the day before. Immediacy, like amber, achieves a certain quality of preservation unmatched by more distant commemorative expression. The same is true for singularity. As David Herbert Donald remarked of the substantial cultural impact of Ellsworth's death as the first casualty of the Civil War, "The tragedy . . . would have gone almost unnoticed in later years, when deaths were reported by the thousands."[7]

With this in mind, let me return to the first of our time passages. I quoted David Feinberg because it is imperative that we remember AIDS in history, historicize its memorialization, and strive for an immediacy that will conjure, if necessarily imperfectly, the mourning time(s) em-bodied in the Quilt.[8] It is no longer the case, as Thomas Yingling insight-fully observed, that "discourse on AIDS invariably invokes the notion of history," which is all the more lamentable because, according to Cindy Patton, "Only when we stand and face the unnarratable horrors can we appreciate the modes of redress that have been left in abeyance because the story of AIDS we now tell leads us to misrecognize the utter contin-gency of the political responses we have known."[9] The tragedy of AIDS is in an important sense a tragedy of public memory: on the whole it cannot be said that communities remember the first wave of the epidemic, the first display of the AIDS Quilt, *as if it were yesterday.* The reasons for this are varied, including the deaths of original memory agents, generational and demographic changes, the cocktail of antiretroviral drugs that has dramatically altered the meanings and experience of this now "chronic" illness, and the lack of a will to history and distorted narratives by and about the stigmatized peoples primarily taken in those dark nights of the AIDS ascendancy. We must retrieve those "horrible times" in order to query about mourning in an epidemic and Feinberg's representative ambivalence about the Quilt as an extraordinary manifestation of that epidemic mourning.

Feinberg, in his assessment that "eventually all will be reduced to nothing but a litany of names chanted at the Quilt, panels of cloth the size of a coffin," was both right and wrong, and spoke about both the memorial and activist impulses that animated engagements with the AIDS Quilt in its early years. Any reckoning with this history must begin in the despair and disorientation Feinberg expresses. The breathtaking body count, in the cumulative tally and the speed with which it mounted in the 1980s, overwhelmed infrastructure and psyche.[10] At grounds zero in San Francisco and New York, Los Angeles and Miami, one typically stood terrified and powerless at the edge of what was once the safe harbor, watching, denying, raging, as the tidal wave swept through. Moreover, the intimacy of the epidemic—as the term more precisely suggests but cannot adequately convey—exacerbated the loss. One's physical body, whether in decline or in fear of diagnosis and death, and one's extended amative body of lovers, friends, community, and culture, recently unfettered, was now at the last of the tether. I am reminded of David Rabe's play *Streamers,* the title of which refers to those in free fall whose parachutes won't open.

To make matters worse, most Americans, which of course means straight Americans, didn't flinch as the bodies hit the ground. Out of apathy or hatred, the "general population," as it was then invidiously and disastrously called, and every institution of power at every level, moralized, demonized, ostracized, neglected, and stalled. The defamation was only slightly less devastating than the silence, both enveloping. We might define this ugly, harrowing context according to the presidency that constituted and governed it. Dennis Altman explained:

In a different sort of society AIDS would be perceived as a crisis of public health rather than a gay issue. In the United States in the first half of the 1980s the coincidence of a weak public health sector and a strong emphasis on community identity has helped shape the particular form the epidemic is taking. Once again the sort of research undertaken, the provision of health care, the response of hospitals and the medical profession, the way in which education of both the public and the "risk groups" is conducted, are all affected by political and cultural factors. The halfhearted response of governments, the considerable stigmatization of those struck by the illness and the politicization of the disease as revealed in the general assumption that AIDS is "the gay plague" all help to give the epidemic certain characteristics of Reaganism.[11]

Thus it was not the illness alone that diminished Feinberg's mourning process. As Douglas Crimp memorably observed, "during the AIDS crisis there is an all but inevitable connection between the memories and hopes associated with our lost friends and the daily assaults on our consciousness. Seldom has a society so savaged people during their hour of loss."[12] Lawrence Howe called it "the most monumental instance of American social neglect since Jim Crow."[13] It is understandable, then, that Feinberg lamented that the inexorable deterioration and degradation of all those cherished lives would end in tiny fragments of name and cloth—terrible metonymy, *memento mori*.

Given this context, the AIDS Quilt constituted an extraordinary rhetorical turn, a reversal and transformation of signification, of meanings, of vision. The narrative of its inception and instantiation between 1985 and 1987 is best left to its creator, Cleve Jones, whose fragments of memoir commence this volume as prologue.[14] It is enough here to emphasize that out of homophobic violence, personal and collective loss, his own HIV diagnosis, and hate and anger and despair emerged Jones's memorial of love and courage and hope. The AIDS Quilt consists of three-by-six handcrafted panels, sewn together in twelve-by-twelve blocks. At the first display in October 1987 at the National March on Washington for Gay and Lesbian Rights, 1,920 panels blanketed the National Mall. The basic functions of what would become the largest community art project in the world were therapeutic and performative. Crimp characterized it as the *ritual of mourning,* "the private mourning ritual of a person or group in-volved in making a panel and the collective mourning ritual of visiting the quilt to share that experience with others," and the *spectacle of mourning,* "the vast public relations effort to humanize and dignify our losses for those who have not shared them."[15] The latter also entailed the prospects of AIDS education, prevention, and fund-raising.

As so many critics, including this volume's contributors, have ex-plained, the rhetorical power of the AIDS Quilt is enacted precisely in the "litany of names" (both seen as well as read aloud as part of the ritual event) and "panels of cloth" that Feinberg cast as reduction. From ex-iguous gravelike inscriptions to excessive productions reminiscent of the carnivalesque, the panels embody names as signatures, as lives. Richard Mohr wrote, "the represented, lightening-quick, single-frame narratives of the Quilt are . . . probes of distinctness. They target, seek out, and display the named individual's personality—his center of narrative gravity, the orchestral tone of his being, life as his gesture. The panels are snapshots of the soul as posed in memory."[16] Magnificent metonymy, *memento vitae.*

But the panels' "sheer specificity" and "democratizing effect," achieved by affording "equal status to all panels regardless of elaboration, style, or uniqueness," only half accounts for the AIDS Quilt's strength.[17] The unfolding whole of those striking parts is striking in its own right: the tragic induction of collective evidence exhibited and the sublimity of its awful magnitude. As Peter Hawkins astutely observed:

> Private identity is held up as monumental; the intimate stretches as far as the eye can see. In fact, by overdramatizing intimacy, by taking small gestures of domestic grief and multiplying them into the thousands, the Quilt makes a spectacular demonstration of the feminist dictum: the personal *is* political. . . . the Quilt redescribes the entire nation in terms of the epidemic—it says, America has AIDS. Here sorrow would knit together the social fabric and personal loss to become the common bond of citizenship: we're all in this together.[18]

Jones' Quilt enacted in crisis a queer transformation of another dictum: *e pluribus unum.*

The mourning ritual and spectacle of the AIDS Quilt, with all their familial and national appeal, however, did not touch everyone, and could not, some believed, adequately confront the epidemic as a health crisis, as a political crisis.[19] Although David Feinberg was at first "blown away by it," the second time around, despite more tears, he ended up making out on the Quilt with a Californian named Bill, "as an act of social disobedience." "The textile responses to the AIDS crisis leave me cold," Feinberg wrote. "I prefer my ACT UP button that says 'ACT UP, FIGHT BACK, FIGHT AIDS' and have people on the subway cringe when they read the last word on it."[20] Feinberg illustrated vividly the prominent activist critique of the Quilt as domesticating and depoliticizing and acquiescing to the epidemic.[21] Anger, not tears, organizing and direct action, not quilting and reading names, should be the response to AIDS grief. While mourners wept on the Mall, Senator Jesse Helms was finalizing his amendment to proposed federal legislation for AIDS funding, a vicious amendment presented only three days after the inaugural display of the Quilt that would "'prohibit the use of any funds provided under this ACT . . . to provide AIDS education, information, or prevention materials and activities that promote, encourage, or condone homosexual sexual activities or intravenous use of illegal drugs.'"[22] We should not forget that in 1987 ACT UP was also created.[23] Indeed, given their simultaneity and historical significance in response to the epidemic, the AIDS Quilt and ACT UP perhaps should, despite their opposition, always be remembered together.

Nor was the political critique the only critique of the AIDS Quilt. Despite the gender-specific roots of quilting as a cultural practice, and the epicene quality of the panels, some noted the paucity of women represented in the AIDS Quilt, or, put differently, the dominance of attention to gay men.[24] Ironically, others argued that the AIDS Quilt "de-gayed" the epidemic in its attempt at generating wide empathy and reaching out to mainstream America. One version of the objection argued that the AIDS Quilt sanitized gay sex through "lies of omission," a particularly egregious betrayal given that so many were mourning not only lovers but the very sexual culture that had liberated them.[25] Still others asked, as Marita Sturken powerfully put it, "Is it a privilege to be able to mourn in the middle of an epidemic?" She argued, "much of the rhetoric [of the NAMES Project] is geared specifically at middle-class communities, gay and straight, rather than at inner-city Latino, black, and other poor communities affected by AIDS. The rhetoric of healing and redemption may, in fact, be one of privilege. Is the AIDS Quilt the product of only one part of the community of AIDS in the United States—that is, the people that have the time and resources for spiritual growth and mourning?"[26]

These are pointed and resonant criticisms that rightfully qualified or demystified the AIDS Quilt, and continue to do so. It is important, however, even as we acknowledge these shortcomings and seek their redress, to once again place them and the AIDS Quilt in time. Christopher Capozzola argued, "Despite all its weaknesses, despite all its limits, during the years between 1985 to the mid-1990s, the Quilt managed to resolve those tensions in positive ways. The form of the memorial mattered a great deal: its creation, display, and ultimate meaning were radically inclusive, and its framework of memory was consistently democratic in ways that could encompass its multiple constituencies and their varying definitions of politics."[27] Cleve Jones, in responding to the activist critique, insisted that "the political message is that human life is sacred."[28] This fundamental claim best captures the emotional depth and moral authority that made the AIDS Quilt a transformative epidemic text. As Mohr concluded, "elegy making and mourning are especially worthy activities, for they, perhaps more than anything else, remind us, presses to both consciousness and conscience, why, in a world where suffering regularly dwarfs well-being, life is worth living in the first place. In valorizing, even sacralizing, the mourned person in his individuality and uniqueness, The NAMES Project and elegy in general manifest why the goal of stopping AIDS warrants screaming in the streets and more as means to that end."[29]

Today

If we could first know where we are, and whither we are tending, we could then better judge what to do, and how to do it.
—Abraham Lincoln, "House Divided Speech," June 16, 1858

Listen carefully and you can hear a survivor of the first wave of the AIDS epidemic sardonically exclaiming, "Look how far we've come!" In the second of our time passages, I recalled Cleve Jones being "taken aback" by news of the twentieth anniversary. Among the plausible explanations for his momentary disorientation might have been a horrifying recognition that, despite the passing of more than two decades since the first display of the AIDS Quilt, despite the massive death and its personal and cultural aftershocks, the epidemic—the pandemic—persists, stronger than ever, a fiasco of magnificent proportions: global, national, local, individual. Richard Kim's grim evaluation in 2002, on the occasion of the twentieth anniversary of AIDS, can be repeated virtually without editing nearly a decade later:

> Any assessment of the epidemic was bound to be an indictment, and not the sort we generally like to read about, in which the guilty are absolutely so, and the innocent many and untainted. Any writer willing to connect the dots would conclude that the systemic political response to AIDS has been a signal failure. . . . The current demographics of AIDS, marked as they are by severe economic and racial inequality, were not preordained. AIDS is a preventable and treatable disease, and it exists as it does because it was allowed to unfold this way, through the same kind of gross political negligence that permitted the disease to become an epidemic in the first place.[30]

According to the UNAIDS/WHO *Report on the Global AIDS Epidemic* (2008) and CDC *HIV/AIDS Surveillance Report* (2007), data reveals that in 2007 an estimated 33 million globally were living with HIV, there were 2.7 million new infections, and 2 million AIDS-related deaths. Women accounted for half of all infections. In the United States (estimates according to thirty-four states and five dependent areas), HIV infection increased 15 percent during 2004–2007. African Americans accounted for 51 percent of new infections in 2007. Men who have sex with men (MSM) comprised 53 percent of new cases in 2005, 2006, and 2007. By the end of 2007, 583,298 Americans had died of AIDS in the fifty states and Washington, D.C.[31] Where are we, and whither are we tending?

The AIDS Quilt, too, has grown exponentially since 1987, evidencing at the same time both its success and failure. The NAMES Project reports that as of November 2008 there were over 46,000 panels, 5,789 blocks, and more than 91,000 names in the AIDS Quilt, representing only approximately 17.5 percent of AIDS deaths in the United States. Given these numbers and the 18,000,000 visitors, one would have to conclude that as a ritual of mourning, the AIDS Quilt has thrived remarkably as a rhetorical text. As a spectacle of mourning, however, even granting the $4 million raised for direct services to people with AIDS, the Quilt arguably has flagged or faltered, if we judge it simply with regard to its goals of awareness and prevention.[32] In addition to the infection rates surveyed above, we might take note that an estimated one-quarter of people living with HIV do not know that they are infected with the virus.[33]

The question of empathy also remains open. Despite discourses decrying imbalanced attention to gay men since the beginning of the epidemic, HIV/AIDS still is concentrated in that demographic, noting a rise of 11 percent in infections among MSM between 2001 and 2005, and noting again that the majority of new diagnoses in the United States for 2005–2007 occurred among MSM.[34] Crimp's perspective is not beyond the pale: "That many in our society secretly want us dead is to me beyond question. And one expression of this may be our society's loving attention to the quilt, which is not only a ritual and representation of mourning but also stunning evidence of mass death of gay men. It would, of course, be unseemly for society to celebrate our deaths openly, but I wonder if the quilt helps make this desire decorous."[35] Further, if we take the current disproportionate rates of infection in communities of color and among women within the contexts of racism, sexism, classism, etc., then the appalling bumper sticker from the first wave of the epidemic remains telling: "AIDS: Killing All the Right People."[36]

These familiar binaries, however, are not the only sites of the ongoing divided house of the epidemic. Beginning in 2001 (if not before), a public battle erupted over proprietorship and purpose of the AIDS Quilt when, plagued by debt and desiring to reconfigure its focus in relation to shifting demographics, the NAMES Project moved from San Francisco to Atlanta. A year later, the NAMES Project also revised its relationship with the network of local affiliate chapters, requiring greater centralized control over promotional materials and issuing a ban on local direct-mail fund-raising while at the same time mandating increased responsibility for shipping fees. For reasons both symbolic and financial, nearly a third of the local chapters disbanded in 2002, including the founding local chapter in San Francisco and one of the largest in Washington, D.C.[37]

Cleve Jones, who had been on the payroll as founder and spokesperson since he stepped down as director for health reasons in 1990, was also embroiled with his colleagues at the NAMES Project. Jones had criticized the organization for not displaying the AIDS Quilt in full on the National Mall in 2004 to dramatize AIDS as an issue in the presidential election. This largely precipitated his firing by the NAMES Project in 2003. A protracted legal battle ensued between 2004–2006 over Jones's termination, emotional harm, and possession of 280 panels, or thirty-five blocks, of the AIDS Quilt. In 2007 the NAMES Project claimed that Jones violated the terms of the 2005 settlement by gaining sponsorship of his nonprofit San Francisco Bay Area Friends of the AIDS Memorial Quilt from the Tides Center in San Francisco. As of this writing, it does not appear that panels have returned to San Francisco.[38]

The larger question is one of purpose and the means to achieve it. Jones seems to believe that the AIDS Quilt must continue to function as ritual of spectacle in the largest sense, namely as a sublime rhetoric that makes magnitude apparent to all in deeply resonant national spaces, most specifically in Washington, D.C. He also has criticized the "warehousing" of the AIDS Quilt in Atlanta instead of taking it to the "front line of activism," to "hot zone[s]" of the epidemic.[39] In speaking of continued infection rates among young gay men, for example, he observed in 2003, "What a horrible condemnation of our culture that all these years after people like Martin Luther King and Harvey Milk gave their lives, we are still producing these children, who when they look in the mirror do not see what we see when we look into their eyes. They don't see the beauty. They don't see the promise of the future. They see nothing. . . . And people want to say it's not political."[40] In short, Jones argued in early 2007, the AIDS Quilt "is not intended as a passive memorial."[41]

The NAMES Project believes that it remains an active agent in the fight, on the frontlines—indeed, on the many fronts, demographically speaking, especially in the African American and Latino communities— of the fight against the AIDS epidemic. Executive director Julie Rhoad responded to criticism by observing that, although lacking the resources to display the Quilt in its entirety, more than half of the panel blocks were displayed in local communities each year 2004–2006, dwarfing display totals at the end of the AIDS Quilt's time in San Francisco.[42] Moreover, the NAMES Project created the Historically Black Colleges and Universities Initiative, with these stated goals:

- Raising awareness of HIV/AIDS as a public health issue that disproportionately affects African-American young people
- Complementing existing HIV prevention programs with The Quilt's proven efficacy as an HIV prevention tool and through the leadership of campus peer educators
- Encouraging African-Americans and youth to access HIV testing and treatment
- Promoting AIDS Memorial panel making within the African-American community in order to bring communities together, promote remembrance and healing, and to address the silence around AIDS by facilitating informed dialogue

Other programs include the Communities of Faith Display Initiative and the National Youth Education Program, which "brings the Quilt to youth around the country in schools and community organizations, raising awareness of HIV/AIDS in a context-sensitive way that is found in the displays of The Quilt that we curate every day."[43] Clearly, then, the NAMES Project would argue that it continues to thrive both as a ritual of mourning and a spectacle of mourning. Authors in this volume offer powerful evidence that this is so.

Still others, especially more radical AIDS activists, continue to question the AIDS Quilt as a movement tactic. As Michael Petrelis observed, "The quilt was very effective in the late '80s and early '90s for AIDS awareness. On the other hand, there's hundreds and thousands of people that need a housing subsidy, just trying to keep a roof over their head. Should we be putting our time into another vigil? I don't know."[44] Knowing where we are and whither we are tending remains a conflict about causes and motives, means and vision. As Crimp rightly suggested many years ago: "Activist antagonism to mourning hinges, in part, on how AIDS is interpreted, or rather, where the emphasis is laid, on whether the crisis is seen to be a natural, accidental catastrophe—a disease syndrome that has simply struck at this time in this place—or as the result of gross political negligence or mendacity—an epidemic that was allowed to happen."[45]

Tomorrow

It is rather for us to be here dedicated to the great task remaining before us; that from these honored dead we take increased devotion to that cause for which they gave the last full measure of devotion; that we here highly resolve that these dead shall not have died in vain.

—Abraham Lincoln, "Gettysburg Address," November 19, 1863

Vito Russo's most remembered discourse was, in its own right, Lincolnesque: "AIDS is a test of who we are as a people. And when future generations ask what we did in the war we're going to have to tell them that we are out here fighting. And we have to leave a legacy to the generations of people who would come after us."[46] One difference here, of course, is tense, and therefore audience. For Lincoln, those in the present answered to those already fallen; Russo and his compatriots answered to those not yet born. Both men, however, fought for life in freedom. Neither man lived to see the culmination of that vision.

Another difference seems to be that of memory. In Lincoln's case the performance of memory is thwarted by the task at hand. For Russo, the performance of memory is activated as essentially the task at hand: "remember, that some day, the AIDS crisis is going to be over." David Román offers an insightful reading of Russo's call to memory:

Russo asks his audience to remember essentially a belief that has no basis in historical fact but is determined by what can only be understood as the political will of the people whom he addresses. He hopes people will align around this shared feeling, which will motivate and inspire change. . . . [He] also imagines that AIDS will be remembered. It runs on the presumption that the historical archives of AIDS and its activism will be preserved so that future generations will know what transpired and how "a brave group of people stood up and fought and in some cases died," sparing them the terrible reality of what Russo and others experienced throughout the early to late 1980s.[47]

Russo's future perfect vision—"a day when we can stop adding panels to this quilt and put it away, as a symbol of a terrible thing that happened and that's now over"—is simultaneously heartening and wrenching given our retrospective location. But the presumptions Román discerns, namely that an archive of AIDS, specifically the Quilt, should be preserved and mobilized as a usable history, serve well as prompts and provocations as we imagine our own versions of the future time of the epidemic. As Sarah Brophy put it, "What we are brought to bear witness to in viewing the quilt is a strange archive, one in which melancholic incorporation (and its attendant disrespect for boundaries) intermingles with more nostalgic tendencies, and with an idealized connection across gender, sexuality, and desire, as well as across familial and national structures."[48] Or we might put it, as does Roger Hallas, in terms of an "archival imperative": "The question of the archive is thus in the end not whether it succeeds in preserving the past from oblivion but how the past that eventually emerges from it can potentially produce a revelatory historical consciousness of our present."[49]

Within contemporary contexts of the pandemic, it is important to ask, as do the authors in the last section of this volume, whether AIDS memory, embodied in the Quilt, is boon or bane to the ongoing struggle against the disease, and how so. One could reasonably claim that, despite the ongoing spread of HIV, the conditions Jeff Nunokawa described have expired: "The understated, understood, remedial urgency of efforts of remembrance such as the NAMES Project, efforts of remembrance that emerge from the gay community itself, describes a pressure that persistently attends the work of remembering such casualties, a pressure to mark deaths that the majority culture is simply not disposed to notice."[50] While the majority culture hasn't changed in its indifference, the disposition of the gay community in particular seems to have changed with the dissipation of that sense of urgency. Both physically and temporally, and consequentially, AIDS has been invented as "chronic." Therefore, perhaps AIDS has been rendered, in a flattened sense, chronological, and perhaps memory work is the morbid lot of those complicit in the death narratives that contemporary HIV rhetorics of manageability, longevity, and health strive to displace and dispel.

Although I fully embrace queer disruption of all defeatist, disciplinary, and discriminatory discourses that have constituted AIDS since its inception, as well as champion those discourses of living that have innumerable beneficial material effects, I also strongly endorse, in various forms, the remembrance, legacy, and archive that Russo bequeathed as obligation. We might consider here memory as ongoing political will as well as the politics of AIDS remembrance. Put differently, "The Quilt embodies a consciousness not just of the political *nature* of commemoration, but of the political *potential* of these acts as well."[51] As a letter on the AIDS Quilt suggests: "By the time this letter is read to you, I will have gone on to my new life. . . . In the future, when you look at the history books that will be written about AIDS, you will find that one of the highlights of the book will be a chapter on one of the good results of the disease—that is—humanity became more compassionate. From that compassion the world became a better place. And you, my friends, will be the history makers."[52] The voice from the Quilt resonates as we reflect on Judith Butler's observation: "If we stay with the sense of loss, are we left feeling only passive and powerless, as some might fear? Or are we, rather, returned to a sense of human vulnerability, to our collective responsibility for the physical lives of one another? . . . To grieve, and to make grief itself into a resource for politics, is not to be resigned to inaction, but it may be understood as the slow process by which we develop a point of identification with suffering itself."[53]

The Quilt's ongoing political potential will be activated by embodied memories in various forms of mobility, as artifacts and ongoing individual and cultural performances, as well as by its influence on other commemorative modes and artifacts, some seemingly unrelated to the AIDS Quilt. In constituting memory as ongoing political will, its materialization and enactment, I have in mind the necessity of AIDS memory, queer memory and history, as prolegomenon and provenance to all GLBTQ activism, common grounds of GLBTQ communities. This is a renewal of Simon Watney's rally cry from 1994: "When so few value us in life, it is especially important to record our everyday experiences of the epidemic from the perspective of those who cannot simply go away. We must define this history, or it will not survive us."[54] Likewise, we must define ourselves in terms of that history; we will not survive without it. As Watney wrote elsewhere,

> Whilst martyrology is distasteful, especially if it lends a posthumous sense of purpose to the accidents of epidemic disease, it is none the less salutary to record and recall the political history of the HIV epidemic. . . . For if we accept that gay identity is not fixed or given, but a complex historical result, it becomes apparent that it is at the level of popular understanding and memory of the epidemic that gay identity will be re-shaped and re-directed.[55]

Such a project would emulate what Lucas Hilderbrand, in his discussion of ACT UP memory, including James Wentzy's commemorative video *Fight Back, Fight AIDS* (2002), calls "retroactivism." Hilderbrand advocates "intergenerational nostalgia," a form of cultural memory that "accounts for generative historical fascination, of imagining, feeling, and drawing from history."[56] In a similar vein, Alexandra Juhasz observes that the mission of what she calls "queer archive activism" is "not merely to get stuck in remembering AIDS images but rather to relodge those frozen memories in contemporary contexts so that they, and perhaps we, can be reanimated."[57] Though the Quilt might not fit with Hilderbrand and Juhasz's desire for nostalgia's mobilization of more radical queer community, the potential of such memory work is broadly applicable and inspiring, for as Hilderbrand concludes, it "not only records a social movement but also regenerates it."[58]

This imperative entails a simultaneous interrogation of history and memory that results, for instance, in an intersectional account of the past instead of one that is exclusively or predominantly gay. Following Kyra Pearson's query in this volume about how to have history in an epidemic, such an interrogation would result in rethinking not only the relationship between AIDS history and the present, but also AIDS history and its preceding pasts. The damage done by what Christopher Castiglia has called "counternostalgia," or "a look back in fury at the sexual 'excesses' of the immature, pathological, and diseased pre-AIDS generation," can only be undone by memory work that might reconfigure individual and collective shame, rage, and other feelings.[59] Provocatively, a number of theorists have recently espoused deep exploration, embrace, and application of "queer negativity." As Heather Love concludes, "the question really is not whether feelings such as grief, regret, and despair have a place in transformative politics: it would in fact be impossible to imagine transformative politics without these feelings. Nor is the question how to cultivate hope in the face of despair, since such calls tend to demand the replacement of despair with hope. Rather, the question that faces us is how to make a future backward enough that even the most reluctant among us might want to live there."[60] At the same time, we would do well to join Hilderbrand in resisting an exclusively traumatic framework, acknowledging and encouraging instead an "affective spectrum and its potential implications for subsequent generations."[61]

We might contemplate in relationship to the Quilt, for instance, the late activist Michael Lynch's ire in the early 1980s at gay men chastising and policing sexual culture, who in his judgment sought "to rip apart the very promiscuous fabric that knits the gay male community together and that, in its democratic anarchism, defies state regulation of our sexuality."[62] We might also engage in countermemories that extend a tradition of altering the terms of the death narrative, one instantiation of which would entail the juxtaposition of Quilt panels against a revival version of ACT UP's installation "Let the Record Show . . ." featuring a backdrop of the Nuremberg trials with foregrounded headstones for Ronald Reagan, Jerry Falwell, Jesse Helms, William F. Buckley, as well as contemporary homophobic, AIDSphobic bigots.[63] Or a visual display featuring familiar images of lovers grieving at the Quilt juxtaposed with the image of Nancy Reagan weeping as she rested her hand on her husband's coffin. And, of course, we could continue to make panels for the Quilt, for those recently deceased and for those long gone but unaccounted for, especially for those who for too long have been underrepresented.

Finally, let me reflect on Russo's hope that there will be "a day when we can stop adding panels to this quilt and put it away."[64] Although the panels continue to accumulate unabated in only partial representation of the epidemic, the Quilt has, in a sense, been put away. I neither affirm nor deny Cleve Jones's claim that the AIDS Quilt has been "warehoused." But storage of historical texts across time passages does constitute an archive. Sturken early on registered the pragmatic difficulties in preserving the AIDS Quilt and the adequacy of digital images of the panels.[65] Those important difficulties persist. I offer instead a different perspective, namely that archives are always political spaces. Important questions regarding access, interpretation, and display must always be asked of the NAMES Project archive, even as we recognize its valued stewardship. As I have said before, "The archive . . . should rightly be understood not as a passive receptacle for historical documents and their 'truths,' or a benign research space, but rather as a dynamic site of rhetorical power."[66] We should remember, too, that although archives, like memory and history, are deployed (and indeed must be deployed) less often for their own sake than for their utility in the present and future, those archived panels are still lives and should be remembered in relation to those important projects giving voice to people living with HIV/AIDS.[67] And we should still remember what it means to mourn: "Mourning, like love, is a vector of attention pointed from the moral agent to the particularity of another person. The proper focus of moral concern in mourning is he who is mourned, not he who does the mourning. Only through and in the mourner's sorrow does the missing of the dead really count for anything."[68]

The Essays

In the pages that follow, we find ten superb essays that embody and engage and interrogate the AIDS Quilt. Like the Quilt itself, no single account, or even limited set of interpretations, can fully convey this richly diverse and complicated epidemic text. Indeed, if some of these authors are correct, we never experience the same Quilt twice; we alter with each encounter. Nevertheless, these insightful essays give us yards and yards of materiality and memory to ponder, feel, challenge, and act upon as the next decades of the AIDS Quilt unfold.

Although the Quilt is by design queerly organized, which is to say without prescribed entrances, routes, barriers, or exits, I risk betraying the text here by grouping the essays according to three thematic *topoi* so as to facilitate the reader's engagement. At the same time, the beauty and brilliance of the essays, as will become clear, is that they, like the Quilt, exceed any stable categorization, conceptually and emotionally circulating throughout the other groupings, through each of the other essays, in the volume.

The first section I label "Emergence" because its two essays explore the contexts and traditions out of and in response to which the Quilt was conceived, formed, mobilized, coalesced, stitched, resisted, orchestrated, performed, mediated, and expanded in its formative years. Most prominent and complex of these contexts was the AIDS epidemic itself—viral, visceral, and volatile in transmogrifying bodies, discourses, and spaces constitutive of selves and others in every sense. But the epidemic must be considered in relation to the many other conditions of Reagan's America. Here too we discover the formative rhetorical patterns and swatches that bound up and expressed and transformed lost lives, lives at the limen.

Origin stories, such as that told by Cleve Jones in this volume's prologue, are never the whole story, compelling though they may be. Every beginning text is indebted intertextually to that which came before, and seldom can we predict how that text, in turn, will be transformed by what comes after it. Carole Blair and Neil Michel, in their essay, "The AIDS Memorial Quilt and the Contemporary Culture of Public Commemoration," place the AIDS Quilt in the historical context of collective memory at the time of its emergence. More specifically, they place the AIDS Quilt "in conversation" with its predecessor, the touchstone Vietnam Veterans Memorial, in order to discover how these rhetorical texts departed from commemorative norms of invention, representation, and reception. Blair and Michel understand this moment as a critical juncture in contemporary public commemoration, with the numerous commemorative sites that followed, particularly the Oklahoma City and 9/11 memorials, both enabled and disabled by anxieties and tensions in the AIDS Quilt's rhetoric.

From our historical vantage, it is perhaps difficult for people who did not live through the first wave of the epidemic to understand that, as Gust A. Yep observes in his essay, "The Politics of Loss and Its Remains in *Common Threads: Stories from the Quilt*," those lost to AIDS were culturally and politically constituted as unreal, abject, ungrievable bodies. In recognizing this dimension of loss with Yep, we see that it constitutes, then as well as now, multiple social, political, and aesthetic relations.

Such relationships of loss, he explains, are manifested in its bodily remains, such as subjectivities; spatial remains, such as representation; and
ideal remains, such as knowledges, across time. Yep illustrates this relationship between loss and its remains in the extraordinary, award-winning
1989 documentary *Common Threads,* a film which beautifully produced
bodily, spatial, and ideal remains of five lives lost to AIDS. Through his
reading of the documentary, Yep not only reveals the politics of loss and
its remains during the epidemic's ascendancy, but also identifies for us
the ways in which those remains might meaningfully haunt us still.

I term the second section "Movement." In one sense this designation is temporal insofar as its span stretches from the first wave of the
epidemic to the present; the approach here is generally diachronic. But
more significantly, movement signifies the emotional, intellectual, moral,
political, theoretical awakenings, rendings, epiphanies, traversals and
transitions, tensions and reverberations that the Quilt has engendered.
And continues to engender. Noteworthy here is the effort to essay the
Quilt in the form of the Quilt, the manifest desire to empanel oneself,
the deeply resonant reflections of walking and stitching this text, and the
engagements with others this text inspires and provokes. We are offered
vivid proof of the claims that the Quilt is experiential, material, performative. Movement too names the political will, political judgment, activist
impulse, and action imagined, fomented, and enacted in these essays.

As many who have contemplated the AIDS Quilt point out, the intellectual and emotional experience of its display derives from the radical
particularity of the panels, an experience that isn't mapped but inevitably
reroutes those who encounter it. In that spirit, Kevin Michael DeLuca,
Christine Harold, and Kenneth Rufo provide us with a unique experience of their "Q.U.I.L.T.: A Patchwork of Reflections." Through their
wide-ranging "thought panels," we process loss directly, tour the NAMES
Project headquarters in Atlanta, engage the AIDS Quilt as a representative failure, as public, as sanctuary, as a spectacular sight, as a disorienting surrealist response to funereal aesthetics, as sublime, as cloth, as a
quilting point, as an archive. The creativity of this critical endeavor is
in its own right a memorial to the AIDS Quilt, even as its deconstruction troubles what we thought we knew about this text, its meanings and
promises.

Brian L. Ott, Eric Aoki, and Greg Dickinson, in "Collage/Montage as Critical Practice, Or How to "Quilt"/Read Postmodern Text(ile)s," also "come together" to enact the Quilt by creating a collage/montage of "panels" that bespeak its experiential, material, performative, and theoretical dimensions and force. Striking in these reflections is the sense of engagement, with the Quilt and with each other, and of their interanimation; or, like the Quilt itself, according to their account, they engage in a meaningful "coperformance," "a critical performance that is equally fragmented and unified, communal and individual." After an orientation to the complex manifold history and practice of quilting, Aoki's autoethnography movingly exhibits his intersecting professional and personal efforts to "make peace with the Quilt," to stitch life together again in the wake of his partner Stephen's death from AIDS, and the challenges of stitching Stephen's memory. Dickinson focuses on the material embodiments of walking the Quilt, memorial acts of public (un)stitching of the body politic in a particular "location." He provocatively claims that "the Quilt is a founding mnemonic of late modernity," an experience and constitution of past and present that is "nodal, networked, nomadic, embodied, performative." Ott understands the Quilt as a "living theory" of the text in the Barthesian sense of its ineffability, its radical uniqueness as always a "live performance," its inducement to ecstatic and disorienting experience, its production. "To experience The Quilt," Ott writes, "is, if only temporarily, to unravel—to come undone." Put differently, such a powerful encounter is momentarily, in a "flash of experience," to be unfettered and thus to reimagine, perhaps to reconfigure, self and community.

Evident in these panels, as in Quilt panels, is not only deep intellectual engagement but also trenchant emotional encounters. Jeffrey A. Bennett conceptualizes this dimension in his essay, "A Stitch in Time: Public Emotionality and the Repertoire of Citizenship." Rejecting the division between reason and emotion, Bennett explores the ways in which the Quilt's emotionality offered a meaningful and inventive counterresponse to the rational official discourses and silences that attended and constituted the epidemic in its early years. Moreover, the Quilt as a "peripatetic site of public emotionality" produced "repertoires of public citizenship": emotional performative embodiments across time and space that have engendered stranger relationality, knowledge and memory, political judgment and participation, and moral action—catharsis, belonging, bonding, and empowerment. Although the Quilt's entextualization has in some ways fallen "prey to hegemonic forces," namely discourses of neo-liberalism, it has also resisted them. "Its incomplete narrative," Bennett concludes, "structures the voids that those engaged with the Quilt must fill and prohibits its therapeutic qualities from eliminating possibilities of change."

A final traversal, spatial in a broader sense and temporally most exigent, Daniel C. Brouwer's essay, "From San Francisco to Atlanta and Back Again: Ideologies of Mobility in the AIDS Quilt's Search for a Homeland," focuses on the multifarious formations of mobility; the power, politics, and ideology of home, homeland, travel, tourism, and other instantiations of place and movement. From the beginning, the AIDS Quilt powerfully subverted the epidemiological constructions of movement by its communally affirming mobility. Indeed, as Brouwer observes, the AIDS Quilt functioned best through its "promiscuous mobility." However, the AIDS Quilt's move to Atlanta, what Brouwer calls a "controversial re-routing," and the subsequent firing of Cleve Jones, created a different politics of mobility, one related to notions of home and homeland and inflected especially by race and gender. Here Brouwer discovers "new combinations of memory, fantasy, people, and place as it unsettled long-standing combinations of those elements."

The final section I label "Transformation." Though these essays share with work in the previous section many of the elements of movement, they also chart distinct trajectories into the future. They most directly contemplate the peril and potential of remembering, memorializing, and archiving the Quilt. Does the Quilt still function as a means of survival? For whom? How might it be retrofitted to function as such? Has the Quilt become monumental, which is to say hegemonic, at the expense of more vibrant activist modes? Does remembering the Quilt displace other, equally powerful or perhaps superior, memory work? What are the wages of history, memory, in an epidemic without end?

In "Rhetorics of Loss and Living: Adding New Panels to the AIDS Quilt as an Act of Eulogy," Bryant Keith Alexander seeks to thwart the dominant AIDS death narrative, as well as the inadequate representation of African American gay men in AIDS history and memory, through the ethnoperformative texts of "mourning subjects." While acknowledging the historical significance of the AIDS Quilt, Alexander "resists the historicizing of lives still living in hope," the foreclosure of the experiences of those yet to be, perhaps never to be, quilted. Through what he calls "short stories" or "counternarratives"—powerful narratives including his own reflection on his brother's death from AIDS and the voices of Black gay PWAs [persons with AIDS]—Alexander envisions and enacts "rhetorics of loss and living," a reconfiguration of the genre of eulogy, a "resistant archival process," that mediates ("ruptures" and "sutures" by "stand between persons") between past and present, presence and absence, individual and community, grief and political action. These narratives constitute the AIDS Quilt as "performance of possibilities," functioning "like new panels" to reinvigorate the NAMES Project as a transformed discursive space, political modality, and museum.

It is worth noting again that 2012 will mark the twenty-fifth anniversary of ACT UP. The starkly different approaches these organizations adopted in response to the epidemic produced tensions and debates among various communities that have been exceptionally illuminating. Erin J. Rand, in her essay "Repeated Remembrance: Commemorating the AIDS Quilt and Resuscitating the Mourned Subject," revives and extends this significant engagement by participating in what she astutely calls our "doubled commemoration," commemorating a memorial. Rand examines the ways in which the AIDS Quilt helped to produce gay men as "mourned subjects," those who gained subjectivity, which did not previously exist, by virtue of being codified as those dying of AIDS. Such subjectivity, generated through grief, granted a certain measure of national social recognition and tolerance of this group. However, Rand questions the agency afforded by the constitution of the mourned subject, arguing that instead we should look carefully at anger as a productive alternative response that achieves progress through activism, an alternative embodied in the demos and political funerals of ACT UP. As we ourselves repeat the ritual of memorialization, Rand asks again: mourning or militancy?

Finally and fittingly, Kyra Pearson, in "How to Have History in an Epidemic," queries time—that is, the discourses of history in relation to the rhetorical relevance and constitution of the ongoing epidemic as embodied in and engaged by the Quilt. Or, as she provocatively asks, "What might it mean to have a *history* in an epidemic? *How* might we historicize an epidemic that is now within Western nations considered a 'manageable,' chronic condition (at least for those who can afford treatment)? And *why* might a sense of the past be important now?" Arguing for the centrality of temporality to AIDS activism, Pearson situates the unfolding of the Quilt across time and space within the contexts of inescapable precedent and ephemerality. The Quilt resists both of those powerful "invocations of the past," Pearson argues, by virtue of its functioning as an "artifact of progression" rather than a memorial to progress. As her diachronic analysis of media coverage of the Quilt suggests, however, the irony of this artifact of progression is that it has thus become vulnerable to the charge of obsolescence, mired in a struggle over activist meaning and value. Shaped by time and timing, ambivalence about the Quilt should remind us all that *kairos* is about the past as much as the present and future.

NOTES

1. Eve Kosofsky Sedgwick, "White Glasses," *Tendencies* (Durham, NC: Duke University Press, 1993), 264.
2. Paula A. Treichler, "AIDS, Homophobia, and Biomedical Discourse: An Epidemic of Signification," *How to Have Theory in an Epidemic: Cultural Chronicles of AIDS* (Durham, NC: Duke University Press, 1999), 11–41. See also Susan Sontag, *AIDS and Its Metaphors* (New York: Farrar, Straus and Giroux, 1989); Cindy Patton, *Inventing AIDS* (New York: Routledge, 1990).
3. David B. Feinberg, *Queer and Loathing: Rants and Raves of a Raging AIDS Clone* (New York: Penguin Books, 1994), 198.
4. Christopher Capozzola, "A Very American Epidemic: Memory Politics and Identity Politics in the AIDS Memorial Quilt, 1985–1993," *Radical History Review* 82 (2002): 91–109.
5. Vito Russo, "Why We Fight," in *Common Threads: Stories from the Quilt,* produced by Bill Couturie, Rob Epstein, and Jeffrey Friedman, and directed by Rob Epstein and Jeffrey Friedman (New York: Telling Pictures and the NAMES Project Foundation, 2004).
6. Abraham Lincoln, "To the Father and Mother of Col. Elmer Ellsworth," in C. A. Tripp, *The Intimate World of Abraham Lincoln* (New York: Free Press, 2005),

121–122. Elmer Ellsworth was a dashing and gifted young soldier whom Lincoln had admired and befriended in Springfield, Illinois, between 1859 and 1861. Upon taking the presidency, Lincoln brought Ellsworth with him to Washington, rapidly and pointedly arranging for his placement in the office of the chief clerk of the War Department, then a month later his promotion to adjutant and inspector general of militia for the United States. In the first days of the war, Ellsworth knew that a Confederate flag flying over a hotel in Alexandria, Virginia, distressed Lincoln, who could see it from across the Potomac. While on a nearby mission on May 24, 1861, Ellsworth took his men into the hotel to seize the flag and was killed in the action. Lincoln's grief was severe, so severe, in fact, that his composure more than once failed him in sobbing waves as he attempted to conduct official business. He twice visited Ellsworth's body at the Naval Yard and arranged for funeral services to be held at the Executive Mansion. Ellsworth's death was also precipitous militarily, as David Donald observes, "Up to this point Lincoln had favored delay, but he now ordered an advance against the Confederate army." David Herbert Donald, *Lincoln* (New York: Random House, 1995), 306. See also Tripp, *Intimate World,* 109–124; Ruth Painter Randall, *Colonel Elmer Ellsworth: A Biography of Lincoln's Friend and First Hero of the Civil War* (Boston: Little, Brown and Co., 1960).

7. Donald, *Lincoln,* 306.

8. For a similar call to historicize AIDS, see David Román, "Remembering AIDS: A Reconstruction of the Film *Longtime Companion*," *GLQ: A Journal of Lesbian and Gay Studies* 12 (2006): 281–301.

9. Yingling explained, "research suggests a 'natural history' of the virus (ten-year-plus incubation periods); gay and lesbian rhetoric links the fight against AIDS to Stonewall and to the entire question of gay and lesbian history; PWA [person with AIDS] rhetoric states that the ethics of our historical moment will be judged by its response to AIDS; journalists and experts alike project 'the next ten years' or re-hearse the present and past in a narrative behind which always hovers a specter of apocalypse in which AIDS functions as the demonic counterpart to the beneficent 'end of history' coded in myths of America." Thomas Yingling, "AIDS in America: Postmodern Governance, Identity, and Experience," in *Inside/Out: Lesbian Theories, Gay Theories,* ed. Diana Fuss (New York: Routledge, 1991), 297–298; Cindy Patton, *Globalizing AIDS* (Minneapolis: University of Minnesota Press, 2002), 6.

10. For accounts of the first wave of the epidemic in the United States, see Dennis Altman, *AIDS in the Mind of America: The Social, Political, and Psychological Impact of a New Epidemic* (New York: Anchor Books, 1987); Cindy Patton, *Sex and Germs:*

The Politics of AIDS (Boston: South End Press, 1985); Randy Shilts, *And the Band Played On: Politics, People, and the AIDS Epidemic* (New York: St. Martin's Press, 1987); Paul Monette, *Borrowed Time: An AIDS Memoir* (San Diego: Harcourt, Brace, Jovanovich, 1988); John Preston, ed., *Personal Dispatches: Writers Confront AIDS* (New York: St. Martin's, 1988); George Whitmore, *Someone Was Here* (New York: New American Library, 1988); James Kinsella, *Covering the Plague: AIDS and the American Media* (New Brunswick, NJ: Rutgers University Press, 1989); *Tongues Untied,* directed by Marlon Riggs (Berkeley, CA: Frameline Films, 1989); Patton, *Inventing AIDS; Longtime Companion,* screenplay by Craig Lucas, directed by Norman René (Santa Monica, CA: Samuel Goldwyn, 1990); David Wojnarowicz, *Close to the Knives: A Memoir of Disintegration* (New York: Vintage, 1991); ACT UP/NY Women and AIDS Book Group, *Women, AIDS, and Activism* (New York: Between the Lines, 1991); Sarah Schulman, *My American History: Lesbian and Gay Life during the Reagan/Bush Years* (New York: Routledge, 1994); Larry Kramer, *Reports from the Holocaust: The Making of an AIDS Activist,* rev. ed. (New York: St. Martin's Press, 1994); Steven Epstein, *Impure Science: AIDS, Activism, and the Politics of Knowledge* (Berkeley: University of California Press, 1996); David Román, *Acts of Intervention: Performance, Gay Culture, and AIDS* (Bloomington: Indiana University Press, 1998); John-Manuel Andriote, *Victory Deferred: How AIDS Changed Gay Life in America* (Chicago: University of Chicago Press, 1999); Cathy J. Cohen, *The Boundaries of Blackness: AIDS and the Breakdown of Black Politics* (Chicago: University of Chicago Press, 1999); Dudley Clendinen and Adam Nagourney, *Out for Good: The Struggle to Build a Gay Rights Movement in America* (New York: Simon and Schuster, 1999); Patton, *Globalizing AIDS;* Andrew Holleran, *Chronicle of a Plague, Revisited* (New York: Da Capo Press, 2008).

11. Altman, *AIDS in the Mind of America,* 29.

12. Douglas Crimp, "Mourning and Militancy," *Melancholia and Moralism: Essays on AIDS and Queer Politics* (Cambridge, MA: MIT Press, 2002), 136–137.

13. Lawrence Howe, "The AIDS Quilt and Its Traditions," *College Literature* 24 (1997): 109.

14. For background on Jones, see Cleve Jones, with Jeff Dawson, *Stitching a Revolution: The Making of an Activist* (San Francisco: HarperSanFrancisco, 2000); Randy Shilts, *The Mayor of Castro Street: The Life and Times of Harvey Milk* (New York: St. Martin's, 1982); Shilts, *And the Band Played On;* Clendinen and Nagourney, *Out for Good.*

15. Douglas Crimp, "The Spectacle of Mourning," *Melancholia and Moralism: Essays on AIDS and Queer Politics* (Cambridge, MA: MIT Press, 2002), 198.

16. Richard D. Mohr, "Text(ile): Reading The NAMES Project's AIDS Quilt," in *Gay Ideas: Outing and Other Controversies* (Boston: Beacon Press, 1992), 109.

17. Peter S. Hawkins, "Naming Names: The Art of Memory and the Names Project AIDS Quilt," *Critical Inquiry* 19 (1993): 770; Marita Sturken, "Conversations with the Dead: Bearing Witness in the AIDS Memorial Quilt," *Tangled Memories: The Vietnam War, the AIDS Epidemic, and the Politics of Remembering* (Berkeley: University of California Press, 1997), 193.

18. Hawkins, "Naming Names," 777.

19. Among the many valuable analyses, Crimp best articulates ambivalence toward the AIDS Quilt. See "Mourning and Militancy" and "The Spectacle of Mourning." In the latter, for instance, he concluded, "In an epidemic that didn't have to happen, and whose continuing to this day to spread virtually unabated is the result of political neglect or outright mendacity, every death is unacceptable. And yet death itself can never finally not be accepted. We have to accept death to continue to live. But the difference, and the resulting ambivalence, is precisely this: the difference between those of us who must learn to accept these deaths and those who still find these deaths acceptable. And who can say whether or not the Names Project quilt might cut both ways." Crimp, "The Spectacle of Mourning," 202.

20. Feinberg, *Queer and Loathing*, 37–38, 184. Deborah Gould's study suggests that Feinberg's reaction was consonant with ACT UP's organizational response to the Quilt: "As part of its mobilization for the FDA action, ACT UP passed out a leaflet at the quilt showing. One side blared, '"SHOW YOUR ANGER TO THE PEOPLE WHO HELPED MAKE THE QUILT POSSIBLE: OUR GOVERNMENT."' Text on the reverse read, '"The Quilt helps us remember our lovers, relatives, and friends who have died during the past eight years. These people have died from a virus. But they have been killed by our government's neglect and inaction. . . . More than 40,000 people have died from AIDS. . . . Before this Quilt grows any larger, turn your grief into anger. Turn your anger into action. TURN THE POWER OF THE QUILT INTO ACTION."' Deborah B. Gould, *Moving Politics: Emotion and ACT UP's Fight Against AIDS* (Chicago: University of Chicago Press, 2009), 225–226.

21. For more on this activist critique, see Mohr, "Text(ile)," 114–117; Sarah Brophy, *Witnessing AIDS: Writing, Testimony, and the Work of Mourning* (Toronto: University of Toronto Press, 2004), 45–51.

22. Quoted in Douglas Crimp, "How to Have Promiscuity in an Epidemic," in *AIDS: Cultural Analysis, Cultural Activism*, ed. Douglas Crimp (Cambridge, MA: MIT Press, 1991), 259.

23. For accounts of ACT UP, see ACT UP's Web site: http://www.actupny.org/; Joshua Gamson, "Silence, Death, and the Invisible Enemy: AIDS Activism and Social Movement 'Newness,'" *Social Problems* 36 (1989): 351–367; Douglas Crimp and Adam Rolston, *AIDS DemoGraphics* (Seattle: Bay Press, 1990); Douglas Crimp, "Right On, Girlfriend!" in *Fear of a Queer Planet: Queer Politics and Social Theory,* ed. Michael Warner (Minneapolis: University of Minnesota Press, 2003): 300–320; Kramer, *Reports from the Holocaust;* Andriote, *Victory Deferred;* Benjamin Shepard and Ronald Hayduk, eds., *From ACT UP to the WTO: Urban Protest and Community Building in the Era of Globalization* (New York: Verso Books, 2002); Ann Cvetkovich, *An Archive of Feelings: Trauma, Sexuality, and Lesbian Public Cultures* (Durham, NC: Duke University Press, 2003); *AIDS RIOT New York, 1987–1994: Artist Collectives Against AIDS* (Grenoble, France: Magasin, 2003); T. V. Reed, "ACTing UP against AIDS: The (Very) Graphic Arts in a Moment of Crisis," in *The Art of Protest: Culture and Activism from the Civil Rights Movement to the Streets of Seattle* (Minneapolis: University of Minnesota Press, 2005), 179–217; Gould, *Moving Politics.*

24. See Sturken, "Conversations with the Dead," 202–206; Hawkins, "Naming Names," 767–770. See also Cindy Patton, *Last Served: Gendering the HIV Pandemic* (London: Taylor and Francis, 1994); Flavia Rando, "The Person with AIDS: The Body, the Feminine, and the Names Project Memorial Quilt," in *Gendered Epidemic: Representations of Women in the Age of AIDS,* ed. Nancy L. Roth and Katie Hogan (New York: Routledge, 1998), 191–204.

25. See Sturken, "Conversations with the Dead," 208; Mohr, "Text(ile)," 121; Crimp, "Mourning and Militancy," 140–141.

26. Sturken, "Conversations with the Dead," 209, 211. See also Phillip Brian Harper, *Are We Not Men? Masculine Anxiety and the Problem of African-American Identity* (New York: Oxford University Press, 1996); Cohen, *The Boundaries of Blackness;* E. Patrick Johnson, *Appropriating Blackness: Performance and the Politics of Authenticity* (Durham: University of North Carolina Press, 2003); Horacio N. Roque Ramírez, "A Living Archive of Desire: Teresita la Campesina and the Embodiment of Queer Latino Community Histories," in *Archive Stories: Facts, Fictions, and the Writing of History,* ed. Antoinette Burton (Durham, NC: Duke University Press, 2005): 111–135; Eric Darnell Pritchard, "'This is Not an Empty-Headed Man in a Dress': Literacy Misused, Reread and Rewritten in Soulopoliz," *Southern Communication Journal* 74 (2009): 278–299.

27. Capozzola, "A Very American Epidemic," 93.

28. Jones, *Stitching a Revolution,* 170.

29. Mohr, "Text(ile)," 126. See also Jonathan Weinberg, "The Quilt: Activism and Re-membrance," *Art in America* 80 (1992): 37–39.

30. Richard Kim, "Beyond the AIDS Quilt," *Nation,* December 30, 2002, 28. Assess-ments at the twenty-fifth anniversary remained strikingly consistent. See, for example, Leslie Fulbright, "AIDS at 25: Disease Denial Devastating for African Americans," *San Francisco Chronicle,* June 5, 2006, A1.

31. Joint United Nations Programme on HIV/AIDS (UNAIDS), *Executive Summary: 2008 Report on the Global AIDS Epidemic,* http://data.unaids.org/pub/GlobalRe-port/2008/JC1511_GR08_ExecutiveSummary_en.pdf; Centers for Disease Control and Prevention, *HIV/AIDS Surveillance Report,* 2007, vol. 19 (Atlanta: U.S. De-partment of Health and Human Services, Centers for Disease Control and Pre-vention), http://www.cdc.gov/hiv/topics/surveillance/resources/reports/2007report/pdf/2007SurveillanceReport.pdf (accessed August 12, 2009).

    I want to point out that throughout this volume statistical assessments of the toll of AIDS vary. This "inconsistency" is, on one hand, not uncommon among mul-tiple reputable sources; on the other hand, it strikes me as an important rhetorical effect of the ongoing political struggle over the signification of AIDS.

32. AIDS Quilt facts are taken from the Web site of the Names Project Foundation AIDS Memorial Quilt, http://www.aidsquilt.org/index.htm (accessed August 18, 2009).

33. Centers for Disease Control and Prevention, *HIV/AIDS Surveillance Report.*

34. UNAIDS, *Executive Summary: 2008 Report on the Global AIDS Epidemic;* Centers for Disease Control and Prevention, *HIV/AIDS Surveillance Report.*

35. Crimp, "The Spectacle of Mourning," 201.

36. Quoted by Cleve Jones in the documentary *Then and Now* on the *Common Threads* DVD.

37. See Bob Adams, "A Rip in the AIDS Quilt," *Advocate,* June 25, 2002, 38; Jen Chris-tiansen, "A Rip in the Quilt," *Advocate,* February 26, 2006, 28–35; Jesse McKinley, "A Changing Battle on AIDS Is Reflected in a Quilt," *New York Times,* January 31, 2007, A1, A16.

38. Matthew J. Bajko, "Names Project Delivers New Setback to AIDS Quilt Cre-ator," *Bay Area Reporter,* January 4, 2007, http://www.ebar.com/news/article.php?sec=news&article=1454 (accessed August 18, 2009); Wyatt Buchanan, "San Francisco's AIDS Quilt's Permanent Return to City in Doubt," *San Francisco Chron-icle,* January 4, 2007, http://www.sfgate.com/cgi-bin/article.cgi?f=/c/a/2007/01/04/

BAG31NCNTM1.DTL (accessed August 18, 2009); Christiansen, "A Rip in the Quilt"; McKinley, "A Changing Battle." Currently, there is no update regarding the Quilt on Cleve Jones's Web site, at http://www.clevejones.com. Activist Michael Petrelis, on his blog, has criticized Jones for failing to follow through with his plans for the Quilt as a local resource for HIV prevention in San Francisco. Michael Petrelis, "Cleve's Broken 2005 AIDS Promises to BAR; Indicators of DC March Success?" *Petrelis Files,* August 10, 2009, http://mpetrelis.blogspot.com/2009/08/cleves-broken-2005-aids-promises-to-bar.html. (accessed August 18, 2009).

39. Christiansen, "A Rip in the Quilt"; McKinley, "A Changing Battle."
40. Quoted by Cleve Jones in *Then and Now.*
41. McKinley, "A Changing Battle," A16.
42. Christiansen, "A Rip in the Quilt"; McKinley, "A Changing Battle."
43. AIDS Quilt initiatives are taken from the Web site of the Names Project Foundation AIDS Memorial Quilt, http://www.aidsquilt.org/index.htm (accessed May 7, 2007).
44. McKinley, "A Changing Battle," A1.
45. Crimp, "Mourning and Militancy," 133.
46. Russo, "Why We Fight," in *Common Threads.*
47. Román, "Remembering AIDS," 282.
48. Russo, "Why We Fight," in *Common Threads.* It is important to note that Russo's vision has been remembered from multiple historical locations, with differing effects. Not long after Russo's death, Douglas Crimp wrote, "Vito's death painfully demonstrated to many AIDS activists that the rhetoric of hope we invented and depended upon—a rhetoric of 'living with AIDS,' in which 'AIDS is not a death sentence,' but rather 'a chronic manageable illness'—was becoming difficult to sustain. I don't want to minimize the possibility that anyone's death might result in such a loss of hope for someone, and, moreover, within a two-week period of Vito's death, four other highly visible members of ACT UP New York also died, a cumulative loss for us that was all but unbearable. But I think many of us had a special investment in Vito's survival, not because he was so beloved, but because, as a resolute believer in his own survival, and a highly visible and articulate fighter for his and other's survival, he fully embodied that hope" (Crimp, "Right On, Girlfriend!," 303). Brophy, *Witnessing AIDS,* 49.
49. Roger Hallas, "Queer AIDS Media and the Question of the Archive," *GLQ:A Journal of Lesbian and Gay Studies* 16 (2010): 431, 435. See also Roger Hallas, *Reframing Bodies: AIDS, Bearing Witness, and the Queer Moving Image* (Durham, NC: Duke

University Press, 2009); for a recent example, see Robert McRuer, "Disability and the NAMES Project," *The Public Historian* 27 (Spring 2005): 53–61.

50. Jeff Nunokawa, "'All the Sad Young Men': AIDS and the Work of Mourning," in *Inside/Out: Lesbian Theories, Gay Theories,* ed. Diana Fuss (New York: Routledge, 1991), 319.

51. Capozzola, "A Very American Epidemic," 96.

52. Sturken, "Conversations with the Dead," 217.

53. Judith Butler, *Precarious Life: The Powers of Mourning and Violence* (London: Verso, 2006), 30. See also Cvetkovich, *An Archive of Feelings,* esp. chap. 6; David L. Eng and David Kazanjian, eds., *Loss: The Politics of Mourning* (Berkeley: University of California Press, 2003).

54. Simon Watney, "Acts of Memory," *OUT* (September 1994): 97.

55. Simon Watney, "The Possibilities of Permutation: Pleasure, Proliferation, and the Politics of Gay Identity in the Age of AIDS," in *Fluid Exchanges: Artists and Critics in the AIDS Crisis,* ed. James Miller (Toronto: University of Toronto Press, 1992), 363.

56. Lucas Hilderbrand, "Retroactivism," *GLQ: A Journal of Lesbian and Gay Studies* 12 (2006): 308. The concept of retroactivism is brilliantly embodied in Sarah Schulman and Jim Hubbard's ACT UP Oral History Project at http://www.actuporalhistory.org/.

57. Alexandra Juhasz, "Video Remains," *GLQ: A Journal of Lesbian and Gay Studies* 12 (2006): 320.

58. Hilderbrand, "Retroactivism," 313.

59. Christopher Castiglia, "Sex Panics, Sex Publics, Sex Memories," *boundary 2* 27 (2000): 160. See also Patrick Moore, *Beyond Shame: Reclaiming the Abandoned History of Radical Gay Sexuality* (Boston: Beacon Press, 2004).

60. Heather Love, *Feeling Backward: Loss and the Politics of Queer History* (Cambridge: Harvard University Press, 2007), 163. See also Cvetkovich, *An Archive of Feelings;* Lee Edelman, "Antagonism, Negativity, and the Subject of Queer Theory," in "Forum: Conference Debates. The Antisocial Thesis in Queer Theory," *PMLA* 121 (2006): 821–823; Judith Halberstam, "The Politics of Negativity in Recent Queer Theory," in "Forum: Conference Debates. The Antisocial Thesis in Queer Theory," *PMLA* 121 (2006): 823–825; David M. Halperin and Valerie Traub, eds., *Gay Shame* (Chicago: University of Chicago Press, 2010).

61. Hilderbrand, "Retroactivism," 307.

62. Quoted in Clendinen and Nagourney, *Out for Good,* 479.

63. "Let the Record Show . . ." was created by ACT UP and displayed in November 1987 in the window of the New Museum of Contemporary Art in New York. Although ACT UP rightly refused to put an image of a person with AIDS in the installation as a means of defying the prevailing discourse of the AIDS victim, I believe the juxtaposition of a Quilt panel and a variation of this installation as a hybrid text would now constitute a powerful refutation and repudiation of dominant memory of key figures in AIDS history. See Richard Meyer, "Vanishing Points: Art, AIDS, and the Problem of Visibility," *Outlaw Representation: Censorship and Homosexuality in Twentieth-Century American Art* (New York: Oxford University Press, 2002), 225–227.

64. Russo, "Why We Fight," in *Common Threads.*

65. Sturken, "Conversations with the Dead," 218.

66. Charles E. Morris III, "The Archival Turn in Rhetorical Studies; Or, the Archive's Rhetorical (Re)Turn," *Rhetoric and Public Affairs* 9 (2006): 115. See also "Forum: Archivists with an Attitude," *College English* 61 (1999): 574–598; Antoinette Burton, ed., *Archive Stories: Facts, Fictions, and the Writing of History* (Durham, NC: Duke University Press, 2005); "Forum: The Politics of Archival Research," *Rhetoric and Public Affairs* 9 (Spring 2006): 113–151.

67. Diana Taylor, *The Archive and the Repertoire: Performing Cultural Memory in the Americas* (Durham, NC: Duke University Press, 2003). In addition to the vision Bryant Alexander charts in this volume, consider in this regard Jean Carlomusto's and Jane Rosett's installations, "AIDS: A Living Archive" and the "Southern AIDS Living Quilt." http://www.jeancarlomusto.com/PortraitGallery.html and http://www.tigoe.net/livingarchive/index.shtml; http://www.livingquilt.org/ (accessed August 24, 2009).

68. Mohr, "Text(ile)," 120.

PART I

Emergence

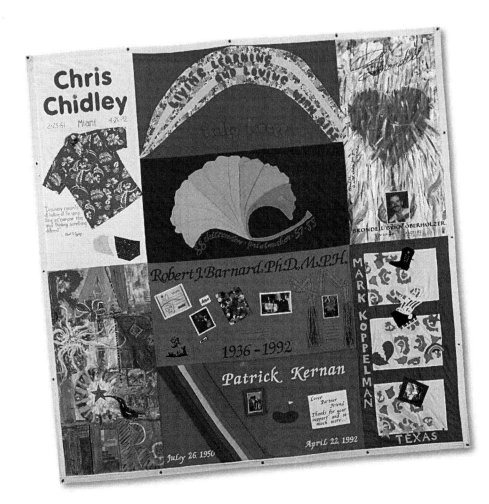

The AIDS Memorial Quilt and the Contemporary Culture of Public Commemoration

Carole Blair and Neil Michel

T he AIDS Memorial Quilt marks the lives and deaths of tens of thousands of individuals. It represents the deaths of hundreds of thousands of others it does not name explicitly. It creates spaces for moving rituals to remember the dead. AIDS Quilt displays often have been attended by events and demonstrations that advocate for those who continue to live with HIV/AIDS. It sometimes moves the otherwise unin- volved visitor to tears.[1] The AIDS Quilt executes, in other words, multiple rhetorical feats and gives rise to a great many others—all of which are important in evaluating the legacy of this unusual commemorative monu- ment. But so too is the place of the AIDS Memorial Quilt in the history of U.S. public commemoration.

The AIDS Memorial Quilt marks an important, tensive moment in the cultural milieu of late twentieth-century public commemorative building practices, a conjuncture of a sort, in which public commemora- tion harbored both the potential for a progressive political practice and the conditions for subversion of that practice.[2] The Quilt neither created nor resolved the conjuncture, but the particularities of its rhetoric display a range of anxieties and tensions that continue to both enable and disable contemporary public commemoration.

The AIDS Memorial Quilt is addressed here as part of an emerging, late twentieth-century culture of public commemoration that began with the Vietnam Veterans Memorial (VVM). The AIDS Quilt appropriated and radicalized the VVM's potent rhetorical patois, and a number of later commemorative sites took up an apparently similar set of issues and rhetorical features but depoliticized them or, perhaps more accurately, repoliticized them, to serve more conservative interests.

The situation of public memory practices is no small matter for politics, for culture, or for rhetoric. The importance of public memory has been recognized by scholars in multiple disciplines, as well as by many in the popular press. Although memory's significance is manifold, most commentators agree about its gravity for the present moment. Public memory is often the very battleground upon which are fought issues of contemporary concern. Because of the pronounced tendency of contemporary public commemoration to take up subject matter that yields to ongoing fractiousness, or at least cultural anxiety, it is more likely that issues of the present will be deliberated by debating memory.[3]

Moreover, with the ever decreasing interval between event and public commemoration, it becomes increasingly difficult to perceive a distance between past and present; if we attend to how rapidly, for example, moves have been made to commemorate the Oklahoma City bombing or the attacks of September 11, 2001, the past seems hardly "the foreign country" David Lowenthal has called it.[4] The formal—and at the time highly unusual—features of the VVM and the AIDS Memorial Quilt, as well as the reception of both memorials, prefigure the issues and divides that characterize more recent attempts to commemorate significant events. The Quilt has been many things, but it certainly may be seen as a barometer of contemporary commemorative culture.

The Vietnam Veterans Memorial and the AIDS Memorial Quilt

The AIDS Quilt has been linked to the VVM by others, most notably by Marita Sturken and by Peter S. Hawkins, and we rely to varying degrees on their observations as well as our own.[5] We are less concerned here with the influence of the VVM than with how the AIDS Quilt appropriated *and* changed its rhetoric. The AIDS Memorial Quilt was an early participant in a groundswell, called by some a "mania," of public memorializing, rivaled in the United States perhaps only by the aftermath of the Civil War.[6] It is arguable that most, if not all, of the public memorial projects undertaken since the VVM have been enabled by it. Certainly the large number of local and state Vietnam veterans memorials were. And there is little question that the VVM provoked the Korean War Veterans Memorial project, which in turn gave rise to the more recent World War II Memorial. But commemorative building projects completely unrelated in substance also were given impetus by the publicity and success that the VVM generated.[7]

Equally important, though, was that many of the memorials following in the wake of the VVM during the final two decades of the twentieth century, and extending into the first decade of the twenty-first, took up elements of its rhetoric, appropriating and adapting it to their own ends. For example, its signature black granite became for the first time a popular primary material for memorial designers. Naming the dead in the 1980s and 1990s also was *au courant*, to such a degree that Abramson labels that practice as well as the use of black granite as "clichés."[8] The naming gesture, of course, did not originate with the VVM, nor is it obvious that the VVM supplied the inspiration for the names on the AIDS Quilt. Indeed, Cleve Jones has identified his principal source as a family quilt.[9] Whatever its source, though, the naming feature of the two memorials—and the ways that it works rhetorically with each—sparks the reading together of the two artworks. There are, however, multiple continuities besides that admittedly important one.

The VVM design probably does not seem very radical to most Americans now, but in the early 1980s it generated a bitter conflict, resolved

only by the addition of Frederick Hart's synecdochic, "realistic" sculpture and a flagpole on the site. That controversy was precisely about its
genre-busting character; the objections raised at the time were all about
the expectations of scale, color, and representational realism that were
produced by experience with other major U.S. memorials. One need only
think of some memorials within the VVM's proximity, like the Lincoln,
Grant, Jefferson, or U.S. Marine Corps memorials, to understand why
it was seen as a departure from the norm. The VVM did not render the
beaux arts–inspired or representational monument irrelevant, but it did
declare both inadequate to the representation of the Vietnam conflict.

The AIDS Quilt extended that challenge to genre even further in a
number of its semiotic features. If the VVM seemed horizontal beside its
earlier predecessors, the Quilt intensified the horizontality, at least in its
full displays in Washington, D.C., where it was laid out on the ground of
the Mall and the Ellipse. If the VVM had darkened the color palette of
memorials in Washington, the AIDS Quilt carnivalized it, with its individual panels screaming out every shade and hue one could imagine and in
combinations perhaps *never* imagined. The VVM's narrative certainly was
fragmented; its chronology of death begins at the apex, breaks at the end
of the east wall, begins again on the west wall, and ends at the apex. The
panels of the AIDS Quilt are linked together in different combinations
for different displays, so if it can claim a narrative at all, it is a protean
one. All of these features essentially changed the subject of classic commemorative form, rendering a major departure from genre and opening
them to charges of inappropriateness or worse.[10]

Although all of these gestures are important to the rhetorics of the
two memorials, we focus our attention principally upon three other issues: the two memorials' modes of democratic representation, their blurring of the contexts of invention and reception, and their coding of the
balance between public and private spheres. Those are central to how
the two memorials "work" rhetorically, but they also shed light on some
troubling issues that have arisen with commemorative sites that have followed them or that are currently under development.

DEMOCRATIC REPRESENTATION

U.S. memory studies have been fairly consistent in the claim that memory practices and representations in this country have become increasingly democratized over time. Michael Kammen is as explicit as anyone in claiming that, at least since the turn of the century, there has been a rather steady move toward democratization. He concludes that "successful monuments, historic places, and museums increasingly had to be compatible with democratic values and assumptions." John R. Gillis appears to take the trend toward democratization of memory as a given. And while John Bodnar does not accept the assumption so readily, his conclusions about the successes of vernacular resistance to official cultural memory makes his conclusions at least consistent with those of Kammen and Gillis. That memory practices, and in particular commemorative art practices in the United States, became more democratic over the course of the twentieth century is difficult to contest.[11]

There can be little question that the VVM was a major contributor to the democratization of national public commemoration. The most prominent memorials within its immediate orbit represented singular governmental and military figures—George Washington, Thomas Jefferson, Abraham Lincoln, Ulysses S. Grant.[12] Even national memorials that honored groups, especially soldiers from various U.S. military conflicts, had settled on the synecdoche or the abstract representation, with a sculptural figure or group standing in for the larger group or an allegorical figure marking the group's ethos. The U.S. Marine Corps Memorial was an example of the former, with the soldiers raising the flag over Mt. Suribachi standing in for the Marine Corps at large. The Second Division Memorial, a few blocks east of the VVM on Constitution Avenue, rendered allegorical tribute to the soldiers of that unit with a sculptural flaming sword.

The VVM names the name of every U.S. soldier killed or missing in action from the Vietnam conflict. The names are recorded in absolutely uniform fashion; the only differences among them are the markers for KIA or MIA. There are no military ranks or units listed, not even military branches. This represents a departure from the representations of the dead in U.S. military cemeteries and on most the walls of the missing from the two World Wars. Military gravestones almost always mark rank,

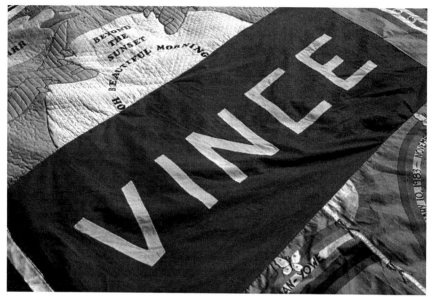

"Quilt Panel: Vince": A panel titled "Vince" on the AIDS Quilt.

unit, and branch of the service, as well as major commendations. Most walls of the missing do the same. At the VVM, though, every individual is represented, and each is marked as absolutely equal in death.[13]

The AIDS Quilt arguably democratizes its representation even further, but its mode of democratization is very different. There is no attempt to name everyone who has died of AIDS. Indeed, the NAMES Project is careful to note in its materials the relatively small percentage of AIDS deaths it marks. For example, the approximately 91,000 names on the Quilt in 2007 "represent approximately 17.5% of all U.S. AIDS deaths" and, of course, a minute percentage of worldwide AIDS-related deaths.[14] Nor is there any uniformity of representation in the Quilt. The democratic trope of the AIDS Quilt is not personal equality but individual difference. Granted, most of the individual Quilt panels name one individual, as well as his or her birth and death dates. And almost all measure three feet by six feet, essentially the size of a coffin. But even those features vary. For example, a number of the earliest panels carry only a first name, protecting the individual's legacy or his surviving partner or family from the stigma of the disease or from being outed (fig. 1). That sentiment is made even more explicit in a panel that says: "I have decorated this banner to honor my brother. Our parents did not want his name used publicly. The omission of his name represents the fear of oppression that AIDS victims and their families feel."

Others name someone in terms of relationship—for example, Daddy or My Brother. In addition, a number of panels name more than one individual. One is dedicated to the San Francisco Gay Men's Choir, another to Federal Express employees who died AIDS-related deaths, and another to members of the wonderfully outrageous Sisters of Perpetual Indulgence.[15] Apparently due to a misunderstanding, a few quilt panels were submitted that measured three by six inches rather than feet; these were attached to a standard sized panel so that they could be displayed.[16] Some panels are double size or even larger, usually those that represent more than one death.

The individual quilts are made of very different materials, from simple cotton sheeting to leather. Some panels are relatively unadorned, spray painted with a name, for example, while others are carefully sewn or decorated with symbols or significant objects from a person's life. The NAMES Project lists some of the materials used in the Quilt:

> 100 year-old quilt, afghans, Barbie dolls, bubble-wrap, burlap, buttons, car keys, carpet, champagne glasses, condoms, cookies, corduroy, corsets, cowboy boots, cremation ashes, credit cards, curtains, dresses, feather boas, first-place ribbons, fishnet hose, flags, flip-flops, fur, gloves, hats, human hair, jeans, jewelry, jockstraps, lace, lamé, leather, Legos, love letters, Mardi Gras masks, merit badges, mink, motorcycle jackets, needlepoint, paintings, pearls, photographs, pins, plastic, police uniforms, quartz crystals, racing silks, records, rhinestones, sequins, shirts, silk flowers, studs, stuffed animals, suede, t-shirts, taffeta, tennis shoes, vinyl, wedding rings.[17]

Objects from individuals' lives adorn most of the panels—a professional uniform, a favorite photograph, a beloved stuffed animal, old blue jeans, even a bowling ball. Many tell stories about the individual's professional, social, or home life.

Some individuals are remembered by multiple quilt panels. At last count, Ryan White had fifteen panels.[18] Michel Foucault is named on at least four. Many are marked as "Anonymous," while others name very famous names, like Rock Hudson, Liberace, Robert Mapplethorpe, or Arthur Ashe. Some are poignant, others tacky, some funny, and still others caustic.[19] The crucial point is that the many and tremendous differences of representation serve a democratizing function, as does the tight focus on the individual as an individual. As Richard D. Mohr suggests, "The moral point of the NAMES Project is the valorizing of the individual life, not necessarily because such a life issues in the honorable, but just because it is unique—the working out, even if stumblingly, of a self-conceived plan of life."[20]

It was not just these memorials' formal features, of course, that democratized. Their subject matter played perhaps an even more important role in the commemorative explosion that would follow. Certainly no one could have predicted that there would be a memorial on the National Mall to the veterans of the most unpopular military conflict the United States had ever engaged in, much less one that the nation lost. The organizers of the effort to build the VVM were careful to designate it as a *veterans* memorial, decidedly not a *war* memorial, to distinguish the warrior from the conflict. Although that distinction has been lost on numerous commentators and even on some scholars, it was a significant one.[21]

Even more improbable was a giant memorial to those stricken down by an epidemic, especially one that manifested first in the gay male community. Neither Vietnam veterans nor gay men, especially gay men with a communicable disease that kills, were the most likely subjects for commemoration in the 1980s. And yet, perhaps because of the ingenious formal characteristics of the VVM and the AIDS Memorial Quilt, these two memorials enjoyed nearly unprecedented cultural success. The positive reception of the VVM has been well documented. But the AIDS Quilt's popular success has been less discussed, perhaps because fewer people have made a deliberate commemorative pilgrimage to a Quilt display than to the VVM. However, it seems quite remarkable that an estimated 18 million people have seen the AIDS Quilt, especially given that most of its displays are small and fragmentary, and that all of its displays are temporary and brief. It has also been a great fund-raising success, generating millions of dollars not only to continue its display journey, but also to provide direct services to people living with AIDS.[22]

CONTEXTS OF INVENTION AND RECEPTION

The standard, if not always accurate, view of public memorials and monuments tends to be about state power, about "official" renditions of the past, about the imposed authorization of heroes who become models for the everyday life of a polity.[23] That view is not always or even frequently accurate, because many of the most prominent memory sites in the United States were the result of citizen efforts, often even funded by popular subscription. Still, as attested by both Mike Wallace's and John Bodnar's very different histories of memory practices in the United States, there have been moments of imposition, of officially sanctioned attempts to "educate" the masses in their patriotic, occupational, and cultural "responsibilities."[24]

As a generalization, it is fair to suggest that most U.S. national memorials, even those projects that have arisen as a result of "grassroots" efforts, have had the benefit of founding support from a group with considerable cultural capital. That is true in the cases of the VVM and the AIDS Memorial Quilt as well. Both projects were initiated by individuals—Jan Scruggs and Cleve Jones respectively—who hardly were shrinking violets. Scruggs was a well-educated and articulate spokesperson who proved quite capable of shaming Americans to open their wallets to contribute to the Vietnam Veterans Memorial Fund (VVMF), to muster the support for a major design competition, and to successfully lobby Congress to supply the prime real estate for the VVM. Jones, who had been a visible gay rights advocate in San Francisco, had the recognition and networks to turn his vision of the Quilt into a reality, by soliciting donations not only of money, but also and more importantly, Quilt panels. By the time of its first Washington, D.C., display in the fall of 1987, the AIDS Memorial Quilt had grown from a single panel, made by Jones for his friend Marvin Feldman (fig. 2), to 1,920 separate panels, a figure that would quadruple in just one year.

These "origin stories" offer only the most narrow understanding of the contexts of invention of these two contemporary memorials, however.[25]

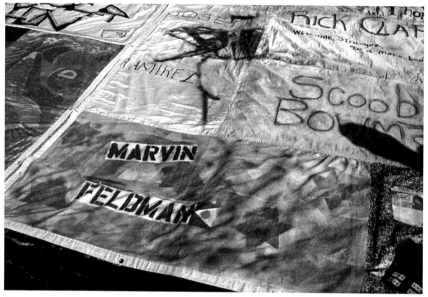

"Quilt Panel: Marvin Feldman": After Marvin Feldman's death, friend Cleve Jones conceived the idea for the AIDS Quilt.

Both of the memorials are cases of the social character of invention, in the most literal of terms.[26] The rhetorical invention of the VVM extended well beyond Jan Scruggs, the VVMF, and VVM designer Maya Lin, in at least two senses. First, the VVM was allowed to be constructed on public land only after a fractious conflict over its design, a conflict played out in public as a result of objections lodged against Lin's design by a handful of Vietnam veterans. Although the conflicts did not result in the sought rejection or alteration of the Lin design, the opponents were successful in forcing a compromise that added Frederick Hart's "Three Fightingmen" sculpture and a flagpole to the site. In turn, that augmentation raised objections that women who had served in Vietnam were not represented adequately by the memorial. The Vietnam Women's Memorial sculpture was added as a further augmentation to the site in 1993. That these sculptural additions have altered the site's rhetoric is virtually undisputed.[27] The ultimate success, if we wish to call it that, of these two attempts to augment the VVM suggest that the U.S. public is not just an audience but also a collective participant in the invention of the site.

In addition to the sculptural amendments to the VVM, visitors to the memorial reinvent its rhetoric daily, in the common practice of leaving "offerings" at the wall—everything from combat boots to poems.[28] Each day those artifacts modify the rhetoric of the VVM, leading visitors to focus on the relationship of artifact to architecture, on the character of a particular person listed on the wall, on a particular event in Vietnam, and so forth. In these senses, the VVM may be declared complete (as it has been by the National Park Service), but its rhetoric is never "complete," as long as it remains open to such inventive augmentation on the part of its visitors.

Still, the VVM—apart from the offerings that adorn it—has an official status, governmental sanction and maintenance, and a fixed location, attributes that distinguish it, as Hawkins points out, from the AIDS Memorial Quilt.[29] Although we may understand—and many people have treated—the VVM as a context for rhetoric more than as a rhetorical object in its own right, it retains in its design a relatively stable rhetorical imprint, especially in comparison to the AIDS Memorial Quilt. Hawkins calls the Quilt "authorless," elaborating this way:

> It is true that Jones "invented" the initial three-by-six-foot panel, which he then imagined as one patch taking its place in a larger patchwork. Since then, however, he has had no control over how the Quilt would look, either in its parts or in its larger configurations, nor has the NAMES Project, beyond requiring specific dimensions for each panel and the name of the person to be remembered. Otherwise, design depends entirely on the quilters.[30]

Of course, the Quilt is not really "authorless," but instead has literally tens of thousands of "authors." Still, Hawkins is correct in observing that there is no author in the classic sense that offers unified interpretive authority. Now, at more than 46,000 panels, the AIDS Quilt has been invented by a massive collection of individuals, most of them strangers to one another. They have each designed a small part of this giant memorial and done so with very different aesthetics, tastes, and goals. As we have already noted, even those strictures of naming and size that Hawkins mentions, have not been adhered to by all of the individual panel "authors."

If the invention and reception contexts of the VVM are complex, with visitors and public advocates reinventing the site, those contexts become even more complicated with the AIDS Memorial Quilt, again in at least three important senses. First, any individual or small group that makes a Quilt panel is already engaged, during that process, in a private mourning activity, one that bears a strong similarity to the memory quilt tradition.[31] Unlike in that tradition, however, the AIDS Quilt panel is not retained by the individual or intimate group, but is relinquished to the NAMES Project for inclusion in the larger, collectivized, public memorial. The intimates of the dead, those who have designed individual Quilt panels, are almost certain to become audience members too, after the fact of relinquishment.[32] Many of them attend AIDS Quilt displays. But they are audience members among a great many others, some Quilt panel makers, others not. So, the relatively private inventional creation of mourning becomes a part of a larger, more public performance, over which the individual panel designer wields no control.

Second, the AIDS Quilt is *literally* not finished. Although no one legitimately expects that all AIDS-related deaths will be acknowledged by the Quilt, the invitation to submit panels remains perpetually open. One of the most disturbing features about the AIDS Quilt's rhetoric always has been its massive growth, an urgent reminder that AIDS continues to claim more lives, despite medical breakthroughs with drug therapy. In the most recent full display of the AIDS Quilt, in Washington, D.C., in 1996, its roughly 40,000 panels covered the National Mall, twice as many panels as in the full display in Washington just four years earlier.[33] Even photos from atop the Washington Monument could not capture its scale, for trees blocked the view of about one-third of the Quilt panels (fig. 3). Each Quilt display became the impetus for new additions to it, again transforming audience members into rhetors. And so it has continued to grow larger, its message elaborated by each addition.

Third, the NAMES Project has actively cultivated visitors' contributions of supplemental discourse to the Quilt at its displays. While no one perhaps anticipated the desire to leave "offerings" in the form of artifacts or messages at the VVM, it was an early expectation at sites of Quilt exhibitions. Signature blocks are set aside for people to write their reactions, and these blocks become part of the Quilt's rhetoric of display.[34]

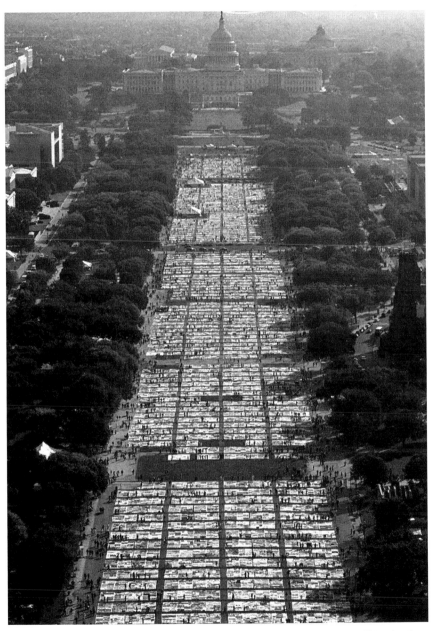

"View from the Washington Monument of Quilt Display on Mall": The last full display of the AIDS Quilt took place in 1996, on the National Mall in Washington, D.C.

Here an invited mode of reception becomes an inventional process, with visitors becoming rhetors. In our experience, these blocks, in turn, receive a significant amount of attention; visitors eagerly read the recorded reactions and messages of other visitors.

PUBLIC AND PRIVATE SPHERES

Almost no matter where one begins in the massive, interdisciplinary literature about "the public," the distinctions and relationships between public and private emerge as crucial issues.[35] We often refer unreflectively to collective memory sites as "public" memorials, when, indeed, they represent differential relationships of publicity and privacy, just as certainly as they occupy public space.[36] But some of these public memorials code those relationships much more explicitly than others. In recent times, the naming memorials have done so most prominently. No matter how much these commemorative works may differ from one another, naming multiple individuals in public space not only nominates those individuals as particularly significant members of the collective, but also marks a specific relationship between individual and collective.

The VVM strikes a relatively precise equilibrium between private and public concerns. Close views reveal the inscription of individual names that, of course, imply much more than the identity "Vietnam veteran." From that close perspective, one must focus on individuals, for the larger view of the wall disappears from view. Still, the names reveal only limited information. They announce that this individual lived, was a U.S. soldier, and died in (or on the way to/from or as a direct result of) the Vietnam conflict; visitors are offered little information beyond that, unless through the supplement of an "offering" left at the wall. Of course, names are symbolic harbingers of individual lives, but this is a rhetoric of implicature. The large majority of the names belong to people who are strangers to any one visitor, and thus visitors cannot know much about them as individuals.

From a more distant vantage point, the individual names disappear, and the massive cost of war comes into view. The visual character of the wall is such that the names of individuals are legible in tight focus, but even in a close-up view the name of one individual cannot be seen in the absence of others names. Moreover, the names share space with the mirror images of visitors; the interpellation is inevitable. Whether or not the visitor has a private relationship with anyone whose name appears on the wall, and whatever the visitor might think about the advisability of the U.S. military involvement in Southeast Asia, a public relationship is forged indelibly by reflection. The names of the dead are "our" representatives, those sent to their deaths under the sign of a national public good.

The relationship of private individual to the public collective shows up very differently in the AIDS Memorial Quilt. There are similarities to the VVM, to be sure. Visitors to an individual Quilt panel see the quilts of other individuals that are grommeted to it, at least in a block of eight, the usual manner of displaying the Quilt groupings. At a larger distance, one sees the massive loss, one giant memorial rather than the thousands of smaller ones. A visitor may focus on the loss of one, but not in the absence of others. Visitors may also attend to the collective loss, but not without consideration of the individuals composing that collective.

But there are also significant differences in the ways in which the two memorials cast the specific lives and their relationships to a larger, public realm. Private lives are rendered visible in the AIDS Quilt much more than in the VVM. Granted, some of the Quilt panels bear only a name, offering little information about the individual. And, of course, those panels honoring "Anonymous" seem to offer even less information than an inscription on the VVM wall. Nonetheless, most of the Quilt panels tell rather than imply stories. Visitors learn about the hobbies, political leanings, cultural status, age, work lives, favorite vacation spots, intimate relationships, personal accomplishments, and aspirations of the individuals represented by the AIDS Quilt. Some individual panels are performances of coming out. Visitors often see photographic representations of the individuals commemorated. In the large majority of the panels, names are named, but the names take on faces, personalities, and personal histories. In sum, private lives are displayed publicly, not by means of commemorative supplement, but by design of the memorial itself.

Some of the panels composing the AIDS Quilt portray the commemorated individuals' public identities. Individuals of high profile often have quilt panels that link their lives to the source of their fame. For

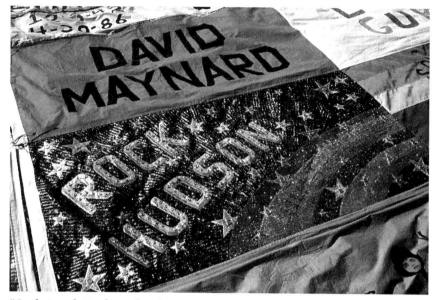

"Quilt Panel: Rock Hudson": Prominent actor Rock Hudson elevated awareness of the AIDS epidemic.

example, Liberace's panel incorporates as its principal visual element a
grand piano. Rock Hudson's panel (fig. 4) is covered with stars, along with
a rainbow that says "Hollywood."

Other Quilt panels, bearing names not so well known, link the individual to public causes. Many of the panels incorporate a rainbow flag or
a smaller representation of one. Some identify their subjects as members
of the military. Some use national or state flags or parts of patriotic symbols as background. Others make claims on public issues verbally. For
example, the Quilt panel for Paul Burdett says: "The San Diego 50 Hour
Prayer Vigil was his creation. Please—More Prayers. More Funding." A
panel in honor of Roger Lyons reads: "I came here today to ask that this
nation with all its resources and compassion not let my epitaph read he
died of red tape." Another Quilt panel, identified as honoring a military
officer, says: "They gave me a medal for killing two men, and a discharge
for loving one." In various ways, then, many of the Quilt panels, however
straightforward or sardonic they may be, render the relationship of the
deceased to a larger, political collective by means of effigy or elegy.

A remarkably high percentage of the AIDS Quilt panels, though, assert the identity of their subjects in terms of personal, rather than public, relationships. Quilt panel makers often sign the panels. Many mark the individual by familial or social role—for example, lover, father, son, brother, child, friend, husband, wife, sister. Some bear messages to the deceased, such as "I didn't get a chance to say goodbye." The much reproduced panel in honor of Jac Wall surrounds a silhouette of the deceased man with these words:

> Jac Wall is my lover. Jac Wall had AIDS. Jac Wall died. I love Jac Wall. Jac Wall is a good guy. Jac Wall made me a better person. Jac Wall could beat me in wrestling. Jac Wall loves me. Jac Wall is thoughtful. Jac Wall is great in bed. Jac Wall is intelligent. I love Jac Wall. Jac Wall is with me. Jac Wall turns me on. I miss Jac Wall. Jac Wall is faithful. Jac Wall is a natural Indian. Jac Wall is young at heart. Jac Wall looks good naked. I love Jac Wall. Jac Wall improved my life. Jac Wall is my lover. Jac Wall loves me. I miss Jac Wall. I will be with you soon.[37]

The marking of identity by interaction and by relationship is such a pervasive feature that it simply cannot be ignored. It is remarkable not only because of the frequency with which it appears in the AIDS Quilt, but also because it so exceeds the norms of public memorializing.

Public memorials clearly are always about relationships. In the absence of survivor memories, there would be no public memorials. Their inventional contexts may even be, in some respects, about personal relationships. For example, veterans groups often are sufficiently motivated by the closeness of their relationships with their GI "buddies" to commemorate them, sometimes even by taking on the wearisome work of advocating for a public memorial to be constructed. But it is not at all within the boundaries of the typical for a public memorial to code the specifics of personal relationships. More than any public memorial before, the AIDS Quilt seems to be as much about the survivors as about the deceased. That is not to say simply (and obviously) that it is *for* the survivors; its rhetoric is very much *about* them. Quilt panels often tell visitors the nature of the panel maker's relationship to the deceased, how he or she felt about the deceased, and what he or she feels about the loss, as in Jac Wall's case. If public memory has always been about the present, and thus more about survivors than the dead, this memorial is more explicit about that than any predecessors we have observed. With the AIDS Memorial Quilt, then, the private-public representation is weighted toward the private.[38]

That is reinforced in an odd way by the fact that these memorials have been characterized in popular interpretation, academic writing, and cultural practice as "therapeutic." For example, Charles L. Griswold asserts, without apparent hesitation or evidence, that "a main purpose of the Memorial is therapeutic, a point absolutely essential for an adequate understanding of the VVM. . . . It was generally understood that what the nation needed was a monument that would heal the veterans as well as the rest of us, rather than exacerbate old wounds and reignite old passions."[39] The AIDS Memorial Quilt is, if anything, referenced in the terms of psychoanalytic metaphors more explicitly, assertively, and frequently even than with the VVM. These typical newspaper headlines demonstrate just how pervasive this terminology became: "AIDS Quilt Comforting U.S. Grief," "The NAMES Project: A Catharsis of Grief," "A Healing of Hearts."[40]

Terms like "therapy," "therapeutic," "rehabilitation," and "healing" are ubiquitous, not appearing very often in the discourse of the VVMF or the NAMES Project, but instead in the popular and academic interpretive milieux. That these memorials should be understood as offering therapy for trauma can be accounted for in any number of ways.[41] The terminology may reach back to the realm of physicality, wherein the figure of both the Vietnam veteran and the person with AIDS represent abject bodies, the wounded soldier and the terminally ill patient in need of therapy and healing. But it more frequently seems to reference psychoanalytic forms of treatment, either literally or metaphorically. Literally, of course, the reference makes sense. Many returning Vietnam veterans were treated for PTSD (post-traumatic stress disorder). With AIDS, especially in urban gay communities, people often have sought out grief therapy to cope with the loss not just of a loved one, but sometimes of whole friendship networks—often within a very short time period.[42]

But there is also a metaphoric use of this terminology, which assigns ill health to the public realm and suggests that the memorials work their

therapeutic processes on the diseased polity. At the very least, most commentators that use the terminology tend to tack back and forth between
the literal sense of individuals seeking therapy and figurative "therapy"
being worked on a larger, political collective. This usage, of course, not
only shifts issues of privacy into the public, but also reinforces the blurring of the contexts of invention and reception discussed earlier, and
in ways that seem to us to be problematic. This unfortunate headline
suggests part of the problem: "Powerful Images: Quilt Softens Pain of
AIDS Deaths."[43] The article that follows is about panel makers working
on a Quilt panel for their loved one, not about an AIDS Quilt display.
The AIDS Quilt, of course, was intended to do precisely the opposite of
the headline; its distinctly political mission was to confront people with
the enormity of loss, to intensify, not "soften," the pain. As Christopher
Capozzola argues, the AIDS Quilt was "intended as a tool of political mobilization and as a weapon in the battle for access to economic resources
that could be used in the fight against AIDS."[44]

Unfortunately, the language of therapy, when the metaphor reaches
too far, depoliticizes the AIDS Memorial Quilt, rendering it as comforting and curative *rather than* as angry and confrontational. The political
climate that inspired the NAMES Project should not be discounted here.
As Capozzola points out, "During the 1980s, many AIDS activists condemned the Reagan administration for its silence on the issue of AIDS;
the President did not even mention the word AIDS publicly until over
21,000 Americans had already died of the disease."[45] It was not until 1996,
in fact, that a U.S. president attended a Quilt display, in spite of the
proximity to the White House of the four prior full displays of the AIDS
Quilt (fig. 5), an absence that was much remarked on in the 1980s and
early 1990s.

As Alan Zarembo concludes, "In the 25 years of the epidemic, no
symbol has managed to capture the sense of rage and loss like the quilt."
Mourning and activism, as Douglas Crimp has pointed out, do not have
to be mutually exclusive. When the language of therapy overwhelms the
political, however, the AIDS Memorial Quilt is diminished. It unbalances
understandings of the Quilt as a vehicle of both productive mourning
(especially, but not exclusively, in its inventional contexts) and political
activism.[46]

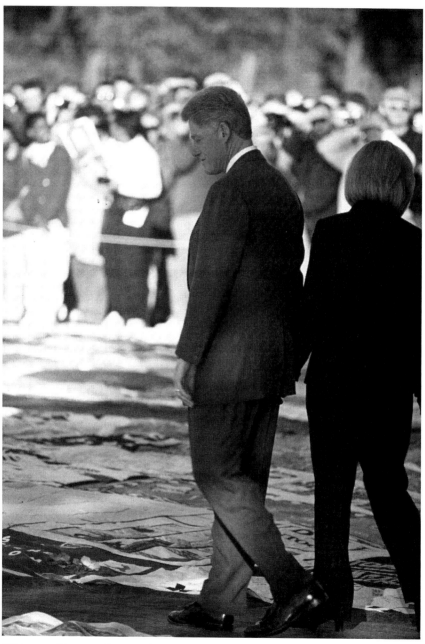

"Clintons Visiting the Quilt": President Bill Clinton and First Lady Hillary Clinton visit the AIDS Quilt during its display on the National Mall in 1996.

That is also the conclusion Zarembo implies, bemoaning what he sees as the Quilt's recent devolution to "a museum piece."[47] He attributes the Quilt's much slower growth, its nearly moribund fund-raising capacity, and its relative lack of attention to a number of conditions, especially the exportation of concern that has occurred "as new drugs have driven down the death rate here and shifted the epicenter of anguish abroad, where the disease kills 2.8 million people a year."[48] He also notes as a factor the shifting demographics of the disease in the United States. But the subtext of the article gets at an important, final issue having to do with the shifting ground of public and private concern: the ownership of the AIDS Quilt.

Since nearly the beginning of the NAMES Project, "ownership" issues have been in play, particularly with respect to questions of the Quilt as a "gay memorial." As AIDS demographics shifted from the "risk groups" of gay men, hemophiliacs, and intravenous drug users to a larger population, there were debates about "de-gaying" the AIDS Quilt. There were conflicts too, from time to time, between the national NAMES Project headquarters and local chapters. But "ownership" is now literally ownership, and the NAMES Project is at odds with Cleve Jones (who was fired from the project in 2004), as well as with many of the local chapters, the ones that are still in existence. This is, in part, a conflict of purpose, with Jones insisting that "everything about AIDS is political," and that "the people with the quilt have a weapon that they have decommissioned."[49] Meanwhile, according to Zarembo, "The [NAMES Project] foundation recently completed writing a two-page strategic plan, saying that the quilt has outgrown its activist roots and should now serve as an inspiration to those living with AIDS."[50] The ownership disputes seem now to have been almost inevitable, given the democratic character of the inventional process and the frequent linkages of AIDS activism and gay identity issues. But they have had the unfortunate result of relegating the Quilt to near repose in its warehouse in Atlanta.[51]

A New Politics of Commemoration?

The VVM is typically credited with, or blamed for, initiating the contemporary culture of commemoration, one in which the issues we have raised here continue to be addressed with a variety of results. Although some claims may be made to the progressive character of this new culture, there are reasons to approach it with a certain degree of skepticism. The VVM is a touchstone; new commemorative works are inevitably compared to it. But we believe that understanding of this contemporary commemorative culture may be enhanced if we consider it against the backdrop of a conversation between the VVM and the AIDS Memorial Quilt—their agreements and disagreements, continuities and discontinuities—about how to commemorate in the contemporary United States. Like many others, we have placed these two important memorials in conversation with one another, not because they always "agree," but precisely because they often do not. Their most important shared attribute, in our view, is an attitude toward public commemoration that is straightforwardly rhetorical, rhetorical in the sense of being accountable to its subject matter, if not always to generic expectation.

Their differential departures from the norms of traditional, Western commemoration were an important source of their success. It is not just formal differences—height, color, and so forth—that distinguish the VVM and the AIDS Memorial Quilt from that tradition. The works display an attitude of sincerity, an attempt at honesty about the difficulties of commemoration, particularly about public commemoration in a sometimes troubled republic. These two memorials focus in different ways on the individual, but they also dignify a spirit of collectivity marked by mutual obligation. The rhetoric of both subverts the (sometimes perhaps disingenuous) claims of their spokespersons that they are "apolitical." Both make the claim that the political collective does not always do right by its citizens, but they insist that it should.

The number of new public commemorative sites of both national and local interest in the United States since 1982 is staggering; indeed, we have no way of enumerating them, because there are so many, and because they continue to spring up. Even the number of national projects is difficult to track, for similar reasons. It is no small matter to plan, design, and build a national memorial, but literally hundreds of groups have made the attempt in recent years, and many of them have succeeded. In addition to the VVM, its sculptural supplements, and the AIDS Memorial Quilt, the following is a sample of those projects that have been completed.

- African American Civil War Memorial (Washington, D.C.)
- Astronauts Memorial (Cape Canaveral, Florida)
- Franklin Delano Roosevelt Memorial (Washington, D.C.)
- George Mason Memorial (Washington, D.C.)
- Indian Memorial (Little Bighorn Battlefield National Monument, Montana)
- Korean War Veterans Memorial (Washington, D.C.)
- National D-Day Memorial (Bedford, Virginia)
- National Japanese American Memorial (Washington, D.C.)
- Oklahoma City National Memorial (Oklahoma City)
- Pentagon Memorial (Arlington, Virginia)
- U.S. Air Force Memorial (Arlington, Virginia)
- U.S. Holocaust Memorial Museum (Washington, D.C.—a dedicated memorial and museum)
- U.S. Law Enforcement Officers Memorial (Washington, D.C.)
- U.S. Navy Memorial (Washington, D.C.)
- Victims of Communism Memorial (Washington, D.C.)
- Women in the Military Services for America Memorial (Arlington, Virginia)
- World War II Memorial (Washington, D.C.)

In various stages of planning, but not yet completed at this writing, are national memorials honoring American Veterans Disabled for Life, Dwight David Eisenhower, John Adams (and family), and Martin Luther King, Jr. Also in process are memorials at each of the two remaining death sites from September 11, 2001; the Pentagon Memorial was dedicated in September 2008. The rash of new projects has led to a number of attempts to limit additional commemorative building, particularly in the monumental core of Washington, D.C. The restrictions so far have been undermined, frequently by the same decision makers who put them in place; congresspersons, presidents, and agency heads have found that the politics of memory is realpolitik.[52]

Not included in these already lengthy lists are memorials that have generated broad national interest but that are not, technically speaking, national memorials, like the Civil Rights Memorial (Montgomery, Alabama), the Witch Trials Tercentenary Memorial (Salem, Massachusetts), the Freedom Forum Journalists Memorial (Washington, D.C.), and the Kent State May 4 Memorial (Kent, Ohio).[53] In any case, the issue is not just how many, but how rapidly, these have appeared. In the United States, it clearly was the VVM that set in motion the rush to commemorate, but Holocaust memory work, especially in the 1990s, fueled the drive further.

It is well beyond the scope of this chapter to outline in any exhaustive way the culture of commemoration these new memorial projects represent. But we take up some fragmentary features of the culture in order to reach back to the conjuncture marked by the AIDS Quilt. Even a cursory glance at the list of new commemorative works must suggest at least the amazing diversity of projects, from those undertaken to honor the "dispossessed" (Japanese American internees during World War II, African American soldiers in the Civil War, women in the military, Native Americans killed at the Little Bighorn, civil rights workers, those accused of witchcraft in seventeenth-century New England, and students killed by the Ohio National Guard in May 1970) to those that acknowledge groups already possessing some cultural capital, like U.S. presidents and statesmen, astronauts, police officers, journalists, and U.S. soldiers from various periods. It is a dizzying array that defies easy explanation.

In a sense, though, an explanation—however incomplete—begins to arise from our examination of the VVM and the AIDS Memorial Quilt. These 1980s memorials reeducated the U.S. political culture about the importance of affect in public life and of the significance of the past to the formation and maintenance of political identities, even when the past sometimes is not what we wish it had been. Following a period of almost forty years in which commemoration was coupled to an affectless public works project mentality (taking the form of "functional" or "recreational" memorials), the 1980s memorials rearticulated commemoration and public art.[54] The popular success of that rebuilt relationship was profound, and it points back to the democratization of public commemoration, discussed by memory scholars and enacted by the VVM and the AIDS Memorial Quilt.

Almost all of these many new additions to the political geography were undertaken by grassroots groups and became national-scope efforts. Some, like the U.S. Navy Memorial and the FDR Memorial, had been proposed years before but gained new impetus in the late 1980s. Others took shape only in the wake of the VVM and the AIDS Memorial Quilt. Still others reflect the increasingly rapid move to commemorate an event. The Oklahoma City Memorial was dedicated just five years after the 1995 Murrah Building bombing. Editorials urging public commemoration of September 11, 2001, began to appear in major newspapers just days after the attacks, sometimes with quite specific suggestions of what the memorials should look like.[55] Initial plans for the Pentagon memorial projected its dedication for the first anniversary of the attacks, but apparently clearer heads prevailed, at least on the issue of how long the project would require.[56]

The establishment of new public commemorative sites in recent years seems to us, on balance, to be a positive contribution to U.S. public memory. Not only has it "recovered" some events from the past that clearly were worthy of commemoration, but it also has begun to further democratize the memory landscape, with heretofore under- or unrepresented groups being recognized. Some of the new memorials, like the VVM and the AIDS Memorial Quilt, raise serious questions about the U.S. political imaginary, about its inclusiveness, its adherence to principle, or the soundness of its policy. The juxtaposed representations in the National Japanese American Memorial of Japanese Americans marching off to military duty in World War II while members of their families were stripped of their possessions and marched off to internment camps is but one example. Others of the new memorials, especially the World War II Memorial, are overtly and unquestioningly nationalistic, offering a counter of sorts to the attitude of commemoration forwarded by the VVM and extended by the AIDS Memorial Quilt.[57] Some new memorials follow slavishly the VVM's stylistic features but do not seem able to capture its capacity to move. Some of the new memorials are exceptional artworks, though, offering not only acknowledgment but also eloquent enhancements to the aesthetic of their settings.

On one hand, then, much of the new culture of commemoration seems to reflect, even advance, the progressive attitude of its progenitors. But there is also another hand, and its character emerged perhaps most obviously with the Oklahoma City National Memorial, and later in the planning and debates about September 11, 2001, commemoration. The issues we have taken up here to characterize the VVM and the AIDS Memorial Quilt, those related to democratization, contexts of invention and reception, and publicity and privacy are all in play with these projects, but they emerge in very different, recombinant form.

Most obvious is a clear rush to commemorate. Placed in historical context, the rapidity of commemorative responses to the terrorist attacks of 1995 and 2001 is breathtaking. Consider, for example, that the USS *Arizona* Memorial was not dedicated until more than twenty years after the attack on Pearl Harbor. It was relatively speedy by contrast to the major presidential memorials on the Mall. The VVM was dedicated in 1982, about seven years after the U.S. withdrawal. The AIDS Memorial Quilt is exceptional, of course, because the NAMES Project was founded not to mark the end of the pandemic but to contribute to the effort to end it.

The Oklahoma City National Memorial was dedicated just five years after Timothy McVeigh's bomb exploded. Planning to "officially" commemorate September 11 was in process within less than a year after the attacks on the World Trade Center and the Pentagon. Although two of those projects—in New York and Pennsylvania—remain incomplete, they all were initiated very quickly. But these projects lacked the overtly urgent demands that brought the NAMES Project into existence; there certainly was no shortage of sympathy or support in the immediate aftermath of the 1995 and 2001 attacks on the part of the U.S. public and the U.S. government.[58] The very early planning to commemorate, regardless of whether there was really such urgency, almost certainly accounts for some of the features of the planning, as well as for some of the decisions made in those processes.

The planning processes for the memorials in Oklahoma City, New York, Pennsylvania, and Virginia, of course, have differed markedly from one another.[59] Nonetheless, reports like Linenthal's careful documentation of the process in Oklahoma City, the thorough press coverage of September 11 commemoration, and the well-maintained Web sites from each of the memorial projects point us toward several notable features.[60] Among them are the related figure of "the survivor" and the "therapy" motive. Linenthal's account of Oklahoma City is the most complete to date. It is also—so far—the most chilling, especially if we heed Sturken's admonition about U.S. culture's tendency to "romanticize trauma."[61] Linenthal discusses the difficulty, for example, of defining "survivor," a task made necessary because the mission statement for the Oklahoma City Memorial had specified that names of survivors appear on the memorial site. As he suggests, "Given the *cultural prestige* of the category of 'survivor,' there was a clear danger that the *allure of being so anointed* could tempt some to claim such *status* inappropriately, thereby trivializing the wrenching experiences of others."[62]

Some of the more compelling images from Linenthal's account are about the conflicts and competitions among family members of the deceased and survivors, many of whom were participating in the Oklahoma City planning process as a mode of therapy.[63] Before the project was off the ground, survivors were engaging in recrimination, fighting with one another about who was more injured than whom, and, in a (probably grief-induced) loss of perspective, insisting that the memorial to the 168 people who died there should be of the same scale as the U.S. Holocaust Memorial Museum—a museum that commemorates the deaths of six million people.[64] One cannot help but wonder, in reading Linenthal's account, if the process helped to resolve pain or simply inflicted more for those most directly affected. We will leave the question of the quality of the "healing" process here to social workers and psychologists, but its effectiveness seems to be an open question.

Paul Goldberger's general observation, in his assessment of the World Trade Center site, raises additional, related questions: "The monument issue is complicated by a tendency in the last few years to think of public memorials as 'healing' places for families. But great memorials inspire awe, and make it possible to transcend the simply personal meaning of an event."[65] Whether he is correct in implying that awe is what great memorials always inspire, he does at least help us raise the question of whether the participation in the inventional process of those closest to

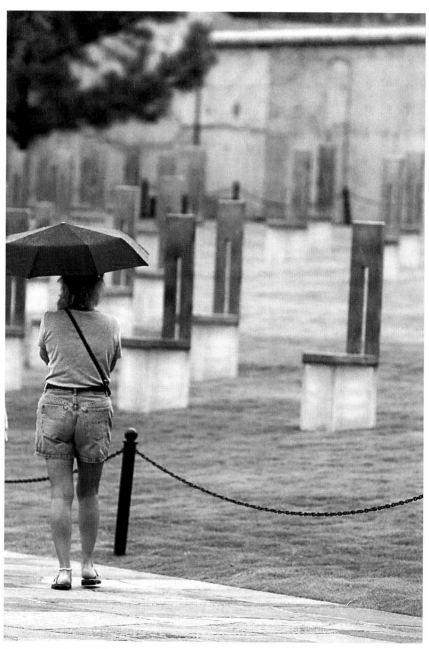

"Visitor at the Oklahoma City National Memorial": A visitor to the Oklahoma City Memorial views "chairs" representing victims of the bombing.

the tragedy are very likely to produce the conditions for great public art. With due respect to the bereaved, it is a question worth posing, for memorials often play a major role in an ongoing public process of negotiating and renegotiating the meaning of an event for generations to come. Nikki Stern, whose husband was killed on September 11, makes the case starkly: "Does losing someone in a terrorist attack make one an expert on terrorism or memorial design? Obviously not."[66]

The second issue raised by Goldberger's statement, however inadvertently, is especially ironic, given our understanding here of the AIDS Memorial Quilt as a harbinger of some of these issues. That is the issue of "family" as the preferred way of referencing survivors. As tempting as it might be, we do not point to that terminology to scold Oklahoma City or New York for not being more like the Castro in San Francisco, where the NAMES Project was initiated. The point is how the boundary between invention and reception has been further breached, with family/survivors fully engaged in the planning and decision-making processes.

The family/survivor also reconfigures the relationship of public and private as they are marked in the memorials' designs. "Special" areas will be restricted to family members of the deceased in the September 11 memorials, a feature that is shared by the Oklahoma City National Memorial. There, only family members are allowed access to the area called the "field of chairs," where each of the 168 stone and glass chairs names one of the individuals killed in the bomb blast (fig. 6).

This area of the memorial, probably the most recognizable from press accounts, clearly was intended as the centerpiece of the site. But the family-only interdiction is enforced by a chain enclosure and by security guards. If a family/survivor is present, her or she is incorporated by visibility as part of the commemorative site, to be gazed upon as another accoutrement of the memorial. Other visitors, members of the public, are denied contact with the memorial's representation of the individual victims—in other words, to the most significant symbol of the site. There are several effects of this decision, not the least of which is to render "family/survivor" as spectacle, but another is a literal dis-location of the public at allegedly public memorial sites. This is a very serious "ownership" issue, of more consequence than various groups' attempts to control a commemorative artwork. Oklahoma City's restrictions, as well as the planned "private" areas at the September 11 memorials, raise the question of whether these really are public memorials at all, or whether they are private memorials that merely tolerate public spectators. It is a new development in commemorative design, and it is a rather troubling one.

Conclusion

The VVM may have been the model, the prototype, or the enabler for these new memorial projects. But we believe it is the AIDS Memorial Quilt that most clearly signaled some of the developments in new commemorative works. Of course, the NAMES Project, Cleve Jones, and the panel makers are not responsible for the developments. Nonetheless, we might understand the Quilt's rhetoric as having been an early sign of things to come. It did its rhetorical work first, with its bold and fractious departures from traditional generic expectations. It pushed the boundaries further even than the VVM had done before it, particularly in its foregrounding of difference as a legitimate marker of democracy and its particular mode of blurring reception and invention contexts without completely erasing the line between them. Important and unprecedented too was its weighting of the public-private dialectic toward privacy, but without defacing the public. It initiated the inscription of the survivor as an explicit figure of commemorative work. Along with the VVM, it prefigured the motifs of therapy and healing that have become so pronounced in more recent years, for good or ill.

We believe the AIDS Memorial Quilt still has the potential to be more than "a museum piece." Whatever its *fate* in the years to come, though, we believe a part of its *legacy* will (and should) be as an important commemorative artwork in its own right. Another will be its capacity, particularly in its initial decade, to move visitors to tears and to open their wallets for medical research and for support of people living with HIV/AIDS. A sincere and stirring tribute to the dead, it was also a provocative political instrument. We hope that another part of the legacy of the AIDS Memorial Quilt will be to caution those who plan and design public commemorative artworks, in two senses. The first warning is, in Marita

Sturken's words, that "cultural memory is not in and of itself a healing process."[67] And, second, public commemoration is unlikely to survive the dis-placement of the public.

NOTES

The authors would like to express their appreciation to Chuck Morris for his invitation to participate in this project and to Bill Balthrop for reading and offering suggestions on a draft of this essay. Great appreciation is also due the two anonymous reviewers of this volume for their thoughtful readings and comments.

1. E. G. Crichton put the case well: "The NAMES Project Quilt has an unusually large [audience]: hundreds of thousands of us across the nation who have walked amidst the panels, stood in the sea of colorful memories, cried, found panels of people we've known, hugged strangers—in general been awed, moved, and inspired by the power of the total vision. . . . The NAMES Quilt bridges the gap between art and social consciousness. Art is too often peripheral to our society, seen as superfluous fluff. Political activism, on the other hand, is often perceived as uncreative and separate from culture. The Quilt is a rare successful integration of these two worlds." E. G. Crichton, "Is The NAMES Quilt Art?" *OUT/LOOK* (Summer 1988): 7–8. That is not to suggest that everyone agrees with her assessment. The project has been tarred with labels like "kitsch" and snubbed for promoting exploitative commodification. See Daniel Harris, "Making Kitsch from AIDS," *Harper's Magazine,* July 1994, 35. Regardless of whether one thinks of the AIDS Memorial Quilt as art or as kitsch, it has enjoyed remarkable public success in terms of popularity (as measured by the number of exhibits and attendees) and press coverage.

2. See Lawrence W. Grossberg, "Does Cultural Studies Have Futures? Should It? (Or What's the Matter with New York?): Cultural Studies, Contexts, and Conjunctures," *Cultural Studies* 20 (2006): 1–32. We are not certain that our understanding of a "conjuncture" matches Grossberg's. The commemorative "conjuncture" is not of the same scale as in his use of the term to describe macrocultural phenomena. Though what we describe here as a conjuncture is "small" by contrast, it is culturally significant in its impact on collective memory practices.

3. For example, Brown et al. argue that the national debate over issues of race in the

contemporary United States turns on the "profound disagreement over the legacy of the civil rights movement." Michael K. Brown, Martin Canoy, Elliott Currie, Troy Duster, David B. Oppenheimer, Marjorie M. Shultz, and David Wellman, *Whitewashing Race: The Myth of the Color-Blind Society* (Berkeley: University of California Press, 2003), 1.

4. David Lowenthal, *The Past Is a Foreign Country* (New York: Cambridge University Press, 1985).

5. Marita Sturken, *Tangled Memories: The Vietnam War, the AIDS Epidemic, and the Politics of Remembering* (Berkeley: University of California Press, 1997), and Peter S. Hawkins, "Naming Names: The Art of Memory and the NAMES Project AIDS Quilt," *Critical Inquiry* 19 (1993): 752–779. The original inspiration for this chapter, however, comes from Enrico Pucci Jr. and Marsha S. Jeppeson. Their insights about the relationships between the Vietnam Veterans Memorial and the NAMES Project AIDS Quilt have been instrumental in shaping our views of the continuities between the two memorials. Also see Timothy P. Brown, "Trauma, Museums and the Future of Pedagogy," *Third Text* 18 (2004): 247–259, and Christopher Capozzola, "A Very American Epidemic: Memory Politics and Identity Politics in the AIDS Memorial Quilt, 1985–1993," *Radical History Review* 82 (2002): 91–109. These and many other sources take the VVM as a touchstone for the AIDS Quilt and/or place them in critical conversation with one another.

6. See, for example, "Washington's Memorial Mania," *Newsweek*, May 27, 1991, 25, and George F. Will, "The Statue Sweepstakes," *Newsweek*, August 26, 1991, 64. More recently, scholar Erika Doss has picked up this thread in a new book, suggesting that "much of today's memorial making is excessive, frenzied, and extreme—hence manic." Erika Doss, *Memorial Mania: Public Feeling in America* (Chicago: University of Chicago Press, 2010), 13.

7. These have enabled, in turn, still others. See Carole Blair, "Contemporary U.S. Memorial Sites as Exemplars of Rhetoric's Materiality," in *Rhetorical Bodies*, ed. Jack Selzer and Sharon Crowley (Madison: University of Wisconsin Press, 1999), 16–57. See also Patrick Hagopian, *The Vietnam War in American Memory: Veterans, Memorials, and the Politics of Healing* (Amherst: University of Massachusetts Press, 2009).

8. Daniel Abramson, "Maya Lin and the 1960s: Monuments, Time Lines, and Minimalism," *Critical Inquiry* 22 (1996): 679.

9. Hawkins, "Naming Names," 756–757.

10. Carole Blair, Marsha S. Jeppeson, and Enrico Pucci Jr., "Public Memorializing in Postmodernity: The Vietnam Veterans Memorial as Prototype," *Quarterly Journal of Speech* 77 (1991): 279.

11. Michael Kammen, *Mystic Chords of Memory: The Transformation of Tradition in American Culture* (New York: Knopf, 1991), 702; John R. Gillis, "Memory and Identity: The History of a Relationship," in *Commemorations: The Politics of National Identification*, ed. John R. Gillis (Princeton: Princeton University Press, 1994), especially 14, 17; John Bodnar, *Remaking America: Public Memory, Commemoration, and Patriotism in the Twentieth Century* (Princeton: Princeton University Press, 1992).

12. Both the Franklin Delano Roosevelt Memorial and the George Mason Memorial, also nearby, were constructed after the VVM.

13. See Blair, "Reflections on Criticism and Bodies: Parables from Public Places," *Western Journal of Communication* 65 (2001): 278–283.

14. NAMES Project Foundation, http://www.aidsquilt.org/quiltfacts.htm (accessed February 23, 2009).

15. Anyone not familiar with the Sisters might wish to access the Sisters of Perpetual Indulgence, Inc., http://www.thesisters.org/. Its mission statement reads as follows: "The Sisters of Perpetual Indulgence, Inc. is a leading-edge Order of queer nuns. Since their first appearance in San Francisco on Easter Sunday 1979, the Sisters have devoted themselves to community service, ministry and outreach to those on the edges, and to promoting human rights, respect for diversity and spiritual enlightenment. The Sisters believe all people have a right to express their unique joy and beauty and use humor and irreverent wit to expose the forces of bigotry, complacency and guilt that chain the human spirit."

16. Cindy Ruskin, *The Quilt: Stories from the NAMES Project* (New York: Pocket Books, 1988), 126.

17. NAMES Project Foundation.

18. Ryan White was an Indiana boy diagnosed with AIDS in 1984, at age thirteen. His fight to continue to attend a public school brought international attention to him and his cause. He died in the spring of 1990.

19. For example, a Quilt panel for Roy Cohn, infamous for his role in the Ethel and Julius Rosenberg trial and for his public homophobia (although he was homosexual), bears simply his name and the words "Bully," "Coward," "Victim." Another for Cohn inscribes his name on a flag of the Soviet Union. See the AIDS Memorial Quilt

Archive, http://www.archive.aidsquilt.org (accessed January 8, 2007).

20. Richard D. Mohr, *Gay Ideas: Outing and Other Controversies* (Boston: Beacon Press, 1992), 110–111. Although we are uncomfortable with Mohr's diremption of the moral and the political, his reading of the Quilt is an important one, and on the issues he raises on mourning and the moral, we are indebted to his work.

21. See, for example, Mark Gottdiener, *The Theming of America: Dreams, Visions, and Commercial Spaces* (Boulder, CO: Westview Press, 1997), 122–123. Gottdiener recognizes the distinction at first, in his description of the effort to build "a memorial to the veterans of the Vietnam War" (122) but then, without comment, abandons it; in further discussion it becomes the "Vietnam War Memorial" (123, 170).

22. NAMES Project Foundation.

23. See, for example, Henri Lefebvre, *The Production of Space,* trans. Donald Nicholson-Smith (Oxford: Blackwell, 1991), 220–228. Also see Malcolm Miles, *Art, Space and the City: Public Art and Urban Futures* (London: Routledge, 1997), 58–83.

24. See Bodnar, especially his chapter "The National Park Service and History" in *Remaking America,* 169–205. See also Mike Wallace, *Mickey Mouse History and Other Essays on American Memory* (Philadelphia: Temple University Press, 1996). Especially pertinent on this point is his essay "Visiting the Past: History Museums in the United States," 3–32.

25. See Sturken, *Tangled Memories,* 71, 185–186.

26. Karen Burke LeFevre, *Invention as a Social Act* (Carbondale: Southern Illinois University Press, 1987).

27. See, for example, Christopher Knight's astute assessment of the impact of the Vietnam Women's Memorial. Christopher Knight, "Politics Mars Remembrance," *Sacramento Bee,* November 7, 1993, Forum 1. For the origins of the second sculpture augmentation, see Karal Ann Marling and John Wetenhall, "The Sexual Politics of Memory: The Vietnam Women's Memorial Project and 'The Wall,'" *Prospects* 14 (1989): 341–372.

28. See Thomas B. Allen, *Offerings at the Wall: Artifacts from the Vietnam Veterans Memorial Collection* (Atlanta: Turner Publishing, 1995); Kristin Ann Hass, *Carried to the Wall: American Memory and the Vietnam Veterans Memorial* (Berkeley: University of California Press, 1998); and A. Cheree Carlson and John E. Hocking, "Strategies of Remembrance at the Vietnam Veterans Memorial," *Western Journal of Speech Communication* 52 (1988): 203–215.

29. Hawkins, "Naming Names," 762.

30. Ibid., 763–764.

31. Ibid., 766–767; Sturken, *Tangled Memories,* 191–194.

32. This "relinquishment" may be the most difficult part of the process. Both Kerewsky and Krouse address the fact that panel makers often have a hard time letting go of the their contributions. Shoshana D. Kerewsky, "The AIDS Memorial Quilt: Personal and Therapeutic Uses," *Arts in Psychotherapy* 24 (1997): 431–438, and Mary Beth Krouse, "Gift Giving, Identity, and Transformation: The AIDS Memorial Quilt," *Journal of Gay, Lesbian, and Bisexual Identity* 4 (1999): 241–256.

33. Allegedly because of the major expense and massive organizing effort required, and the difficulty of finding a location large enough to display the full Quilt, 1996 was the last full display. To our knowledge, there have been no plans on the part of the NAMES Project to attempt it again. The AIDS Quilt weighs more than fifty-four tons, and spread out horizontally with walkway fabric, it would cover 1,293,300 square feet. See NAMES Project Foundation, http://www.archive.aidsquilt.org/quiltfacts.htm (accessed 3 January 2007).

34. The important nuances of the idea of a "rhetoric of display" are elaborated effectively by Lawrence J. Prelli, "Rhetorics of Display: An Introduction," in *Rhetorics of Display,* ed. Lawrence J. Prelli (Columbia: University of South Carolina Press, 2006), 1–38.

35. See, for example, Robert Asen and Daniel C. Brouwer, eds., *Counterpublics and the State* (Albany: State University of New York Press, 2001); Nancy Fraser, "Rethinking the Public Sphere: A Contribution to the Critique of Actually Existing Democracy," in *Habermas and the Public Sphere,* ed. Craig Calhoun (Cambridge: MIT Press, 1992); G. Thomas Goodnight, "The Personal, Technical, and Public Spheres of Argument: A Speculative Inquiry into the Art of Public Deliberation," *Journal of the American Forensic Association* 18 (1982): 214–227; Jürgen Habermas, *The Structural Transformation of the Public Sphere: An Inquiry into a Category of Bourgeois Society,* reprint ed. (Cambridge: MIT Press, 1991); Gerard A. Hauser, *Vernacular Voices: The Rhetoric of Publics and Public Spheres* (Columbia: University of South Carolina, 1999); Richard Sennett, *The Fall of Public Man* (New York: Alfred A. Knopf, 1977); and Michael Warner, *Publics and Counterpublics* (New York: Zone Books, 2002).

36. We take seriously efforts to rethink the public sphere as a spatialized notion, but such spatialization calls even more attention to the relationship of public and private. See Setha Low and Neil Smith, eds., *The Politics of Public Space* (New York: Routledge, 2006).

37. Hawkins, "Naming Names," 774.

38. Also bearing this out is the practice of submitting a letter along with a Quilt panel to the NAMES Project. See Joe Brown, *A Promise to Remember: The NAMES Project Book of Letters* (New York: Avon, 1992).

39. Charles L. Griswold, "The Vietnam Veterans Memorial and the Washington Mall: Philosophical Thoughts on Political Iconography," *Critical Inquiry* 12 (1986): 712. Also see Kim Servart Theriaut, "Re-membering Vietnam: War, Trauma, and 'Scarring Over' after 'The Wall,'" *Journal of American Culture* 26 (2003): 421–431.

40. Gary Abrams, "AIDS Quilt Comforting U.S. Grief," *Los Angeles Times*, March 22, 1988; Gerry Gentry, "The NAMES Project: A Catharsis of Grief," *Christian Century*, May 24–31, 1989, 550; and Tom Dixon, "A Healing of Hearts," *Frontiers*, April 6–20, 1988, 60. Such usage has been just as pervasive in academic discourse. See, for example, Brown, "Trauma, Museums and the Future of Pedagogy"; Hawkins, "Naming Names"; Kerewsky, "The AIDS Memorial Quilt"; Krouse, "Gift Giving, Identity, and Transformation"; and Sturken, "Tangled Threads." See also Jacqueline Lewis and Michael R. Fraser, "Patches of Grief and Rage: Visitor Responses to the NAMES Project AIDS Memorial Quilt," *Qualitative Sociology* 19 (1996): 433–451; and Gregg Stull, "The AIDS Memorial Quilt: Performing Memory, Piecing Action," *American Art* 15 (2001): 84–89.

41. See Brown, "Trauma, Museums and the Future of Pedagogy."

42. One often reads accounts of gay male urban dwellers attending a funeral every month or even more frequently. Cleve Jones's report of his experience is hardly atypical: "I wasn't just losing friends, but also losing all the familiar faces of the neighborhood—the bus drivers, clerks and mailmen. . . . When I walk up 18th Street from Church Street to Eureka Street, a distance of eight blocks, just looking at all these houses and knowing the stories behind so many of the windows, makes me feel so old. To know that's where Shane died, that's where Alan died, that was Bobby's last house, that's where Gregory died, that's where Jimmy was diagnosed, that's the house Alex got kicked out of" (quoted by Ruskin, *The Quilt*, 18).

43. Rochelle D. Lewis, "Powerful Images: Quilt Softens Pain of AIDS Deaths," *St. Petersburg Times*, March 31, 1989, 1D.

44. Capozzola, "A Very American Epidemic," 93.

45. Ibid., 98.

46. Alan Zarembo, "Once a Mighty Symbol of Love and Loss: The Tribute to Victims of AIDS Has Gone from Large to Largely Forgotten," *Los Angeles Times*, June 4, 2006, A1. Douglas Crimp, "Mourning and Militancy," *October* 51 (1989): 3–18.

47. Zarembo, "Once a Mighty Symbol of Love and Loss," A1. If his position seems

rather unfair, it is worthwhile to contemplate the NAMES Project's own account of itself. On the back of the 2007 NAMES Project Foundation's calendar, sent out each year to donors, is this self representation: "The NAMES Project Foundation, Inc.,—the international, non-governmental organization that is the custodian of The AIDS Memorial Quilt—was established in 1987. The mission of the NAMES Project Foundation is to foster healing, heighten awareness and inspire action in the age of AIDS. At the close of 2005, The NAMES Project Foundation/AIDS Memorial Quilt was awarded a prestigious Save America's Treasures Federal Grant. The Quilt is now recognized as part of America's priceless historic legacy, an enduring symbol that helps define us as a nation."

48. Zarembo, "Once a Mighty Symbol of Love and Loss," A1.

49. Qtd. in ibid.

50. Ibid.

51. Ibid. The NAMES Project moved from San Francisco to Atlanta in 2001. Cleve Jones was fired by the foundation in 2004.

52. To resist, for example, the pressure to build the World War II Memorial, even in the face of bitter reaction against its location and design, would have been a major political risk. And indeed, Congress and the president finally just ordered it built, bypassing any further hearings or reviews.

53. It also does not include the establishment of "virtual memorials," like the one announced on January 18, 2007, in Robert Greenwald's blog and Brave New Films' Web site: "In thinking of how we at Brave New Films can contribute, and inspired by the AIDS Quilt, the Vietnam memorial, and the *New York Times* biographies of the 9/11 victims, we decided to create a living online memorial to U.S. soldiers killed during the Iraq War" (http://www.robertgreenwald.org/2007/01/announcing_the_iraq_veterans_memorial.php [accessed January 19, 2007]). The virtual memorial may be found at http://iraqmemorial.org.

54. Andrew M. Shanken, "Planning Memory: Living Memorials in the United States during World War II," *Art Bulletin* 84 (March 2002): 130–147. Also see Carole Blair and Neil Michel, "The Rushmore Effect: *Ethos* and National Collective Identity," in *The Ethos of Rhetoric*, ed. Michael J. Hyde (Columbia: University of South Carolina Press, 2004), 172–175.

55. See, for example, Judy Mann, "Peace on Earth Would Be the Best Memorial," *Washington Post*, September 19, 2001, C11.

56. Information about the Pentagon Memorial may be found at the Web sites of the Pentagon Memorial Fund (http://www.pentagonmemorial.net/home.aspx) or the U.S.

Department of Defense http://www.defenselink.mil/home/features/2008/0708_memorial/.

57. Indeed, some have argued that it is a tribute to American imperialism. See, for example, V. William Balthrop, Carole Blair, and Neil Michel, "The Presence of the Present: Hijacking 'The Good War'?" *Western Journal of Communication* 74 (2010): 170–207; Erika Doss, "War, Memory, and the Public Mediation of Affect: The National World War II Memorial and American Imperialism," *Memory Studies* 1 (2008): 227–250; Erika Doss, *Memorial Mania,* 207; and Christopher Knight, "A Memorial to Forget," *Los Angeles Times,* May 23, 2004, E27. Others simply cast it as nationalistic or authoritarian. See Kirk Savage, *Monument Wars: Washington, D.C., the National Mall, and the Transformation of the American Landscape* (Berkeley: University of California Press, 2009), 297–306.

58. We are aware, of course, that some saw an urgency in the fact that the September 11 sites were functionally "gravesites." However, that cannot account for the Oklahoma City site, where the physical remains of all the dead were recovered. Moreover, even in the case of the World Trade Center site, where physical remains often were not recovered, the desire to commemorate quickly was pragmatically futile, given the massive cleanup efforts and the large number of "stakeholders" in the battle over the site.

59. To keep this discussion reasonably manageable, we discuss here principally the Oklahoma City project and the planning and projections for the memorial at the World Trade Center in New York City. Some of the characterizations here would be parallel, others not as much, if we discussed in more detail the Flight 93 Memorial, planned for Somerset, Pennsylvania, and the Pentagon Memorial, in Arlington, Virginia.

60. See Edward T. Linenthal, *The Unfinished Bombing: Oklahoma City in American Memory* (New York: Oxford University Press, 2001). Also see Lower Manhattan Development Corporation, World Trade Center Site Memorial Competition, http://www.wtcsitememorial.org; Flight 93 National Memorial, http://www.flight93memorialproject.org; and Pentagon Memorial Fund, http://www.pentagonmemorial.net.

61. Sturken, *Tangled Memories,* 257.

62. Linenthal, *The Unfinished Bombing,* 190; emphasis added.

63. Ibid., 4. "In Oklahoma City," he says, "the memorial process involved hundreds of people, and it was consciously designed to be therapeutic."

64. Jesse Katz, "Driving Need for Catharsis," *Los Angeles Times,* Orange County Ed., April 19, 1997, A1+.

65. Paul Goldberger, "Groundwork: How the Future of Ground Zero Is Being Resolved," *New Yorker,* May 20, 2002, 95.

66. Nikki Stern, "Our Grief Doesn't Make Us Experts," *Newsweek,* March 13, 2006, 20.

67. Sturken, *Tangled Memories,* 259.

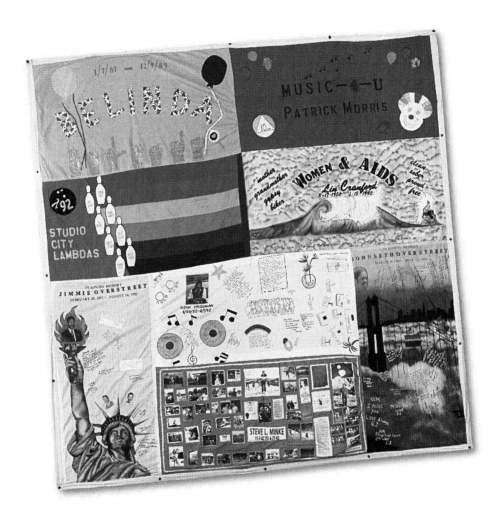

The Politics of Loss and Its Remains in *Common Threads: Stories from the Quilt*

Gust A. Yep

With panels corresponding to the size of a body, coffin, or a grave, the AIDS Memorial Quilt evokes "for many an image of war dead strewn across a now quiet battlefield."[1] With the Quilt operating as a surrogate for the bodies of people who have died of AIDS, viewers, whether they are in a museum, church, school, city hall, or the Washington Mall, are invited to witness and experience the atrocity of the disease and the enormity of the human loss of the AIDS epidemic. First displayed in Washington, D.C., in October 1987 with 1,920 panels, and growing to more than 47,000 in recent years, the Quilt was "a brilliant strategy for bringing AIDS not only to public attention but into the mainstream of American myth, for turning what was perceived to be a 'gay disease' into a shared national tragedy."[2] There is no prescription for viewing and experiencing this tragedy. When visiting a Quilt display, no one tells viewers where to start or finish, what panels to focus on, when to stop or leave, or how to respond to the collage of loss surrounding them. As of April 2009, more than 18 million people have visited the Quilt.[3]

With the easy accessibility and increased availability of mass media products today, anyone can experience the Quilt without traveling to a display. Highly acclaimed and recommended by film critics in the United States and winner of the Academy Award for Best Documentary Feature in 1990, *Common Threads: Stories from the Quilt,* narrated by Dustin Hoffman, tells the story of the NAMES Project AIDS Memorial Quilt by focusing on the lives of five very diverse individuals represented by panels in the Quilt. The documentary is, in Cleve Jones's words, "a beautiful essay" that tells the stories of these five people "struggling with AIDS at a time when hope for survival was nonexistent." In addition to being an important Quilt merchandise and carried by numerous libraries and video rental sites, this documentary has been shown extensively on public television.[4]

In this essay, I examine the politics of loss and its remains in *Common Threads.* To accomplish this, I first discuss the notion of loss and its remains. Next, I provide a brief overview of the film and situate it in its appropriate political and historical context. Third, using the concepts of bodily, spatial, and ideal remains, I analyze the politics of loss in the film. I conclude by examining these politics as we approach the silver anniversary of the inaugural display of the AIDS Memorial Quilt.

Loss and Its Remains

Although the notion of loss has conventionally been relegated to the realm of the psychological or psychoanalytic, Judith Butler contends that loss should be conceived "as constituting social, political, and aesthetic relations."[5] Loss, in this sense, cannot be confined as something that occurred in the past to be left there; on the contrary, loss creates and induces an active tension between the past and the present, and in so doing, it constitutes and transforms the present. As such, the social, political, and aesthetic relations of the present are always already comprised of, and haunted by, loss in its symbolic, ideal, and material forms. This new way of thinking about loss, Butler continues, "seeks to bring theory to bear on the analysis of social and political life, in particular, to the temporality of social and political life."[6] Such a perspective is particularly significant to individuals and social groups, such as gay men, injecting drug users, women and men of color, commercial sex workers, and transgenders affected by the AIDS epidemic. Besides being the most impacted by HIV/AIDS, these individuals and groups are already among the most disenfranchised in U.S. society.[7] These lives—and losses—are, as Butler argues, unintelligible and "unreal" in the national imaginary, thus, making them "ungrievable." An ungrievable life, Butler notes, "is not quite a life; it does not qualify as a life and is not worth a note," for "it is already the unburied, if not the unburiable."[8] A new perspective of loss engages in an analysis of social and political life, including those deemed unreal, ungrievable, unburied, and unburiable.

Loss cannot be cut off and detached from its remains. As David Eng and David Kazanjian aptly observe, "We might say that as soon as the question 'What is lost?' is posed, it invariably slips into the question 'What remains?' That is, loss is inseparable from what remains, for what is lost is known only by what remains of it, by how these remains are produced, read, and sustained."[9] Engaging loss from the perspective of remains animates the past through the creation of bodies, subjectivities, and subjects (bodily remains); spaces, representations, and new meanings (spatial remains); ideals, potentialities, and knowledges (ideal remains).[10] These three realms of remains might be seen as active rather than reactive, creative rather than insipid, prophetic rather than nostalgic, social rather than solipsistic, confrontational rather than reactionary. The panels of the AIDS Memorial Quilt, including the ones in *Common Threads,* are powerful bodily, spatial, and ideal remains—and riveting reminders—of the lives lost to AIDS.

Reading Common Threads

Common Threads: Stories from the Quilt is a significant cultural artifact associated with the AIDS Memorial Quilt. This artifact was widely distributed by the NAMES Project Foundation, the national organization that provides funding and oversees the display of the Quilt. Based in part on the book *The Quilt: Stories from the NAMES Project,* written by Cindy Ruskin, photographed by Matt Herron, and designed by Deborah Zemke,

Common Threads is a feature-length documentary released in 1989, two years after the first display of the entire AIDS Memorial Quilt on the National Mall in Washington, D.C.[11]

The film focuses on the lives of five people memorialized by panels in the Quilt. They are Dr. Tom Waddell, an Olympian, founder of the Gay Games, and a white gay man whose story is told by his friend and mother of his child, Sara Lewinstein; David Mandell Jr., a white young boy with hemophilia whose story is told by his parents, David and Suzi Mandell; Robert Perryman, an injecting drug user and heterosexual African American man whose story is told by his widow, Sallie Perryman, an African American woman; Jeffrey Sevcik, a white gay man whose story is told by his partner, Vito Russo, a film historian and a white gay man; and David Campbell, a white gay man whose story is told by his partner, Tracy Torrey, a U.S. Navy veteran and a white gay man who became his own storyteller as he succumbed to AIDS during filming.

Interspersed with the life narratives of the five men from early childhood to death, the documentary presents a parallel history of the U.S. government's neglect and lack of political response to the growing epidemic and the emergence and creation of the AIDS Memorial Quilt. Using statistics to detail the number of U.S. Americans diagnosed with, and killed by, AIDS, the film provides coverage of the early years of the epidemic (1981–1989) and concludes with a powerful and solemn sequence of names read aloud on the Washington Mall.

Situating Common Threads *in a Political and Historical Context*

The film's (re)presentation of the early years of the AIDS epidemic is a chronicle of, and reaction to, the social, cultural, and political climate of the United States at that moment in history. AIDS is actually an amalgamation of two parallel epidemics—biomedical and cultural—mutually influencing each other. AIDS, the biomedical epidemic, is a narrative of an infectious disease and the search for a cure. AIDS, the cultural epidemic, is an ongoing social and political struggle over scientific, sexual, and social processes of signification associated with the biomedical epidemic.[12]

Indeed, cultural struggles over definitions and meanings started at the onset of the biomedical crisis. The definition of AIDS itself has evolved and changed over the years. In 1981 medical researchers called the newly identified medical condition GRID (gay-related immunodeficiency). The process of coupling a medical condition with a sexual identity served to create, maintain, and perpetuate discursive dichotomies and social hierarchies in the United States (for example, homosexual and the "general population"; us and them; guilty and innocent; moral and immoral; perpetrator and victim; love and death; anus and vagina; normal and abnormal).[13]

As disease and marginal groups in society (such as gays, injecting drug users, commercial sex workers) became endlessly and inextricably linked by the dominant biomedical discourse of AIDS, the notion of "high-risk" groups emerged. As the name suggests, "high-risk" groups focus on identity—who people are personally, socially, and culturally—rather than behavior—what people do that might put them at risk for HIV infection.[14] This focus maintains a safe distance between the mainstream (i.e., white heterosexuals) and the disenfranchised (i.e., white homosexuals and drug users of color) in the United States. It is therefore hardly surprising that the U.S. government, dominated by the ultraconservative politics of the Reagan era, remained silent about the exploding AIDS epidemic in its early years. This point is made more poignantly by Jan Zita Grover about Reagan's silence: "Gary Bauer, president Reagan's assistant, told *Face the Nation* that the reason Reagan had not even uttered the words AIDS publicly before a press conference held late in 1985 was that the Administration did not until then perceive AIDS as a problem: 'It hadn't spread into the general population yet.'"[15] It is painfully clear that the lives of people in the "general population" are infinitely more valuable. As Judith Butler reminds us, they are "highly protected, and the abrogation of their claims to sanctity will be sufficient to mobilize the forces of war," while the lives that are socially and culturally marked do "not even qualify as 'grievable.'"[16]

It was during this grim and frightening—the lack of effective biomedical treatment to keep people living with HIV/AIDS alive—and shameful and embarrassing—the government's silence and neglect of people living with HIV and dying of AIDS—period of U.S. history that the AIDS Memorial Quilt was conceived and created and *Common Threads* was produced and distributed. It was a time of hopelessness, desperation, terror, and despair.[17]

Although Cleve Jones's AIDS Memorial Quilt draws on the U.S. tradition of quilting, it is, as Christopher Capozzola accurately observes, "largely an invented tradition" designed to challenge the conservative discourse of nation and traditional definitions of the family prevalent during the Reagan years. Through this contestation, it demanded that marginalized groups in U.S. society, such as gays and injecting drug users, be included in what it means to be American. The Quilt, Peter Hawkins notes, "redescribes the entire nation in terms of the epidemic—it says, America has AIDS," and in the process it attempts to persuade the government to act with compassion toward its citizens.[18] Ironically, to ensure the inclusion and sympathetic treatment of gay men in the discourse of "America has AIDS," Cleve Jones and the NAMES Project staff disavowed the Quilt's close ties to the gay community. In fact, Jones admitted that he and his staff "deliberately adopted a symbol and a vocabulary that would not be threatening to nongay people." Although the process of "de-gaying" the Quilt was not necessarily uncontroversial, this was nevertheless the political and historical context in which *Common Threads* was produced and circulated.[19]

The stories of the five lives memorialized in the AIDS Memorial Quilt and presented in *Common Threads* serve to "maintain contact with the dead," thus enacting an active tension between the present and the past and loss and its remains.[20] These are the lives that are, in Judith Butler's words, "unreal" and have "already suffered the violence of derealization" by the powerful and invisible dynamics of normativity in U.S. culture. Such lives, Butler adds, "have a strange way of remaining animated," and by engaging with them in *Common Threads*, we can embark on an analysis of their bodily, spatial, and ideal remains.[21]

Engaging the Politics of Loss and Its Remains in Common Threads

The process of viewing attempts to create a sense of identification between the viewer and the subject, and viewing *Common Threads* enacts the relationship between the viewer and the remains of lives lost to AIDS. As Simon Watney suggests, the process of identification works in two ways: "the transitive one of identifying the self in relation to the difference of the other, and the reflexive one of identifying the self in a relation of resemblance to the other."[22] Loss and its remains resulting from AIDS enter the realm of public visibility in the transitive mode, with the condition that any possibility of identification with it is thoroughly refused. What are the politics of this engagement with loss and its remains? What are the potentials of this engagement? What are the new possibilities suggested by this engagement?

BODILY REMAINS

Bodily remains activate the relationship between the past and the present through the creation of bodies and subjects.[23] This relationship attends to the ways unreal and ungrievable, abject and unlivable bodies are haunted by creative possibilities whose meanings emerge from making sense of their material remains. Based upon a close reading of *Common Threads,* I focus on two bodily remains: the AIDS body and the sexuality of such bodies.

Moving away from abstract AIDS statistics to concrete images of people with AIDS during the early years of the epidemic, the media created, maintained, and perpetuated a particular representation of the AIDS body. Such a representation has become so familiar in the popular imagination that most people do not question its hegemonic status. The AIDS body, in this dominant and pervasive representation, is "ravaged, disfigured, and debilitated by the syndrome," and the subjects with the condition are "generally alone, desperate, but resigned to their 'inevitable' deaths."[24] Presenting the lives of five people with AIDS, *Common Threads* complicates this hegemonic representation of the AIDS body by reinforcing it at times and challenging it at other times.

At first glance, it appears that the images in the documentary reinforce many of the familiar representations of the AIDS body. There are pictures of the "before and after" to provide evidence of the ways HIV ravages the body and destroys the person. Tom Waddell is shown as an athlete who competed in the Olympic Games in Mexico City in 1968. David Mandell

Jr. is described by his mother as a "life eater" while he is playing in a yard. Robert Perryman is seen with his wife, both healthy-looking and dressed in formal attire. Jeffrey Sevcik is shown as a healthy young man in a black-and-white photograph. David Campbell and his partner, Tracy Torrey, are seen in pictures as professional young men at work. The "after" pictures show Tom Waddell alone and looking out a window, David Mandell Jr. looking emaciated in a photo with his brother, Robert Perryman looking thin and forlorn, Jeffrey Sevcik lying in bed, and Tracy Torrey looking wasted and speaking to the camera in bed alone. The disfigurement is particularly noticeable in images of Mandell and Torrey, and bottles of medicine—another indication of disease and illness—are prominent visual elements of their narratives. The inescapability of death of the AIDS body is particularly poignant when Tracy Torrey makes his own quilt panel and tells his deceased partner, David, through the rolling camera, "Hang in there, buddy. It won't be long before we are together again."[25]

Common Threads also appears to reinforce hegemonic representations of the AIDS body through race, class, gender, and sexuality. The five lives presented in the documentary are three white gay men, an African American heterosexual male drug user, and a young white hemophiliac, representing the three major "risk groups"—homosexuals, injecting drug users, and hemophiliacs—identified by the medical establishment. Such a selection reinforces the popular media image that gay men are "always presumed to be white and middle class," and injecting drug users are presumed to be straight "poor people of color."[26] By keeping these "risk groups" separate and independent, gay men of color, white injecting drug users, white women and women of color, among others, become unseen, obscured, and unintelligible in terms of funding; educational, medical, and social services; and the popular imagination. Although Sallie Perryman tests positive for HIV, she remains a narrator of her late husband's life, and her own psychological and material realities of living with the virus are ignored in the name of focusing on the life of her dying partner. The gay men in the film—Waddell, Sevcik, and Campbell, along with Russo and Torrey—and the young hemophiliac and his parents—the Mandells—are signaled by their speech, self-presentation, profession, and surroundings as distinctively middle class. Perryman, the African American man, is established right at the onset as a heterosexual male, and discussion of his struggle with drugs confirms his identity as a drug user. When his wife, Sallie, says, "He didn't take my furniture out of my house. He didn't rob me. He didn't rob anybody," she appears to be challenging the ubiquitous image of the drug user with AIDS—the inner-city poor, criminal, heterosexual of color.[27] The statement, however, appears peculiar in this context. We do not typically imagine a husband robbing his wife, and by conjuring up this prevalent image, it ends up reactivating and affirming it in the popular imagination.

Although the film reinforces some of the hegemonic representations of the AIDS body, it also challenges them in important ways. During the Reagan era, dominant conceptions of nationhood and the family certainly did not include AIDS and the populations it affected. AIDS seemed so "un-American," and many people and communities in the United States actively avoided it symbolically and materially.[28] These hegemonic discourses of nation and family are brought into crisis in *Common Threads.* Calling it "truly an All-American family," Sara Lewinstein discusses how she, a lesbian, and Tom Waddell, a gay man, decided to become a family and have their daughter, Jessica. Tom "was everything I would want for my child to grow up with," exclaims a smiling Lewinstein. When they decided to have a child, she recalls what she said to Waddell, "You are wonderful. You are athletic. You are smart. You are a doctor. My mother would have no complaints."[29] The idea that a lesbian and a gay man are so perfectly matched emotionally, intellectually, and psychologically to form a family and have a child confronts and resists the traditional heteronormative model of family.

Defying popular stereotypes of drug users, the documentary shows Robert Perryman as a dedicated and responsible father. Sallie, his wife, recalls, "Rob wanted to be the best father that he could and he was so nurturing and caring about his daughter. He bathed her, he washed her, he took her for walks, he rolled the stroller, he changed diapers."[30] These images open up new discursive horizons for thinking about families and family life in the United States in the late 1980s.

As I discussed earlier, popular images of the AIDS body is one of death and decay; it is certainly not one of life and vitality. Although some of the images depicted in *Common Threads* are in hospital rooms, a common site where AIDS bodies are located, one sequence involving Tom

Waddell tampers with popular expectations. In the scene, Waddell is in a hospital room, not as a patient, but as a visitor and a proud and expecting father. Lewinstein has just delivered Jessica, their daughter, and Waddell looks radiant and ecstatic. While the popular imagination expects AIDS bodies to be ravaged and waiting for death, Waddell's image is glowing from bringing life to the world.

The AIDS body is not conceived as sexual in the popular imagination. With the exceptions of Waddell and Perryman, who produced children, *Common Threads* depicts its subjects as essentially devoid of sexuality. The absence of discourse about their desires, fantasies, and activities literally edits their sexual lives off the screen, or, as Richard Mohr puts it, "sex is bleached right out."[31] However, sex and sexuality are fundamental dimensions of human experience and subjectivity, and this seems to be particularly true of gay men who are socially and culturally defined by their sexual identity.[32] That Waddell's and Perryman's sexuality remain on the screen while others' were edited out is worth noting. Perryman is a heterosexual man, and Waddell is a gay man who had a child with his best friend, a lesbian. The showcasing of procreative sexuality at the expense of silencing other forms of erotic engagement continues to reinforce a particular hierarchy of human sexual expression that is damaging to gay men, lesbians, and other sexual minorities.[33] However, the visual and discursive presence of two gay men and their partners—Jeffrey Sevcik and Vito Russo, David Campbell and Tracy Torrey—and their discussion of the physical attraction between them at least suggest an unseen, yet palpable, nonprocreative and nonheteronormative sexuality that is resistive, resilient, and undeniable.

SPATIAL REMAINS

Spatial remains animate the relationship between the past and the present through the creation of spaces and representations.[34] Such a relationship attends to the intersections between subjectivity and space and the representation and temporalization of loss. I focus on two spatial remains, based on my reading of *Common Threads*. The first is the association of AIDS with large gay meccas and inner cities in the United States, which creates the connection between physical geography and AIDS. The second is the construction and institutionalization of the sequelae "HIV-positive = AIDS = Death," which uses the chronological presentation of events in the film to create a discursive space to interpret the biomedical and cultural epidemic.

When the biomedical establishment and the government instituted and institutionalized the notion of "high-risk" groups, they essentially attached AIDS to a social identity. As AIDS became inextricably linked to gay men and injecting drug users, a spatialization of the disease was also cemented: the association of AIDS with large gay meccas and inner cities in the United States. This spatialization of AIDS is largely supported and preserved in the film.

The connection between AIDS and large metropolitan centers with substantial gay populations, such as San Francisco and New York City, is made in the documentary. Three of the gay men—Waddell, Sevcik, and Russo—lived and died in either San Francisco or New York City. Waddell lived, and died, in San Francisco. The Golden Gate Bridge, a familiar landmark of the city, is featured when Tom and Sara decide to become a family and have a child. Sevcik was shown in a street interview during the Gay Parade in New York's Chelsea District. His partner, Vito Russo, originally lived in New York City. Living to his commitment of "we are going to do this together," Vito moved to San Francisco to take care of his partner after Jeffrey was diagnosed with AIDS.[35] In addition to these life stories, many of the news reports—interviews with physicians, street reports, coverage of community events—were also set in San Francisco.

The inner city is a racially coded space to signify people of color with limited financial resources, opportunities, and life chances. That inner cities and drug users are associated in the larger AIDS national imaginary is not surprising. Although this connection is not explicitly made in the depiction of Robert Perryman in the film, there are subtle visual cues that point the viewer in that direction. When his wife, who was presumably being interviewed in her home, is onscreen, the viewer sees a room with a refrigerator and a small table with a sewing machine on top. One is left to wonder if this is a small kitchen or very small living quarters. When Robert decides to die in the hospital, the camera shows his room, and through his window the viewer can see roofs of shabby buildings, the visual signifiers of a poor neighborhood.

In contrast, David Mandell Jr., the young white hemophiliac, is shown in what his mother, Suzi Mandell, calls "our middle American home."[36] The house appears spacious, and young David has many places in which to play. Some of the visual cues seem to confirm that they live in the suburbs. After David's death, Suzi recalls her response to an invitation to go to the local Gay and Lesbian Community Services Center to make a quilt panel for her son: "I gulped. I said I have to ask my husband. We had not ventured very far from our middle American home into that area of the city." But they decided to go. After arriving, Suzi recalls, "It seems like five minutes later that David [her husband] was very, very busy helping them out with the mailing and I was very busy stitching letters into a person's panel." She then came to the powerful realization that, "suddenly, for the first time since my son's death, it was okay to laugh, really laugh."[37] In this scene, new promises for connection and community and new possibilities for political engagement can be imagined when the spatialized boundaries of AIDS are crossed, and perhaps temporarily torn down.

Through the narrative structure of the documentary, another form of spatialization is produced. This one creates a temporalization of loss—a chronology—that establishes the discursive space for the formula "HIV-positive = AIDS = Death." It is important, however, to situate it in a larger context: HIV was not labeled a causal agent of AIDS until 1984, and an HIV-antibody test was not licensed until a year later.[38] Although the chronology remains somewhat unclear, it appears that some of the people in the film were diagnosed with AIDS either before an HIV-antibody test was licensed or the antibody test was meaningless in the presence of AIDS-related symptoms and illnesses. Sara Lewinstein recalls Waddell's negative results for a number of medical tests he ordered. He was diagnosed with AIDS shortly after Sara noticed his weight loss and Tom discovered white patches on his tongue. Both were "signs of AIDS" at that time. Vito Russo discovered a spot on his leg that later turned out to be a kaposi sarcoma lesion, a rare form of skin cancer that people with AIDS were developing during the early years of the epidemic. In these narratives HIV and AIDS become conflated, reflecting the limited biomedical knowledge about the condition at that time. Because the five lives depicted in the film end in death, the HIV-AIDS-death sequelae is established. The separation of HIV—the virus—from AIDS—the medical condition—becomes clearer when Sara Lewinstein and her daughter test negative for HIV. In another scene, Sallie Perryman reveals that she had already been HIV-positive for more than two years at the time of the filming. Seemingly hopeful and realistic, she says, "In my mind, I decided that I am not going to get sick. I don't have to get sick. I am not going to let worrying about it make me sick. That's how I've been coping. Whether this works or not, time will tell. But I feel great."[39] The documentary does not conclude with a voiceover, as most viewers had become accustomed to hearing in those days, announcing Sallie's death. Whether this was because Sallie was alive or the producers elected not to reveal Sallie's death at the time the documentary was released is unknown, but the lack of a voiceover opens up a space to imagine hope and to challenge the inevitability of the temporalization of loss based on the formula "HIV-positive = AIDS = Death."

IDEAL REMAINS

Ideal remains activate the relationship between the past and the present by invoking potentialities, knowledges, and new ways of becoming. The lives lost to AIDS represent blocked potentials of ideals and meanings; the process of engaging with ideal remains can "unblock their political and social potentials and to create an openness to the world in the interest of imagining alternative strategies of becoming."[40] Based on my reading of *Common Threads,* I discuss two remains: the ideal of the uniqueness of the individual and the ideal of justice, activism, and affective life.

The documentary suggests that each of the five lives portrayed on the screen, and in each Quilt panel, are unique. Seeing the "Quilt as evidence" of this uniqueness, Cleve Jones observes, "For all the beauty and tenderness of each panel, the hard fact was that someone of value had to die to make it happen."[41] Their lives—the amalgamation of genealogy, history, biography, psychology, and geography—are like no other. The focus on the individual, Richard Mohr reminds us, reflects the primary central claim of liberalism. He further notes that "it asserts the individual, not groups, classes, or society in toto, as the locus of human value" and in turn interprets this prime value to be "the permission for a person to make plans of her own and to carry them out to a degree compatible with other people having a similar permission."[42]

The process of naming names and remembering individual lives not only makes such lives irreplaceable, it also engages the viewer in a relationship between the past and the present to unblock the potentials of such lives. The opening sequence of the film, slowly showing photographs of several faces, from children to adults, against a backdrop of news reports on AIDS, invites the viewer to wonder about the trajectory of these lives if AIDS hadn't arrived. The scene continues with the camera moving to the AIDS Memorial Quilt display in Washington, where individual loss and national devastation, unrealized plans and blocked potentials, are witnessed en masse.

The uniqueness of the five lives featured in the documentary is captured and reported in some detail. Waddell is characterized as a high achiever—an Olympian and an ultra-competitive athlete, a leader who founded the Gay Games, a respected activist, an intellectual with a doctorate degree—and a loving human being—a great friend, sensitive man, dedicated father. Perryman is presented as a thoughtful husband, devoted father, giving friend, and supportive counselor. Mandell is characterized as a strong and active child, a "life eater," and a courageous soul. Sevcik is described as innocent and childlike, gentle and sensitive, playful and theatrical, spiritual, passive, pessimistic, and nervous in large gatherings. Campbell is described as a handsome man, and both Torrey and Campbell are presented as successful professionals—one in the Navy and the other in landscape architecture. Dustin Hoffman, the narrator of the film, tells us, "these lives take very different roads to the same fate," their death from AIDS.[43]

The sense of "being different" is evident in some of the film's protagonists. Sevcik and Campbell, both gay men, and Mandell, a hemophiliac, are aware of their difference in the social world. Russo described his partner, Sevcik, as "too gentle to live among wolves." These men express the ideal of, and wish for, equality in treatment in different ways. For example, Torrey tells us that Campbell, his partner, realized his homosexuality at an early age, and "he would have become an interior designer if it weren't for the great stigma attached to that occupation, and therefore, decided to become a landscape architect instead." In an attempt to realize the ideal of equal treatment, Campbell did not pursue his professional dream. Mandell's father, aware of his son's difference as a hemophiliac and the violence perpetrated on them in the early years of the epidemic, notes in the film that "I felt that it was important for David to have as much freedom and abilities without us putting restrictions on him so that he could have a normal life." The struggle for "normality," which I read as an investment in the ideals of inherent personal value and equal and fair social treatment, is particularly salient for individuals whose lives are "disposable," valueless, and unreal.[44]

Witnessing some of the injustices resulting from an oppressive social body, an inhumane and unresponsive government, a homophobic and sex-negative medical establishment, and a sensationalistic and invasive media, the documentary provokes and stirs powerful affective responses, including anger and rage, sadness and grief, empathy and compassion. The last scene, set at an AIDS Memorial Quilt display in Washington, has the camera scanning thousands of panels as names of the deceased— men and women, sons and fathers, daughters and mothers, brothers and sisters, adults and children, relatives and friends from all walks of life— are read aloud by different people and in different sections of the display. After reading a list of names aloud, including that of her own son, David, Suzi Mandell walks through the massive display and reminds us:

> Too many people . . . too many people . . . too much love gone . . . too much tragedy. I took David's story . . . and multiply that by the number of panels and it was all so horrendous. Every one of those persons that is represented by a panel is a person who was loved by somebody and that loss, the tremendous loss . . . and I kept thinking of the possibilities for David, what he could have been, what his promise was, and how cut short it was, and again multiply that by the number of panels . . .[45]

If the number of lives lost appears impossible, unbearable, and unfathomable, the viewer is brought in to witness the enormity of the loss one final time with a panoramic view of the Quilt.

The process of witnessing "the naming of the dead" and emoting over these losses does not necessarily constitute progressive political action, as it might give the viewer the fantasy of participation and concern.[46]

Elaborating on this point, Michael Musto suggests that there should be a warning sticker on the Quilt that reads "Don't feel that by crying over this, you've really done something for AIDS."[47] While viewing the lives—and their loss—in *Common Threads* might provide the viewer with the personal and collective context to experience grief and mourning, some AIDS activists, such as Douglas Crimp, argue that it is not enough:

> The fact that our militancy may be a means of dangerous denial in no way suggests that activism is unwarranted. There is no question but that we must fight the unspeakable violence we incur from the society in which we find ourselves. But if we understand that violence is able to reap its horrible rewards through the very psychic mechanisms that make us part of this society, then we may also be able to recognize—along with our rage—our terror, our guilt, and our profound sadness. Militancy, of course, then, but mourning too: mourning *and* militancy.[48]

In this sense, mourning and activism are more intertwined than opposed. Just as mourning takes on many forms—individual and collective, public and private—so does activism—social, cultural, political, and academic, to name a few.[49] Together they can generate energy for continuing political work.

Postscript

Common Threads was released in the midst of a period of hopelessness, desperation, terror, and despair. The AIDS epidemic was—and still is—advancing at an alarming rate in some of the most disenfranchised communities in the United States, leaving few lives untouched and killing many. The slow government response and the homophobia apparent in biomedical research and AIDS-related services fueled and maintained potent social stigma imposed on people with AIDS. With a focus on loss, I examined the creative and political potentials of bodily, spatial, and ideal remains of the lives depicted in the documentary. While it reinforced and maintained some disempowering notions of the AIDS body, it also opened up new possibilities for thinking about more inclusive, less heteronormative, and more queer conceptions of the family.[50] With the exception of procreative sexuality, the AIDS body was desexualized but always haunted by its unseen possibilities. The film also maintained the spatialization of AIDS, particularly the association of AIDS with large gay meccas and U.S. inner cities. Although at times it preserved the formula "HIV-positive = AIDS = Death," there were also moments of disruption of such inevitability. The documentary depicted the five lives living with AIDS as unique and valuable, which challenges the "unreality" and "ungrievability," to invoke Judith Butler's terms again, of such lives.[51] In addition, by showing the enormity of loss due to AIDS, *Common Threads* opens up possibilities for the viewer to mourn and engage in progressive political action.

In spite of the declaration of its "nonpolitical" nature by its creator Cleve Jones, the AIDS Memorial Quilt is a political project engaged in the naming of the unnameable—the lives lost to AIDS—in an era of public silence, social discrimination, and government complicity.[52] Similar to the Quilt's conversion of "bodies of people with AIDS, coded as frightening, untouchable, and contaminating" into "embraceable and tactile forms that evoke warmth and attraction," *Common Threads* transforms the lives with AIDS from a statistical abstraction to embodied multidimensional human beings with all their fragility, character, and potential.[53]

What are the creative and political potentials of the documentary at the end of the third decade of the AIDS epidemic? With the introduction of highly active antiretroviral therapies (HAART) in the mid-1990s, AIDS has changed from a frequently fatal disease to a manageable "chronic health condition," at least in wealthy nations on the Western Hemisphere.[54] People are still dying of AIDS, but many individuals with HIV/AIDS are living longer and healthier lives. Although the epidemic continues to profoundly affect gay communities in the United States, it is rapidly spreading in communities of color and the poor and killing many of their constituents.[55] Given the simultaneous systems of oppression based on race, class, gender, and sexuality in this country, women, people of color who are also gay, men who have sex with men but do not identify as gay, trans-identified individuals, commercial sex workers, and prisoners, among others, continue to be acutely affected by the epidemic. But AIDS is not simply an epidemic affecting disenfranchised groups in wealthy nations. AIDS is, and has always been, a devastating disease with a global reach.[56]

In the current biomedical, political, social, and cultural landscape of AIDS, some of the radical images in *Common Threads* are quite simply not that radical anymore.[57] For example, the radical notion of family depicted by Tom Waddell and Sara Lewinstein—a gay man and a lesbian having a child together—is more visible and commonplace today, at least in large metropolitan centers in the United States. At the same time, the emaciated and ravaged AIDS body has less cultural resonance today. On the other hand, the disruption of the sequelae "HIV-positive = AIDS = Death" has gained greater strength, a product of the combination of medical treatment advances and aggressive pharmaceutical advertising. Finally, the sexuality of AIDS bodies remains highly controversial in the current U.S. cultural landscape. It invokes powerful images of fear and terror. As evidenced by the emergence of topics such as "barebacking," "bug chasing," and "the down low," these images are also endlessly fascinating in the popular imagination. The sexuality of AIDS bodies also reactivates the homophobic fantasy that Simon Watney compellingly describes: "the spectacle of AIDS calmly and constantly entertains the possible prospect of the death of all western European and American gay men from AIDS—a total, let us say, of some twenty million lives—without the slightest flicker of concern, regret, or grief."[58]

Reading *Common Threads* at this moment of history is a journey to the early years of the AIDS epidemic, the quiet activism of the AIDS Memorial Quilt, the ambivalence of witnessing the remains of AIDS that remind viewers of their own personal vulnerabilities and losses, and the "archive of emotions" of the fight against AIDS—both the biomedical and the cultural epidemics.[59] It is also a journey of continuing reanimation of past losses in terms of what remains—bodily, spatial, and ideal—to engage their creative and political potential.

NOTES

I wish to thank Olga Zaytseva for her research assistance and Drs. John P. Elia and Emma L. Negrón for their loving friendship and unending support. This essay is dedicated to the memory of my parents. Their untimely deaths prompted me to examine the meanings of loss and its remains. Finally, I thank Dr. Donald Arquilla for his clarity and encouragement as I continue to engage with these losses.

1. Marita Sturken, *Tangled Memories: The Vietnam War, the AIDS Epidemic, and the Politics of Remembering* (Berkeley: University of California Press, 1997), 196.

2. Cleve Jones with Jeff Dawson, *Stitching a Revolution: The Making of an Activist* (San Francisco: Harper, 2000), 251–266. Current figures can be found in NAMES Project Foundation, "Quilt Facts," at http://www.aidsquilt.org; Peter S. Hawkins, "Naming Names: The Art of Memory and the NAMES Project AIDS Quilt," *Critical Inquiry* 19 (Summer 1993): 752–779.

3. Hawkins, "Naming Names," 764; figures are from the NAMES Project Foundation, "Quilt Facts."

4. *Common Threads: Stories from the Quilt,* produced by Bill Couturie, Rob Epstein, and Jeffrey Friedman, and directed by Rob Epstein and Jeffrey Friedman, digital video recording, 79 min. (San Francisco, CA: Telling Pictures and the NAMES Project Foundation); Jones, *Stitching a Revolution,* 148; Sturken, *Tangled Memories,* 212.

5. Judith Butler, "Afterword: After Loss, What Then?," in *Loss: The Politics of Mourning,* ed. David L. Eng and David Kazanjian (Berkeley: University of California Press, 2003), 467.

6. Butler, "Afterword," 467.

7. Walter Bockting and Eric Avery, ed., *Transgender Health and HIV Prevention: Needs Assessment Studies from Transgender Communities across the United States* (Binghamton, NY: Haworth Press, 2005); Douglas Crimp, *Melancholia and Moralism: Essays on AIDS and Queer Politics* (Cambridge, MA: MIT Press, 2002); William N. Elwood, ed., *Power in the Blood: A Handbook on AIDS, Politics, and Communication* (Mahwah, NJ: Lawrence Erlbaum, 1999); Nancy L. Roth and Linda K. Fuller, ed., *Women and AIDS: Negotiating Safer Practices, Care, and Representation* (New York: Harrington Park Press, 1998); Nancy E. Stoller, *Lessons from the Damned: Queers, Whores, and Junkies Respond to AIDS* (New York: Routledge, 1998).

8. Judith Butler, *Precarious Life: The Powers of Mourning and Violence* (London: Verso, 2004), 32–33, 34.

9. David L. Eng and David Kazanjian, "Introduction: Mourning Remains," in *Loss: The Politics of Mourning,* ed. David. L. Eng and David Kazanjian (Berkeley: University of California Press, 2003), 2.

10. Eng and Kazanjian, "Introduction: Mourning Remains," 1–25.

11. Cindy Ruskin, *The Quilt: Stories from the NAMES Project* (New York: Pocket, 1988); Jones, *Stitching a Revolution,* 251–255.

12. Gust A. Yep, "AIDS/HIV," in *Encyclopedia of Sex, Love and Culture: Vol. 6, Twentieth and Twenty-First Centuries,* ed. James T. Sears (Westport, CT: Greenwood, 2008), 14–18; Paula A. Treichler, *How to Have Theory in an Epidemic: Cultural Chronicles of AIDS* (Durham, NC: Duke University Press, 1999).

13. Yep, "AIDS/HIV"; Jan Zita Grover, "AIDS: Keywords," in *AIDS: Cultural Analysis, Cultural Activism,* ed. Douglas Crimp (Cambridge, MA: MIT Press, 1988), 17–30; Treichler, *How to Have Theory;* Yep, "AIDS/HIV."

14. Grover, "AIDS: Keywords"; Cindy Patton, *Fatal Advice: How Safe Sex Education Went Wrong* (Durham, NC: Duke University Press, 1996); Yep, "AIDS/HIV."

15. Grover, "AIDS: Keywords," 23.

16. Butler, *Precarious Life,* 32.

17. For a historical overview of the Quilt, see, among others, Christopher Capozzola, "A Very American Epidemic: Memory Politics and Identity Politics in the AIDS Memorial Quilt, 1985–1993," *Radical History Review* 82 (Winter 2002): 91–109; Hawkins, "Naming Names"; Jones, *Stitching a Revolution;* Sturken, *Tangled Memories.*

18. Capozzola, "A Very American Epidemic," 96–100; Thomas E. Yingling, *AIDS and the National Body,* ed. Robyn Wiegman (Durham, NC: Duke University Press, 1997); Hawkins, "Naming Names," 765, 777.

19. Hawkins, "Naming Names," 777; Sturken, *Tangled Memories,* 207–208; Cleve Jones, quoted in Capozzola, "A Very American Epidemic," 99.

20. Hawkins, "Naming Names," 766.

21. Butler, *Precarious Life,* 33.

22. Simon Watney, *Practices of Freedom: Selected Writings on HIV/AIDS* (Durham, NC: Duke University Press, 1994), 52.

23. Eng and Kazanjian, "Introduction: Mourning Remains," 7–12.

24. Crimp, *Melancholia and Moralism,* 86; Simon Watney, *Policing Desire: Pornography, AIDS and the Media,* 3rd ed. (Minneapolis: University of Minnesota Press, 1996).

25. *Common Threads: Stories from the Quilt.*

26. Crimp, *Melancholia and Moralism,* 102.

27. *Common Threads: Stories from the Quilt.*

28. Capozzola, "A Very American Epidemic," 97.

29. *Common Threads: Stories from the Quilt.*

30. *Common Threads: Stories from the Quilt.*

31. Richard D. Mohr, *Gay Ideas: Outing and Other Controversies* (Boston: Beacon, 1992), 121.

32. Michel Foucault, "Power and Sex," in *Michel Foucault: Politics, Philosophy, Culture: Interviews and Other Writings, 1977–1984,* ed. Lawrence D. Kritzman, trans. David J. Parent (New York: Routledge, 1988), 110–111; Mohr, *Gay Ideas,* 121.

33. It could be argued that perhaps the producers of *Common Threads* were concerned about the production of what Douglas Crimp calls "phobic images"—that is, pictures "of the terror at imagining the person with AIDS as still sexual." The power of this terror might indeed turn presumably heterosexual viewers away from the documentary and confirm and uphold their homophobic and sex-negative attitudes and prejudices toward non-heteronormative erotic fantasies and practices. See Crimp, *Melancholia and Moralism,* 106.

34. Eng and Kazanjian, "Introduction: Mourning Remains," 17–23.

35. *Common Threads: Stories from the Quilt.*

36. *Common Threads: Stories from the Quilt.*

37. *Common Threads: Stories from the Quilt.*

38. Cindy Patton, *Inventing AIDS* (New York: Routledge, 1990); Yep, "AIDS/HIV."

39. *Common Threads: Stories from the Quilt.*

40. Eng and Kazanjian, "Introduction: Mourning Remains," 12–17.

41. Jones, *Stitching a Revolution,* xiv–xv, 138.

42. Mohr, *Gay Ideas,* 107.

43. *Common Threads: Stories from the Quilt.*

44. *Common Threads: Stories from the Quilt*; Watney, *Practices of Freedom,* 58.

45. *Common Threads: Stories from the Quilt.*

46. Sturken, *Tangled Memories,* 186.

47. Michael Musto, quoted in Sturken, *Tangled Memories,* 213.

48. Crimp, *Melancholia and Moralism,* 149.

49. Gust A. Yep, "The Dialectics of Intervention: Toward a Reconceptualization of the Theory/Activism Divide in Communication Scholarship and Beyond," in *Transformative Communication Studies: Culture, Hierarchy, and the Human Condition,* ed. Omar Swartz (London: Troubador, 2008), 191–207.

50. John P. Elia, "Queering Relationships: Toward a Paradigmatic Shift," in *Queer Theory and Communication: From Disciplining Queers to Queering the Discipline(s),* ed. Gust A. Yep, Karen E. Lovaas, and John P. Elia (Binghamton, NY: Harrington Park Press, 2003), 61–86.

51. Butler, *Precarious Life,* 19–49.

52. Capozzola, "A Very American Epidemic," 91.

53. Sturken, *Tangled Memories,* 197–198.

54. Yep, "AIDS/HIV," 16.

55. See, for example, Cathy J. Cohen, *The Boundaries of Blackness: AIDS and the Breakdown of Black Politics* (Chicago: University of Chicago Press, 1999); Brett C. Stockdill, *Activism Against AIDS: At the Intersections of Sexuality, Race, Gender, and Class* (Boulder: Lynne Rienner, 2003); Stoller, *Lessons from the Damned*; Yep, "AIDS/HIV."

56. Stockdill, *Activism Against AIDS*; Stoller, *Lessons from the Damned*; Cindy Patton, *Globalizing AIDS* (Minneapolis: University of Minnesota Press, 2002).

57. When I write about change, I am not suggesting a progress narrative presuming that "things are getting better" in a seemingly linear and unidirectional fashion. Here I stress the importance of locating change in the dense particularities of its context.

58. Crimp, *Melancholia and Moralism,* 106; Perry N. Halkitis, Leo Wilton, and Jack Drescher, ed., *Barebacking: Psychosocial and Public Health Approaches* (Binghamton, NY: Haworth, 2005); Gust A. Yep, Karen E. Lovaas, and Alex V. Pagonis, "The Case of 'Riding Bareback': Sexual Practices and the Paradoxes of Identity in the Era of AIDS," *Journal of Homosexuality* 42, no. 2 (2002): 1–14; Michael Shernoff, *Without Condoms: Unprotected Sex, Gay Men and Barebacking* (New York: Routledge, 2006); Yep, "AIDS/HIV," 17; Keith Boykin, *Beyond the Down Low: Sex, Lies, and Denial in Black America* (New York: Carroll and Graf, 2005); Watney, *Practices of Freedom,* 58.

59. See, for example, David B. Feinberg, *Queer and Loathing: Rants and Raves of a Raging AIDS Clone* (New York: Viking, 1994), 37–38; Ann Cvetkovich, "Legacies of Trauma, Legacies of Activism: ACT UP's Lesbians," in *Loss: The Politics of Mourning,* ed. David L. Eng and David Kazanjian (Berkeley: University of California Press, 2003), 437.

PART 2

Movement

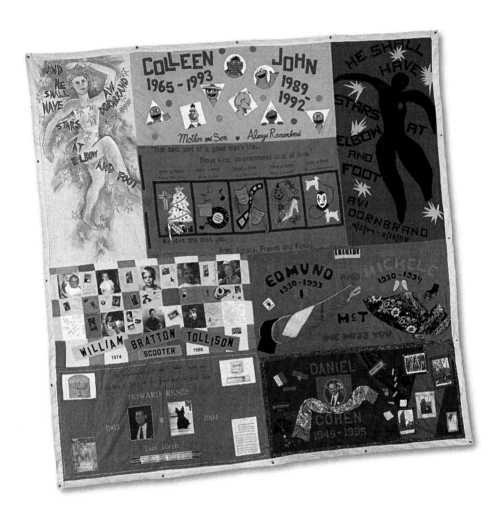

Q.U.I.L.T.: A Patchwork of Reflections

Kevin Michael DeLuca, Christine Harold, and Kenneth Rufo

Haiku in Process: Repetition Sans Resolution

UNCLE JOHN, 1944–1987

I remember lost
keys, your smile, and so much love.
Now, an empty page.

UNCLE JOHN, 1944–1987

I remember lost
keys, your smile, deep love. Now, the
empty, empty page.

UNCLE JOHN, 1944–1987

I remember lost
keys, your smile, deep love. Now, an
empty, empty page.[1]

Ginny's Panel

My brother died of AIDS twenty years ago.

I still cry and I am still pissed.

I sat with John in Sloan Kettering Hospital in New York City the night before he died. "Is it okay for me to go now?" he asked.

I lied and said yes.

I still want to sit outside with him, gossiping endlessly about everyone we love and what we feel and what they feel and what they should do and how we should eat right and exercise more and save the environment and create world peace.[2]

John R. DeLuca died of complications due to AIDS July 18, 1987. He was forty-three years old. I was thirty-four.

Today, his oldest son, Shawn, is married to Mia and John's first grandchild, Isabella turned two in December. His daughter, Kirsten, is married to Victor and lives in John's college town, Burlington, VT. His son, Todd, will be married to Haidee this summer.

They are all doing well, I would tell him. Very well.

And so am I.

So am I.

Our brother Ken died, I would tell him. And I really want to talk with you, I would say, about how guilty I feel about not saving him from booze and cigarettes. I think he took your death very hard. And, oh, I got divorced (that was a scene) and now am remarried and I think you would really like him. And, Dad made it to 83 and was still arguing politics when he died. And, can you believe it, our kids are all in their thirties, and they all hang out together and plan vacations together—all that cousin bonding that we hoped for is still in place. And I really wish you . . . Well there is really way too much.

I am John's fifty four year old sister, still crying in my morning coffee for my brother who died of AIDS twenty years ago and I think—this is what all those numbers of AIDS dead mean. This is what it means when our polices allow this disease to ravage the poorest and most vulnerable in the world. It means millions of sisters (and brothers and children and parents and partners and . . .) weep for years. Our relationships with our dead do not end with their dying.

I did not have my brother, John, in my life for these past twenty years and my life is much less for that.[3]

An Unfolding History

The AIDS Memorial Quilt has been displayed in its entirety only five times in its twenty-three-year history (all in Washington, D.C.). The Quilt was first displayed in 1987, a pivotal year in AIDS awareness. Ronald Reagan gave his first major (and, for many Americans, woefully belated) speech addressing the crisis, calling it "public enemy number one." *San Francisco Chronicle* journalist Randy Shilts published *And the Band Played On,* his hugely influential chronicle of the spread of HIV and AIDS and the U.S. government's seeming indifference to what many considered a "gay plague." That same year, the direct action group ACT UP (AIDS Coalition to Unleash Power) was founded, calling attention to the AIDS crisis by, among other actions, protesting the prohibitive prices the pharmaceutical behemoths were charging for antiviral drugs like AZT. The Quilt's inaugural display was part of a National March on Washington for Gay and Lesbian rights. That weekend in October 1987, nearly half a million people viewed the Quilt, then comprised of 1,920 panels, a space larger than a football field.[4] Approximately 16,488 Americans died of AIDS-related illnesses that year.[5] In 1992, the year of the fourth display of the Quilt, two persons with AIDS—Bob Hattoy and Elizabeth Glaser—were invited to speak at the Democratic National Convention. The previous year, rock star Freddie Mercury of Queen died of an AIDS-related illness, and popular basketball star Earvin "Magic" Johnson told the world he was HIV-positive. In 1992, a reported 41,849 Americans died of AIDS-related illnesses.

The last time the AIDS Memorial Quilt was displayed in its entirety was in October 1996, over fifteen years ago. That year, approximately 38,074 Americans died and 61,124 were diagnosed with the disease. Although 1996 did see the beginnings of what would become a significant drop in AIDS cases and deaths, thanks to the widespread use of combination antiretroviral therapy (sometimes called an "AIDS cocktail"), the numbers of people living with and dying of AIDS globally today are staggering. The number of people living with HIV worldwide is approximately 40 million. Last year (2006), nearly 3 million people died of the disease.

The Quilt has continued to expand along with the disease to which it responds. Today, the AIDS Memorial Quilt includes approximately 46,000 individual panels and the names of more than 83,440 people who have died of AIDS-related illnesses. If it were to be displayed in its entirety, the Quilt would cover 1,293,300 square feet (the equivalent of 185 NCAA basketball courts). If the panels were laid out end to end, it would form a 52.25 mile trail of fabric. The Quilt weighs over fifty-four tons. Today, its sheer size makes it impossible for the Quilt to be displayed in its entirety. Few public spaces could accommodate it. Yet, despite its enormity, the Quilt names a mere 17.5 percent of all AIDS-related deaths in the United States alone. As a text representing visually the atrocity AIDS has wreaked on the world, the Quilt fails miserably.

Visiting, One Immersion

A gray building on the margins. Marginal. Hardly visible. 637 Hoke Street. In fact, you cannot get there from Mapquest. The directions skip Bishop Street. No religious link to get us to the home of the AIDS Memorial Quilt. The Mapquest directions to the NAMES Project lack a name, a Bishop, authority, so we are lost. It is a gritty part of town, industrialized and decaying, home to flotsam and jetsam of buildings and people. The gray concrete building is colorless, nondescript, and out of the way, only a plain banner notes its contents, its mission as home of the world's largest memorial, so large it cannot be seen, cannot be visible in its entirety, cannot be whole. The center of Atlanta is in the distance. Yet the place is apt. Margins, boundaries, and wholeness are what AIDS puts at stake and what AIDS activism and the AIDS Quilt question.

Inside, the place is eclectic, haunting photos and quotes of those lost mingle with pop culture kitsch, like Day-Glo teddy bears and feather boas. But the raw wooden barracks dominate, accommodating the memories made material of the people lost, fifty-four tons of colorful quilt stacked in rows from five to nine levels high. The folded quilt panels stuffed into the barracks echo the photographs of the victims of the Holocaust—gaunt, thin, and stacked in bare barracks. Though here the bodies are nowhere to be seen, memories are salvaged in colorful cloth, juxtaposed mementos, pop culture artifacts, image portraits, and heartrending words. Fifty-four tons is the weight of sadness, of loss, of memories of lives dead.

Some twelve-by-twelve-foot blocks of the Quilt are hanging from the barracks, the three-by-six-foot panels often arranged randomly on a block, the juxtapositions jarring. One poem gets at the ethos of the place and the fight against AIDS: "Be strong, / No matter how / Deep the / Entrenched

Wrong, / No Matter how / Hard the Battle, / No Matter how long, / Faint not, Fight on, / For tomorrow / Comes the song."[6]

Yet tomorrow never comes. Both the fight against AIDS and the fight to preserve the Quilt have become salvation projects, Sisyphean fates. "The gods had condemned Sisyphus to ceaselessly rolling a rock to the top of a mountain, whence the stone would fall back of its own weight. They had thought with some reason that there is no more dreadful punishment than futile and hopeless labor. . . . But Sisyphus teaches the higher fidelity that negates the gods and raises rocks. He too concludes that all is well. This universe henceforth without a master seems to him neither sterile nor futile. . . . The struggle itself toward the heights is enough to fill a man's heart. One must imagine Sisyphus happy."[7]

My character is not Sisyphean. The pathos of the place overwhelms me. The fifty-four tons of sadness. I am constantly on the verge of tears, only not crying in order to obey social conventions. These people reduced to a photograph staring at me, and a quote, and a panel stacked somewhere in the barracks. What do they want from me? These images, these panels, beseech me to pay attention. Attention, the most precious commodity in our speed-addicted, distracted realm. But these faces, these faces of others compelling me to pay attention, to look, are not of the restricted economy of capital but the more general economy of death, the economy of the graveyard. These images, these panels, the size of coffins, attempt to shelter the dead from the ravages of death. The Quilt as graveyard answers "the need to shelter the dead, not only to inter them, but also to shelter them from the oblivion that time itself brings. As when, at the site of a grave, in memory of the one dead and gone, those who survive place a stone."[8]

Visiting, A Second Immersion

On a typical day in February, my colleague and I spent the morning at the NAMES Project headquarters in Atlanta. We were greeted warmly by Janece, the director of communications who, like her colleagues, was eager to share with us the profound responsibility of caring for and promoting the Quilt. The small handful of dedicated people who work full time for the NAMES Project truly love *and live* the Quilt. For a place dedicated to archiving memorials to the dead, this was a surprisingly joyful place. As we entered the space (a freestanding, industrial-looking building off the beaten path in West Atlanta; the inside still carrying the hip, brushed chrome aesthetic of the dot-commers who vacated only months earlier), Janece lead us through a small visual history of the Quilt—faces of children as they poured over felt panels in a grassy football field, an old sewing machine, bits of cloth and string, letters documenting the idiosyncrasies of loved ones. As we turned a corner we entered the heart of the place—a room encircled by the huge shelving units on which the Quilt "blocks" are stored. Deneice, who runs the "warehouse" (although the word fails to capture the warmth of the colorful, softly lit space), easily pulled out one of the units, aided by wheels and tracks, to show us a row of panels. They were stacked neatly, in heavy rows and columns, one on top of another, folded in perfect uniform by Deneice's expert hands. The floor in the middle of the warehouse just barely fit one block—a twelve-by-twelve section of the quilt made up of four three-by-six individual panels. Deneice unfurled for us one after another, the cumbersome folds of memorabilia. We kicked off our shoes as we tiptoed along the thin aisle around each edge so as not to mar the cloth.

I spent the bulk of my time with one panel in particular, one honoring Jimmy Finzel. Finzel had died exactly seven years earlier, in February, his life documented through the eyes of his life partner. Finzel's panel gave some sense of what kind of man he was—an outgoing, Midwestern charmer. But more clear was the pain felt by his partner for having lost him so early. Included on the panel was the handmade program for their commitment ceremony, featuring two clip-art grooms in bow ties and, so that viewers could get a deeper look into the lives of these two men, an eight-by-ten booklet of plastic sleeves containing stained restaurant menus and cocktail napkins, small mementos of an all-too-short romantic history. The final page marks, in an almost quotidian way, the events that would end that history. A page torn from what looked to be an ordinary kitchen calendar, with five hand-scrawled entries:

- February 1: Jim's B-day
- February 15: Jim's suicide
- February 23: Jim disconnected life support
- February 27: Jim's viewing, Michigan
- February 28: Jim's burial, Michigan

This calendar page documented the last days of one life ended by AIDS. The NAMES Project serves as an archive for thousands of such documents. That surprisingly small and colorful space in Atlanta houses not only the Quilt but also countless letters, videos, paintings, teddy bears, and other items that families and friends want to have stored with their panels. For many, the NAMES Project, more so than a grave in some cold cemetery, is the symbolic resting place for their loved ones. There remains something hopeful about this alternative, stitched in fabric rather than buried in the ground, manifest as a lovingly sewn and cared-for comforter.

A Representative Failure

Earlier we suggested, in a purposely provocative statement, that "as a text representing visually the atrocity AIDS has wreaked on the world, the Quilt fails miserably." Such a provocation demands further attention. The "failure," or fault, lies not in the Quilt, but in ourselves, in the expectations produced by our epistemological entrenchment in representation. Taken literally, representation promises that something will be *made present again,* usually throu to symbolize the loss so that we can know it fully, if only through some gh rhetorical figures such as metaphor, intended poetic capture of its essence. But the relationship between the Quilt and AIDS cannot be understood through the figure of metaphor—one is not *like* the other, as children are said to be angels, or communism a cancer. One response to this may be "okay, then, if not metaphor, then metonymy," implying that although the Quilt and AIDS may not be similar, the former stands in for the latter by way of approximation or association. In this view, the Quilt represents the protean face of the global AIDS crisis thanks to the diversity of its subjects—the Quilt as pastiche.

However, the Quilt does not *represent* AIDS, it *responds* to it. Response cannot be understood through mechanisms of substitution. Indeed, most of the panels are not about AIDS at all, but the individual personalities of people lost to it, an important difference. The panels and blocks that comprise the Quilt are idiosyncratic and random. No rhyme or reason governs its aesthetic or its growth. Monuments are metonymic, but this is a schema that cannot account for the power of the Quilt. Let us resist the temptation to ascribe any rhetorical trope to the Quilt. Let us try, instead, to understand how its "failure" to represent is precisely why the Quilt succeeds as a gathering point for AIDS awareness and compassion where traditional memorials might not.

The AIDS Memorial Quilt is a response that cannot be said to *correspond* to AIDS. To "correspond" is to answer by way of agreement, in accordance and conformity *with*. Its goal is harmony between terms or events. As the AIDS crisis has grown, so indeed has the Quilt, but the Quilt could not possibly be up to the task of answering AIDS in some harmonious correlation—one life, one panel. Despite its enormous proportions, the number of names on the Quilt is still only about 17.5 percent of all AIDS-related deaths in the United States alone. That is phenomenal as far as representations go, but, ultimately, as representation the Quilt is doomed to failure. But this "failure," we submit, is its success.

Not only can the Quilt not re-present AIDS, make it present in a way that makes viewers able to fully apprehend it, but the Quilt itself can quite literally not be made present. It is simply too big, too unwieldy, too expensive to display in its entirety. Even those who know the Quilt intimately cannot know it through seeing it. They know it only through its bits and pieces.

The We That Remembers

A quilt. A patchwork. An improvised creation from odds and ends, the left-overs, detritus, the stuff at the margins, not really needed but made useful. The AIDS Quilt. A public monument to a private illness that became a social cause. A public monument that questions the very concepts of public and monument. A public monument without a plan, an architect, a place, an ending. A public monument as *arriangiasti,* a making-do in public with the materials available. A public monument so large that it is invisible, panels placed in anonymous buildings, sometimes seeing the light, touring regions; panels archived electronically, lurking on the Web, accessed accidentally, randomly. A public monument that mutates, fragments, changes constantly, interrupting a reading, a meaning, a public memory.

Public monuments and public memory have become entwined, the monument a solidification of the memory, an ossification of public memory, official memory, both responding to and constituting the memory of Vietnam, of the Korean War, of the Civil Rights Movement, and so on. But, of course, the very phrase "public memory" assumes we know what we mean by "public" and "memory," never mind the two juxtaposed. While many blithely go on doing public memory studies, a questioning has begun. Edward Casey suggests such a questioning in an essay trying to categorize memories, entitled "But What, Then, Is Public Memory?," asserting that "Remembering is always *je meines* ('in each case mine')."⁹ Though Casey goes on to posit a public memory, his question haunts—since memory is a function of an individual human entity, "public memory" affects a misplaced metaphor, extending an individual attribute to a collective function at work in all of society. Society comes to be understood as an aggregation of individuals that somehow forms one large organism so that society is akin to a person with many of the same functions, including memory. This public memory is then excreted in the form of large stone droppings, sedimentations of the society mind.

But who is this public? Though purportedly the object of numerous studies, the public remains an elusive beast. As John Hartley opens his book on the public and publicity, "This book is about the search for something which, from one point of view, does not exist. Looked at another way, it is something so obvious that its existence is usually taken for granted. It cannot be interrogated, inspected, observed or investigated directly. . . . It has no bodily form, but it is powerful."[10] Michael McGee writes of the public as "the people," which he finds to be just as nonexistent: "'The people,' therefore, are not objectively real in the sense that they exist as a collective entity in nature; rather, they are a fiction dreamed by an advocate and infused with an artificial, rhetorical reality."[11]

Memory proves an equally elusive part of the public memory equation. Charles Scott suggests memory as something that is always already about something that is never present, that memory's not about something that happened but, instead, is itself a happening: "The basic meanings of memory in this context are those of presencing with a loss of original presence, continuation with absence of guaranteed continuity, and return to beginnings with absence of a primary origin. . . . public memory occurs as an appearing event."[12]

Of course the problem with all of this is the singularity of both "the public" and "memory." Such singularity erases politics and denies life in favor of a static, stone-cold vision. At the very least, if public memory remains, it must be publics' memories. As McGee concludes, "'the people' exist, not in a single myth, but in the *competitive relationships* which develop between a myth and antithetical visions of the collective life."[13]

A Source of Sanctuary

We often think of sanctuaries as "safe houses," holy in nature, where the persecuted can find refuge from judgment, hospice from an inhospitable public *out there*. Etymological cousins of "sanctuary" include "saint" and, of course, "sanctum," denoting "a private place." The NAMES Project, by choosing to memorialize with a quilt those who have died of AIDS, has provided the dead and their mourners with a sanctuary, however temporary, where they can display private, often inscrutable, information about the individual lives of their loved ones. Often, panel makers choose to offer tiny, quiet details that, for the living, are often relegated to mere ephemera, not worth Remembering. In a colorful panel for James Meade, a handwritten chain of text encircles the image of a yellow-haired man lying under a cozy patchwork quilt, a crescent moon shining through the window above him:

> —Dawn at the window—Birds singing—The cats crying to be fed—Lingering dreams—The light in the tree limbs—Shaving—Putting on a bathrobe—The smell of the coffee—Ironing a shirt—Picking out a tie—Waking up Harry—Feeding the cats—The warmth of the toaster—Oatmeal with raisins—Cleaning the sink—Making the bed—Packing a lunch—Remembering a song—Riding the bus—The weight of a pocketwatch—Telling a joke—Listening to Mozart—Coworkers complaining

and laughing—The breeze in the grass . . . Chow-mein and fortune cook-
ies . . . The kimono hanging on the wall—Fingernail clippings—Reading
in bed—Evening prayer—Stars and sleeping—Dreaming.

These mundane details document, perhaps more powerfully than any
sustained narrative could, a day in a life that was lived. Such details
domesticate AIDS, in that they provide its dead with a home, a dwelling place, a domicile. A sanctuary. For Marita Sturken, this particular
chain of otherwise meaningless signifiers document "a middle-class life
disrupted"; and hence, "the evocation of the daily life of this gay couple
takes on a kind of compelling ordinariness, and small details become
charged with loss."[14] Private though they are, in the context of the Quilt
these small, quiet details only become "charged with loss" through their
display, their *accessibility to a public;* those who presumably know nothing of James Meade's penchant for chow mein or Mozart are affected
by his passing nonetheless. Perhaps this is because the particular, not
the universal, is what connects us as humans. Perhaps this is because
access occurs always already within a sheltering, a gathering together of
panels cared for, united, and constitutive of a new place, a sacred place
inhabitable by those already intimately connected to it, but recognizable
by all.

Limits of Vision

The AIDS Quilt last appeared as a spectacle, as a totalized vision, in October of 1996 on the Mall of Washington, D.C. And it was a spectacular sight, acres of panels swallowing up visitors, immersing spectators in a sea of cacophonous colors, visible as a whole only from a God's-eye point of view. As we have noted, such a vision is now impossible. The question, though, is if it is ever possible. Is it possible to see, to read, to explain any memorial/monument? The Vietnam Veteran's Memorial? Is the visual ever explicable? Meaningful? More than a decade into what W.J.T. Mitchell termed "the pictorial turn," we are still grappling with the visual.[15] Mitchell rightly proffers the term "image/text," but being scribes from Gutenburg's Galaxy, we err on the side of words, turning from the image to context, a linguistic context, a context of words, a context we can read, a context that can tame the madness of images. We forget John Berger's observation: "Seeing comes before words. The child looks and recognizes before it can speak. . . . It is seeing which establishes our place in the surrounding world; we explain that world with words, but words can never undo the fact that we are surrounded by it."[16] Jean Baudrillard warns of the violence of meaning: "Once the hallucination which should properly inhabit the image is buried beneath commentary, walled up in aesthetic celebration and condemned to the plastic surgery of the museum, it is finished. . . . What we have here is quite simply the medium in circulation. And the fundamentally dangerous form of the image gives way to the mere cultural circulation of masterpieces."[17] The necessary move for us is from meaning to force: "The only question is how anything works, with its intensities, flows, processes, partial objects—none of which mean anything."[18] In "The Work of Art in the Age of Mechanical Reproduction," Walter Benjamin offers a productive orientation for engaging images, writing of the audience as "a collectivity in a state of distraction" and asserting that "the tasks which face the human apparatus of perception at the turning points of history cannot be solved by optical means, that is, by contemplation, alone. They are mastered gradually by habit, under the guidance of tactile appropriation."[19] Benjamin is suggesting here, and across his work, the form and objects that mimic his critique, a model for the rhetorical critic to displace the focused gaze with the distracted look of the optical unconscious, the glance of habit, which is tactile in the sense that one is not an observer gazing from a critical distance, but an actor immersed in a sea of imagery, a body pressed upon by the play of images and driven to distraction to survive. The very form of the AIDS Quilt forces this immersion. While with a smaller memorial we can maintain the illusion of the all-encompassing gaze, the capturing with meaning, the acres of the Quilt preclude mastery, visual or linguistic. In the face of the unrepresentable, we want to offer speed, distraction, glances, and immersion as modes of orientation, practices for engaging images, modes of intensities for living among the ceaseless circulation of images of the public screen. Speed, distraction, glances, and immersion suggest not a subject dominating an object but a relationship of simultaneous becoming. Images engaged not as objects of study, corpuses, corpses, but as Deleuzian bodies, modes that introduce relations of speed and slowness into the social and produce affects.

Rupturing the Funereal

The nineteenth-century pataphysicist Alfred Jarry once remarked: "It is conventional to call 'monster' any blending of dissonant elements . . . I call 'monster' every original, inexhaustible beauty."[20] If beauty was for Jarry characterized by a "monstrous" dissonance and inexhaustibility, then he would have found the AIDS Memorial Quilt beautiful indeed. No rules govern its aesthetics; the only requirement is that panels adhere to three-by-six-foot dimensions (the size of a burial plot). As a consequence, the Quilt can only be described as a riotous Mardi Gras parade of color and texture. The panels may roughly symbolize plots, but the Quilt is anything but funereal. Elinor Fuchs writes:

> *Imagine* finding a sublime design of mountains, bordered with "comfort, oh comfort my people" in Hebrew and English right next to a splash of sequins celebrating "Boogie," and directly below a grinning depiction of Bugs Bunny. The Quilt is cemetery as All Fools' Days, a carnival of the sacred, the homely, the joyous and downright tacky, resisting, even *in extremis,* the solemnity of mourning.[21]

It is, in other words, a "carnival of tackiness," but it is precisely this carnivalesque aesthetic that may be "the most moving and at the same time most politically suggestive thing about the quilt: the lived tackiness, the refusal of so many thousands of quilters to solemnize their losses under the aesthetics of mourning."[22] The aesthetics of mourning. In Western culture, with its dominant Judeo-Christian sensibility, mourning is conventionally a somber affair. We are encouraged to honor our dead with an appropriate solemnity. In addition to "staid," "sober," and "sedate," the word "solemn" means "awe-inspiring," or sublime, as in *"solemn beauty."* The funereal aesthetic insists on beauty in the face of death. But, of course, beauty is not a universal category. The beauty of the funereal (black dress, hymns, orations meant to capture the essence of a person or point to transcendental human values) helps us to rationalize death, to make it make sense. It is an understandable and deep-rooted response to the monstrous unknown.

However, might not the *surreal* be a more right and fitting response to the passing from life to death? After all, what is death if not beyond-the-real? Other recent responses to "mass death"—the World War II Memorial, the Vietnam War Memorial, for example—mark the passage from life to death through the classical sense of gravitas, as if memorializing the dead through the weighty medium of stone will anchor life and death, mark the transition with a formal heft that *realizes* it for the viewer in such a way that makes it more recognizable. This is an aesthetic response that hopes to orient the viewer by centralizing death. The Quilt functions quite differently. Although its raison d'être is a serious one, to be sure, its *way of being* can only be described as surreal, committed to the relentless exercise of the imagination—a playful, experimental, dreamlike aesthetic that forms new and unexpected associations. Surrealism, pace funerealism, is decidedly *dis*orienting. Likewise, in the Quilt, a patchwork of otherwise unrelated lives—Christians, Jews, Muslims, Atheists, disco queens, librarians, schoolgirls, truck drivers—are stitched together in a vast and fluctuating tapestry of grief, anger, tenderness, and joy. The Quilt is a surreal monster of inexhaustible beauty; a cacophony of color and texture that allows the mourned and the mourning to speak death with evanescent and glittering breath.

Sublime, Sublated

The AIDS Quilt exceeds sight; it is too large to be seen, to submit to a view. It is too chaotic to be sensible, to be apprehended by reason. Fundamentally, the Quilt is excessive. In its excess it evokes the sublime. The sublime is a long-standing concept in Western thought, with roots in Ancient Greece and developed by Edmund Burke, Immanuel Kant, and, more recently, Jean-François Lyotard.[23] For Burke, the sublime is an intense passion rooted in horror, fear, or terror in the face of objects that suggest vastness, infinity, power, massiveness, mystery, and death.[24] In addition, objects linked to privation are a source of the sublime. "All *general* privations are great because they are all terrible; *Vacuity, Darkness, Solitude,* and *Silence.*"[25] The most sublime object is God, though many objects of nature are often seen as traces of God. There is a sense in Burke that is even more developed in Kant that the sublime is both provoked by nature and unrepresentable. Burke writes of the "passion caused by the great and sublime in *nature,* when those causes operate most powerfully."[26] Kant adds a twist by arguing that the sublime is not actually in nature but in the subject's mind when the subject reaches the limits of representation.

While Kant's move inflates the subject at the expense of the object/nature, we would want to suggest that the sublime emerges in the engagement of the two, with both *becoming* in that relationship. Working from Kant, Lyotard reads the encounter with the sublime, the failure of representation and reason, as a freeing event: "Finally, it must be clear that it is our business not to supply reality but to invent allusions to the conceivable which cannot be presented. . . . Let us wage a war on totality; let us be witnesses to the unpresentable; let us activate the differences and save the honor of the name."[27] In a different take, Charles Scott posits a Dionysian sublime that relates directly to the Quilt and AIDS, for it emphasizes loss and sacrifice: "Nondetermination opens to loss of self and rebirth of different life. . . . His blessing comes after and through dismemberment and the violent touch of uncivilization and in life that is reconstituted and remembered. . . . It is a strange blessing in which the violent loss of 'civilization' is transformed into a way of being civilized out of the ashes of Dionysus' upsurgence."[28] In the encounter with the AIDS Quilt—the excess, the unrepresentable, the chaos, the unfathomable loss—is the sublime.

Stone vs. Cloth

Public monuments. Lincoln Memorial. Washington Monument. FDR Memorial. Vietnam Memorial. Civil Rights Memorial. Stone. The link of monuments to stone seems natural. Stone challenges time. The monuments are made to speak over time, well beyond us, to shape the memories of those yet to come. Stone is elemental. Stone is of the earth. Memory, which is ephemeral, is grounded by stone: "stone is ancient, not only in the sense that it withstands the wear of time better than other natural things, but also in the sense that its antiquity is of the order of the always already. Stone comes from a past that has never been present, a past unassimilable to the order of time in which things come and go in the human world; and that nonbelonging of stone is precisely what qualifies it to mark and hence memorialize such comings and goings, births and deaths."[29] So what do we make of the AIDS Memorial Quilt, a memorial made of the softest of materials—cloth, cotton? Well, first, that time already haunts the Quilt. The Quilt is aging, decaying. It is the patient of preservers, a salvation project. At the cost of millions. Second, the softness of the material sets up a relationship of becoming that the hardness of stone conceals. In butting up against stone, we feel we do not leave a mark, the touches are not reciprocal. Of course, we do leave a mark over time, but it is over a span that exceeds us. Trudging up the steps to St. Peter's Dome, we can see how our steps have worn the stone, shaped it, left a mark. But such a "we" contains millennia and multitudes. We are always touching cloth and cotton. They embrace us all our days.

Quilts encourage us to touch, to embrace, to cuddle. The Quilt is a sensuous experience. It's a relationship of mutually becoming. Our identities transform in the engagement. The quilt takes on my form. My self is extended into the quilt. The quilt is an extension of my skin, of my ability to keep warm. Where I can be is expanded. The Quilt invites me to touch the memories of people I know and do not know. To feel them. To feel the loss. To huddle with the Quilt. Third, and finally, though, perhaps the form of the Quilt, its very material being, the relationships it engenders, what it does in the world, suggest it is not a monument at all. An archive? Perhaps. The archive of the cost of AIDS. An archive of the lives, bodies, experiences lost. Each panel houses the record of a person, inscribed in words, objects, photographs. Not to mention the 500,000 materials housed in a separate room—letters, lists of meds taken, and so on. In the face of a virus that prompted institutional silence and denial, rendering victims invisible, the makers of the Quilt seize the institutional power to name and interpret the event of AIDS. Derrida explains how archive comes from the Greek *arkheion,* the home of the *archon* or magistrate, those with the right and power to interpret the law: "It is thus, in this *domiciliation,* in this house arrest, that archives take place. The dwelling, this place where they dwell permanently, marks this institutional passage from the private to the public."[30] In challenging institutional silence, Quilt makers made manifest the AIDS crisis, made record of it, transforming a private tragedy into a public catastrophe.

The Quilting Point

In their official literature explaining how individual panel submissions are added to the Quilt, the NAMES Project explains:

> After your panel arrives at our main offices . . . it is carefully logged and examined for durability. Sometimes a panel may require hemming to adjust for size, reinforcement, or minor repairs. Next, it is sorted geographically by region. When eight panels from the same region are collected, they are sewn together to form a twelve-foot square. Once sewn, each twelve-by-twelve is edged in canvas and given a number, making it possible to keep track of that block. All the panel, panel maker, and numerical information is then stored in our huge Quilt database.[31]

In this way the patches build, the Quilt grows, and the archive is expanded. What point in this process can be identified with certainty as a rhetorical operation or a moment of signification? Is the rhetorical artifact the individual patches, full of specific meaning and epideictic import? Is the Quilt itself a cohesive and singular artifact, one that manifests a political and rhetorical meaning more than the sum of the patches that comprise it? The answer, we contend, is both/and, and therefore, properly speaking, neither. We believe that while rhetoricians can encounter and engage the Quilt both at the level of individual panels and at the level of a totality, the truly rhetorical moment occurs behind the "scenes," so to speak, in that the essential rhetorical act is not celebrated or made visible in the sense we are accustomed.

This rhetorical moment, the moment when meaning coheres, is named by Jacques Lacan as, coincidentally, the quilting point. Attempting to explain how the subject comes to be structured through language, Lacan contends that there is a *point de capiton,* a quilting point, "at which the signified and the signifier are knotted together."[32] Consequently, he continues: "Everything radiates out from and is organized around this signifier, similar to these little lines of force that an upholstery button forms on the surface of a material. It's the point of convergence that enables everything that happens in this discourse to be situated retroactively and prospectively." Without embracing the discourses and systematicity of psychoanalysis, we can still see in Lacan's formulation the reality that meaning comes about through the ties that bind, the stitches that link a signifier to the signified. In other words, it is neither the signifier of each individual panel that matters most nor the signified of the Quilt-as-totality, from which the Quilt achieves its particular rhetorical force. Rather, it is the act of quilting itself, the never-ending, always expanding, stitching together of panels, batch after batch, and their storage and integration with the archive. The quilting point is, in this instance, quite literally the act of quilting itself.

The Quilt, Archival

When the Quilt moved to Atlanta, it did so under a cloud of controversy. The creator of the Quilt, Cleve Jones, in 2004 sued the NAMES Project in an attempt to keep the Quilt in San Francisco, where activism and awareness of AIDS was, presumably, much higher than in the Georgia capital. Jones feared that the Quilt would simply languish there, essentially locked in a warehouse, stored for future generations but no longer a visible reminder of AIDS. "We have got to constantly be vigilant against the idea that AIDS is over—that's what the quilt can do, particularly for young people who think this is just a treatable chronic condition," he argued. Jones's concerns seem at odds with the evolving nature of the gift he created, and his fundamental distrust of its archiving may have produced more confusion than it did insight. The Quilt is, fundamentally and from its conception *an archive,* an instrument of memory. This instrument does not gain its power, its authority, from its visibility (though early on, when the Quilt was significantly smaller, such visibility did have an important political and rhetorical function). In the beginning, when the Quilt could still hide itself in the role of a monument or conventional memorial, such visibility made sense, but as it grew, and its capacity to function as a discrete, visible object—as a totality—succumbed to its sheer monstrous size, the reality of its archival character became clear.

The archive gains its power from its capacity to alternate between remembering and forgetting; the very fact that much of it remains, if not properly invisible, at least concealed, induces hypomnesia, lowering a particular panel or block below the threshold of memory and hence risking its forgetting. At the same time, the capacity to recall any panel, to search the database, extract the block, and see in that presentation the testimony of the departed, preserved in the archive, engages an anamnesic function, once more thrusting the panel into consciousness.[33] This memory ballet may, at first glance, seem to justify Jones's concerns; a person or organization has to request a panel or request a viewing for the archive to become public. In the absence of such a request, perhaps the risk of forgetting is made real.

But this function of memory, the ambivalent relation that it has to the forgetting and remembering of any particular panel, block, or theme, is a secondary function of the archive. Its primary function is as a site of technology. The capacity of the archive to remember, which stands as antecedent to its capacity to forget, is precisely its particular rhetorical power. For the archive itself will remain visible as a site, a pledge, and a technology of memory long after the cotton threads have worn bare, and long after the public grows tired of viewing a monument, or condemns a memorial to the domestication of tourism.[34] That the archive remains declares there is something to keep, something that is always already contested in the public memory. As such, the archiving of the project in Atlanta may do more for the longevity and rhetorical force of the Quilt than could a lifetime of celebrated displays on the doorsteps of political power.

Sylvester (1944–1988)	Gia Carangi (1960–1986)	Stuart Challender (1947–1991)	Jacques Morali (1947–1991)	Patrick Cowley (1950–1982)	Kiki Djan (1957–2004)	Youri Egorov (1954–1988)	Stephen Oliver (1950–1992)	Louis Potgieter (1951–1993)	Scott Ross (1951–1989)	Roy Cohn (1927–1986)
Peter Adair (1943–1996)	Philly Lutaaya (1951–1989)	Emile Ardolino (1943–1993)	Alvin Ailey (1931–1989)	Michel Foucault (1926–1984)	Steven Grossman (1952–1991)	Howard Ashman (1950–1991)	Kenny Everett (1944–1995)	Colin Higgins (1941–1988)	Richard Hunt (1951–1992)	Alan Bowne (1945–1989)
Amanda Blake (1929–1989)	David Brudnoy (1940–2004)	Néstor Almendros (1930–1992)	Merritt Butrick (1959–1989)	Ian Charleson (1949–1990)	Brad Davis (1949–1991)	Liberace (1919–1987)	Robert Drivas (1938–1986)	Robert Wagenhoffer (1960–1999)	Tom Waddell (1937–1987)	Jerry Smith (1943–1987)
Timothy Patrick Murphy (1959–1988)	Tony Richardson (1928–1991)	Tommy Sexton (1955–1993)	David Oliver (1962–1991)	Denholm Elliott (1922–1992)	Leonard Frey (1938–1988)	Tom Fuccello (1936–1993)	A.J. Antoon (1944–1992)	Kevin Peter Hall (1955–1991)	Rock Hudson (1925–1985)	Alan Wiggins (1958–1991)
Keith Prentice (1940–1992)	Kurt Raab (1941–1988)	Michael Jeter (1952–2003)	Stephen Stucker (1947–1986)	Tim Richmond (1955–1989)	Ondrej Nepela (1951–1989)	Arthur Ashe (1943–1993)	John Curry (1949–1994)	Arvid Noe (1947–1976)	Kimberly Bergalis (1968–1991)	Irving Allen Lee (1948–1992)
John Megna (1952–1995)	Peter Jepson-Young (1957–1992)	Melvin Lindsey (1955–1992)	Roy London (1943–1993)	Gaëtan Dugas (1953–1984)	John Holmes (1944–1988)	Jack Smith (1932–1989)	Richard A. Heyman (1935–1994)	Cookie Mueller (1949–1989)	Marlon Riggs (1957–1994)	Ricky Wilson (1953–1985)
Lance Loud (1951–2001)	Ilka Tanya Payan (1943–1996)	Andy Milligan (1929–1991)	Anthony Perkins (1932–1992)	Ray Sharkey (1952–1993)	Steve Rubell (1943–1989)	Arthur Russell (1951–1992)	Frankie Ruiz (1958–1998)	Michael Kühnen (1955–1991)	Sharon Redd (1945–1992)	Max Robinson (1939–1988)
Joseph Vasquez (1962–1995)	Pedro Zamora (1972–1994)	Fela Kuti (1938–1997)	Murray Salem (1950–1998)	Jorge Bolet (1914–1990)	Robbin Crosby (1960–2002)	Klaus Nomi (1944–1983)	Alan Murphy (1953–1989)	Glenn Burke (1952–1995)	Freddie Mercury (1946–1991)	Billy Lyall (1953–1989)
Tom Fogerty (1941–1990)	Hector Lavoe (1946–1993)	Paul Jabara (1948–1992)	Bernard Kabanda (1959–1999)	John King (1961–1995)	Ray Gillen (1959–1993)	Howard Greenfield (1936–1986)	Nicholas Schaffner (1953–1991)	Randy Shilts (1951–1994)	Karen Dior (1967–2004)	Ofra Haza (1957–2000)
Cazuza (1958–1990)	Bill Sherwood (1952–1990)	Rick Aviles (1952–1995)	Michael Bennett (1943–1987)	Reinaldo Arenas (1943–1990)	Yvonne Vera (1964–2005)	Simon Bailey (1955–1995)	Althea Flynt (1953–1987)	Lucille Teasdale-Corti (1929–1996)	Esteban De Jesus (1951–1989)	Jay Scott (1949–1993)

Methodological Reflection

As is apparent, this essay takes a decidedly nonconventional form. Rather than a series of linear expositions in the service of constructing a larger and conclusive claim, we have chosen to pay homage to that which makes the Quilt such a fascinating and powerful rhetorical artifact: its patchwork of panels, sewn together, each meaningful, and each contributing to something larger than itself. Within the patches of thought that precede this one are the voices of five distinct personalities, and within each of those personalities countless voices more.

Constraining invention in such a fashion makes obvious to author and reader a certain truncated quality, as each panel ends prematurely, its thought processes unfulfilled within the limited space allotted. Like the three-by-six-foot panels of the Quilt, each panel gestures toward something larger than itself; combined they offer a promise of coherence without the steady and reassuring hand of a conclusion. Each thought panel hints at rhetoric at work in the Quilt, but each panel runs up against the limits of its size, and each thereby makes explicit the limits of its own analysis. It is here that the power of the Quilt becomes manifest: like our thought panels, like the Quilt's panels, each life saluted and memorialized within the cotton and canvas blocks ended prematurely, truncated. It is the shared variable of AIDS that unites the record of lives past, but there remains no definitive and unary lesson to be drawn from those deaths, any more than there is to be drawn from the Quilt itself, anymore than there is to be found in the segments of this essay.

What we hope does come across in reading this essay is the sense of its segmentation and the very real limit that such segmentation implies. Like the quilt itself, this essay works, if it works at all, through the stitching together of disparate threads, linked together by a reality that likewise shows no sign of concluding. The Quilt, like our understanding of AIDS, like the reality of AIDS, remains a work in progress.

Thus we come to a close with this, our final panel.

Until the next set of stitches.

NOTES

Celine Nguyen created the quilt panel reproduced in this chapter.

1. Like the construction of this poem, the process of constructing a quilt panel is, for many, a difficult and arduous one. According to those working for the NAMES Project, many panel makers report that the temptation to tinker constantly when trying to capture perfectly the life of a loved one can be overwhelming. Daunted by the process, many wait years before constructing a panel for their loved one.

2. This panel was contributed by Virginia DeLuca.

3. All facts about the Quilt in this panel are from the NAMES Project Web site, "About the Quilt," http://aidsquilt.org/about.htm (accessed February 10, 2007). All AIDS statistics in this panel are from the Avert International AIDS Charity Web site, "Statistics," http://www.avert.org/statindx.htm (accessed February 10, 2007).

4. The poem is by Stephen Vincent and appears on his panel, which is part of Block #05410.

5. Albert Camus, *The Myth of Sisyphus and Other Essays* (New York: Alfred A. Knopf, 1955), 119–123.

6. John Sallis, *Stone* (Bloomington: Indiana University Press, 1994), 18.

7. Edward S. Casey, "Public Memory in Place and Time," in *Framing Public Memory,* ed. Kendall R. Phillips (Tuscaloosa: University of Alabama Press, 2004), 25.

8. John Hartley, *The Politics of Pictures: The Creation of the Public in the Age of Popular Media* (New York: Routledge, 1993), 1.

9. Michael McGee, "In Search of 'The People': A Rhetorical Alternative," in *Contemporary Rhetorical Theory,* ed. John Louis Lucaites, Celeste Michelle Condit, and Sally Caudill (New York: Guilford, 1999), 343.

10. John Hartley, The Politics of Pictures : The Creation of the Public in the Age of Popular Media (New York: Routledge, 1992), 1.

11. Michael Calvin McGee, "In Search of 'The People': A Rhetorical Alternative," *Quarterly Journal of Speech* 61 (1975): 235–249.

12. Charles Scott, "The Appearance of Public Memory," in Phillips, *Framing Public Memory,* 148–149.

13. McGee, "In Search of 'The People,'" 348.

14. Marita Sturken, *Tangled Memories: The Vietnam War, The AIDS Epidemic, and the Politics of Remembering* (Berkeley: University of California Press, 1997), 191.

15. W.J.T. Mitchell, *Picture Theory: Essays on Verbal and Visual Representation* (Chicago: University of Chicago Press, 1995), 11.

16. John Berger, *Ways of Seeing* (New York: Penguin Books, 1972), 1.

17. Jean Baudrillard, *Impossible Exchange* (New York: Verso, 2001), 139.

18. Felix Guattari, quoted in Gilles Deleuze, *Negotiations* (New York: Columbia University Press, 1995), 22.

19. Walter Benjamin, "The Work of Art in the Age of Mechanical Reproduction," in *Illuminations,* ed. Hannah Arendt (New York: Schocken, 1973), 232–233.

20. Alfred Jarry, "L'Ymagier," quoted in Roger Shattuck, *The Banquet Years* (New York: Vintage, 1968), 239–240.

21. Elinor Fuchs, *The Death of Character: Perspectives on Theater after Modernism,* (Bloomington: Indiana University Press, 1996), 195.

22. Elinor Fuchs, "The Aids Quilt," *Nation,* October 31, 1998, 409.

23. Longinus, *On the Sublime,* trans. J. A. Arieti (New York: E. Mellon Press, 1985).

24. See Edmund Burke, *The Works of the Right Honorable Edmund Burke,* vol. 1 February 2005, Project Gutenberg, www.gutenberg.org/ebooks/15043; M. H. Nicolson, "Sublime in External Nature," in *Dictionary of the History of Ideas,* ed. Paul Wiener (New York: Scribner, 1973), 336–337; Stephen Jay Gould, *Dinosaur in a Haystack: Reflections in Natural History* (New York: Harmony Books, 1995).

25. Quoted in Nicolson, "Sublime in External Nature," 337. Also see Jean-François Lyotard, *The Inhuman: Reflections on Time* (Palo Alto, CA: Stanford University Press, 1991), 98–101.

26. Burke, *The Works of the Right Honorable Edmund Burke,* 130.

27. Jean-François Lyotard, *The Postmodern Condition* (Minneapolis: University of Minnesota Press, 1991), 81–82.

28. Charles Scott, *The Time of Memory* (Albany: State University of New York Press, 1999), 81.

29. Sallis, *Stone,* 26.

30. Jacques Derrida, *Archive Fever* (Chicago: University of Chicago Press, 1996), 2.

31. "How Your Panel Becomes Part of the Quilt," in Cleve Jones with Jeff Dawson, *Stitching a Revolution* (New York: Harper Collins, 2000), 270.

32. Jacques Lacan, *The Psychoses 1955–1956: The Seminar of Jacques Lacan Book III* (New York: W. W. Norton and Company, 1993), 268.

33. See Derrida, *Archive Fever,* 10–12.

34. Ibid., 18.

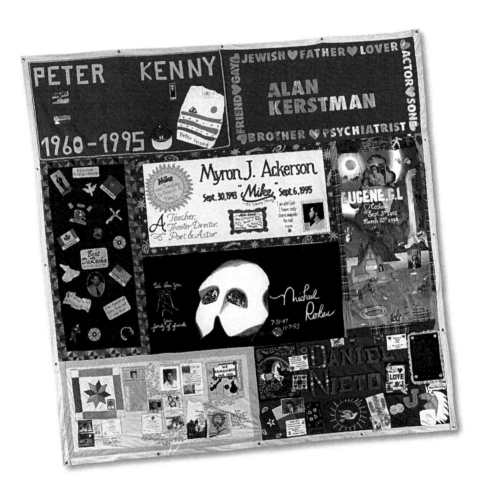

Collage/Montage as Critical Practice, or How to "Quilt"/Read Postmodern Text(ile)s

Brian L. Ott, Eric Aoki, and Greg Dickinson

Both in its creation and display . . . the NAMES Project quilt represents a provocative instance of postmodern cultural politics.

—Van E. Hillard, "Census, Consensus, and the Commodification of Form"

The panels, attached together in groups of eight, are arranged to make space for people to walk between them, so that viewers also become part of the quilt, adding their presence and voices to the composition of the quilt.

—Judy Elsley, "The Rhetoric of the NAMES Project AIDS Quilt"

The cultural politics of the 1980s were especially divisive and contentious. The political and social conservatism of the Reagan administration, with its politics of exclusion and ethos of conformity and moral absolutism, ignited deep-seated fears surrounding difference, fanned the flames of prejudice and bigotry, and produced a toxic atmosphere of intolerance. Meanwhile, progressive movements aimed at multiculturalism, aided by the forces of globalization and the development of information technologies, ushered in an era of unprecedented cultural difference and plurality. It was the height of the U.S. "culture wars," and its battles were vigorously being waged in the arenas of art, education, religion, politics, law, and even the home.[1] As this high stakes fight for the future of America unfolded, traditional boundaries between public/private, individual/collective, and elite/popular increasingly eroded, collapsed, and dissolved, paving the way for new artistic and political forms.

Such was the context that both witnessed and occasioned the emergence of the NAMES Project AIDS Memorial Quilt. The Quilt was and continues to be a poignant and potent rhetorical performance—one that fosters community while honoring individuals, affirms life while invoking death, elicits hope while summoning sorrow, functions politically while appealing aesthetically, challenges the status quo while providing comfort and catharsis, calls for collective action while commemorating personal loss, and envisions a better tomorrow while remembering a painful past. The strange affectivity of the Quilt, as well as its capacity to bridge differences, combat ignorance and intolerance, and speak to diverse audiences, arises from its unusual rhetorical character. Unlike more traditional rhetorical texts, the Quilt is decidedly protean, populist, mobile, material, multivocal, spatial, and fragmentary. It is, simply stated, a *postmodern text(ile)* whose rhetorical consequentiality is as colorful, compelling, and varied as its countless panels.

The Quilt's postmodern (anti)form poses a series of interpretive difficulties and challenges for the would-be critic. How does one assess a text(ile) whose meaning is infinitely diffuse, personal, and mutable? Such a dynamic and ever-changing performance surely cannot be understood, we contend, by traditional manner or method. Commenting on another text of singular eloquence, Lincoln's Gettysburg Address, Edwin Black once cautioned, "sometimes—maybe even all the time—a subject deserves to supersede a method, and to receive its own forms of disclosure."[2] Gregory Ulmer, in an essay titled "The Object of Post-Criticism," goes further still, arguing that postmodern texts resist any critical enterprise aimed at meaning, interpretation, and representation.[3] He proposes, instead, that the critic—following Susan Sontag's call for an erotics of art in place of a hermeneutics of art—attend to the object of study impressionistically, experientially, and sensuously.[4] For Ulmer, this can best be achieved through the device of collage/montage, for it allows the critic to register multiple, even conflicting, sensations and experiences.[5] Such an approach seeks to understand the Quilt not in terms of some generalizable meaning, but in terms of its personal meaningfulness.

In this spirit, we—Eric, Greg, and Brian (the three authors of this piece)—have each written independent accounts, short literary panels, that probe and reflect upon how the Quilt speaks—how it becomes meaningful—to each of us. Although these "panels" are diverse in their content and voice, collectively they provide an entry into the Quilt's wide-ranging affects/effects. It is our hope that readers find value and insight in the distinctiveness of the individual panels, as well as in their essayistic threading together. The panels are arranged alphabetically in an attempt to avoid privileging a particular logic or authorizing a "correct" reading. Indeed, we invite the reader to wander through the essay—to begin wherever he or she likes, to skip ahead and double back, to speed up and slow down in accordance with personal interest and desire—just as one might do in wandering through the Quilt. The reader's chosen path, pace, and movement will, no doubt, create unintended and unpredictable juxtapositions that may, in fact, turn out to be more (or differently) meaningful than anything we intended. Before sharing our individual panels, however, we briefly explore the practice of quilting as a way of introducing the unique form of both the AIDS Quilt and this essay. The essay concludes by discussing the implications and benefits of our approach for criticism.

On the History, Practicality, Aesthetics, and Politics of Quilting

Quilting is a centuries old practice of stitching together multiple layers of cloth. Its history in America is rich and varied. In colonial times, women—though typically only those who were affluent enough to afford household help—would spend their free time engaging in decorative needlework.

But, unlike modern patchwork quilts that involve small pieces of fabric stitched together, early colonial quilts were most often of the whole-cloth variety.[6] Contrary to popular myth, quilting did not, in fact, become a widespread practice in America until the 1800s, and the emergence of quilting bees, or groups of women who quilted together, occurred even later. Quilting's surge in popularity was a consequence, at least in part, of economic and practical necessity. Pioneer women with limited access to (and financial resources for) fabric, for instance, would repurpose swatches of worn-out clothing into quilt squares that could be combined to make quilted blankets and comforters needed to withstand the harsh conditions of frontier life. So, though the history of quilting in America extends back to the Colonies, it did not develop into the practice, as it is understood today, until about the mid-nineteenth century. Since that time, quilts have performed four primary interlocking functions: historical, practical, aesthetic, and political. It is worth briefly reflecting on each of these functions.

"Quilts," in the words of Karen Warren, "are historical records: they capture diverse or distinct cultural traditions and thereby serve collectively to help preserve the past."[7] Quilts are strongly connected to storytelling on multiple levels. The process of quilt making was, by the mid-1800s, frequently a communal activity and also a time for storytelling. For quilters, quilt making provided an opportunity to share one's daily trials and tribulations, as well as her hopes and dreams, with others. No less important than the stories told *by* quilters are the stories told *about* them through their quilts. As Joan Mulholland elaborates, "The sewing of patchwork quilts is a social practice which has developed in America over the last three hundred years into a major discursive genre which provides opportunity for women to engage in special kinds of individual or social speech actions."[8] The discursive character of quilts is evident in friendship quilts, for example, which include some type of signed remembrance. For pioneer women, friendship quilts served as precious memories of the friends and family back home, with whom communication was impractical and infrequent. Through their stories, then, quilts preserved the memories, traditions, and histories of the (mostly) women who made them and the friends for whom they made them. The AIDS Quilt functions similarly. "Each panel tells several stories," comments

Judy Elsley, "first, the story of the person who died of AIDS, and then the story of the person or people who made the block."[9]

As important as quilts are to preserving history, they are designed to serve practical and utilitarian purposes. As Charlotte Pierce-Baker succinctly puts it, "We all understand that a quilt is a blending of disparate pieces to make a whole, and that it is designed for a specific purpose, usually a utilitarian one."[10] The various layers of fabric that comprise quilts function to trap air, which in turn performs an insulating function. Indeed, it is precisely because of quilts' capacity to provide warmth materially that they are often associated with comfort symbolically. No doubt the quilts made as bedding for Union soldiers during the Civil War conveyed a sense of security by evoking the home, where quilts are typically found. However, the comforting character of quilts is more than a metaphor. On the frontier, the ailing were wrapped tightly in quilts to prevent chills and begin healing. Since the comfort and healing that quilts afford is both physical and emotional, the AIDS Quilt provides an ideal vehicle for symbolic action. "In part," Elsley explains, "the panels provide a way for survivors to make a difference. Because caretakers feel particularly helpless in terms of healing those afflicted with the disease, the quilt is something concrete and lasting over which they do have control. . . . Making a panel provides the grievers with a way to begin to deal with their loss."[11]

Anyone who has ever owned or even viewed quilts can recognize their aesthetic value, for "they can be very exciting visually, with precise, varied, and vibrant designs, bold color combinations, and exuberant displays."[12] So, while quilts may be constructed primarily to fulfill practical needs, they also serve as creative and artistic outlets for the persons who make them. According to Jill Schachner Chanen, "Though quilting is a form of needlecraft in which layers of fabric are sewn together with an intricate stitch to create a layered, puffy effect, quilters say it really is an art form."[13] Elaborating on the fact that quilting is not simply a technique, Catherine Amoroso Leslie remarks, "the fineness of the stitches and the way the pattern is executed" involves considerable "artistic skill."[14] Based on their obvious aesthetic appeal, Peter Hawkins notes that, "from the beginning it was clear that the patchwork quilt is our quintessential folk art."[15] Unlike fine art, folk art is produced by ordinary people who have little or no formal artistic training. As a consequence, quilts possess a decidedly local, vernacular, and populist voice—one that is especially well suited to commemorate personal loss. In contrast to official expressions of memory (typical of most public monuments and memorials), which speak *for* "the people," the vernacular expression of the Quilt originates *from* "the people." Thus, the creative, artistic, and aesthetic choices made by panel makers are significant precisely because they are so intensely personal and meaningful.

Like all art, quilts can also be political, for as Van E. Hillard observes, they provide "a vehicle for subverting dominant ideology" and enacting "alternate readings of the world."[16] Elaborating on this point, he adds:

> We should keep in mind that quilts have long been created by marginalized groups: by European-American women, who had few opportunities to express themselves in public discourse and employed their quilts to give expression to private thought and feeling; by African American women who, carrying forward African traditions, practiced the art of salvage and reclamation for utilitarian and expressive purposes; and by African American "quilting slaves," trained to produce quilts for members of the oppressive culture.[17]

One of the most commonly cited examples of quilting's political character is "the freedom quilts that marked the way stations of the Underground Railroad" and "displayed a means for slaves to flee the plantation and journey to freedom."[18] Though there is some question today concerning whether or not quilts actually performed this function (at least as explicitly as has been claimed), scholars agree that the practice of quilting has long utilized *tactics* of symbolic inversion, double coding, and subversive aesthetics.[19] The use of polyrhythmic and nonsymmetrical patterns, as well as looser, broader stitches by African American women, for instance, signals a departure from and challenge to the dominant white European aesthetic. The political import of such practices is less about the specific meaning of these quilts, then, and more about the creation of alternative forms of expression in public spaces. This point is especially noteworthy in the case of the AIDS Quilt, which made visible and public a tragedy that had been and was largely being ignored and disregarded in official and traditional forms of speech.

Highlighting its crucial role in giving voice to the voiceless, Christopher Capozzola notes, "The AIDS Quilt creates an alternative site of memory for many who have been excluded from traditional means of mourning." Central to the power of this "alternative site" is its very public display. Capozzola continues: "Laid out in the symbolic heart of American political culture and cultural memory, within view of the White House, the United States Capitol, and the Lincoln Memorial, The Quilt confronted the exclusions of American political authority and argued for the inclusion of people with AIDS into not just memorial, but political structures from which they had been left out."[20]

In addition to the symbolic significance of the places in which the Quilt has been displayed, there are the very material consequences of its sheer size. Because of the immense volume of space it covers, the Quilt is all but impossible to ignore. Even as the Reagan administration stubbornly refused to acknowledge the AIDS epidemic and its countless victims, the Quilt demanded to be seen. As Hawkins notes, "It leaves the dead to rest in peace, but it does not hesitate to disturb the peace of the living, to force everyone to look beyond the illusion of immunity in order to see a catastrophe that affects us all." In the location (public space), mode (traveling), and manner (immensity) of its display, the Quilt brought "mourning from the margin to center."[21]

Having garnered the public's attention, "The Names Project made extensive use of what its founders called 'traditional American' symbolism in an effort to reach out to 'mainstream' America's hearts and pocketbooks."[22] That symbolism was, as Hawkins elaborates, closely tied to the Stars and Stripes:

> Perhaps the only event similar to it in our national mythology is the making of that other needlework of fabric, color, and pattern that Betsy Ross turned into America's most revered symbol—the American flag. . . . [Cleve Jones] found a brilliant strategy for bringing AIDS not only to public attention but into the mainstream of American myth. He found a way to turn a "gay disease" into a shared tragedy.[23]

This paradoxical invocation of and challenge to traditional American my-thology ultimately makes the Quilt both a compelling and consciousness-raising instance of eloquence—one that "tells a complex story of public and private, personal and political, protest and acquiescence, inclusion and resistance."[24]

Throughout this section we have been suggesting that—like quilting more generally—the Quilt functions historically, practically, aestheti-cally, and politically by telling the stories of those lost to AIDS, provid-ing comfort to those who have lost loved ones, allowing for the creative and artistic expression of panel makers, and challenging the silence and stigmas surrounding this epidemic. But such broad brush strokes, though important, miss how the Quilt "privileges the body [of the viewer/critic] as a site of knowing,"[25] how the Quilt, in addition to being historical, prac-tical, aesthetic, and political, functions as a *(co)performance*—one that is necessarily collective and individual. And if, as Edwin Black argues, "a subject deserves to supersede a method, and to receive its own forms of disclosure," then the Quilt deserves to be engaged on its own terms. As a postmodern text(ile) that is simultaneously fragmented and unified, communal and individual, the Quilt invites a critical performance that is equally fragmented and unified, communal and individual. For this, we turn now to our three experiential panels. There will, no doubt, be some who insist that what follows is not criticism at all. If what is meant by criticism is objectivity, critical distance, and interpretive exhaustion, then we do not disagree, for we scrupulously avoid these dominant regimes of reading in favor of text(ile) immersion, embodied practice, and "an intensely sensuous way of knowing."[26] Through our panels, we seek—to the extent possible in print—to adopt a style that is homologous with the Quilt itself. In short, we engage the Quilt with a quilt of our own.

Panel One: Stitches of Remembrance and Healing

Eric Aoki

As an individual affected by the loss of a romantic partner to AIDS, I know that I have never given the NAMES Project AIDS Memorial Quilt its due attention. Although I have seen blocks of the Quilt on display and felt a sense of humility and emotionality in looking at it, I have never looked for too long or actually allowed myself to be fully vulnerable to the personal and sociocultural healing—the metaphorical *stitching*—for which the Quilt has become so venerated.

Over the past five to six years, my coauthors have been directly connected to my healing process. When I could not speak of the loss of my partner, Stephen, they often sat in silence with me. When I needed to speak of the loss, they listened. When I needed to work, they encouraged. And when I spiraled downward, they lifted me up. My work colleagues, along with the voices of many compassionate students, then, helped to sustain my existence in academia. Over the years, my personal life and work life have become intermingled, often in complex ways, but always in ways that fostered both healing and growth.

So, when I finally engaged the Quilt in a more active way, I found myself in a different mind-set. For the first time in my life, I was ready to learn about the history, hope, and powerful symbolism embedded and embroidered within it. While researching and writing about the Quilt, community friends would approach me at the local cafés I frequent in Old Town, Fort Collins, and ask why I had so many books and materials on quilting. As I shared with them my newfound insights on quilting and, more specifically, the Quilt, I often did so with a telling smile on my face. The smile was present because I had never before envisioned myself writing at a café with a mound of materials about quilts and quilting to both work and heal. Indeed, I found myself increasingly amused by how one's personal life and academic life intersect, how the exigencies created by personal difficulties and scholarly duties can mutually inform and influence one another.

I will, in due course, address my late partner's desire *not* to be a part of the Quilt, as well as the many issues and questions that have arisen because of his wishes. Let me begin, however, simply by noting that Stephen was well aware of my various roles and modes of expression as professor, writer, and artist; Stephen cared not what I did with our stories to educate as a writer, for throughout his own lifetime he educated and advocated as an out and proud gay male. As someone who had AIDS, however, it is fair to say that his path was more challenging. Some of my life stories with him about communicating love and loss are spoken about in my Interpersonal Communication class, and some of his ashes are even embedded in a painting that he knew I would likely do as an artist. Much of our life together, as he knew would be the case, is shared in articles I have written over the years—of course, with selected discretion and privacy on matters and life moments distinctively kept just for us.[27] This manner of expression is the one in which his memory and spirit are primarily carried on in my own work and voice, a space less communal/collective than the Quilt, yet a space more to his wishes. And, yet, in the midst of reading through academic writings on the Quilt, I experienced a sense of disconnection from a memorial that I know holds moving and powerful associations.

In the remainder of this panel, I share a series of autoethnographic reflections about how I have come to make peace with the Quilt—a quilt I know to be so vital to the voice of a community affected by AIDS and a society working to remember and heal. In the end, my voice is meant to celebrate the personal and cultural healing of everyday people who have engaged its *material* and responded.

More than anything else, I remember seeing all the names. At the time that I came in contact with the impressive and eclectic blocks of the Quilt on my own university campus in the early 2000s, seeing all the names was different than the first time I had seen blocks of the Quilt in San Francisco, in the mid- to late 1980s. On this second viewing, my life had changed. I was now someone who had lost a partner to the disease; I was now someone who understood differently the lives affected by the stitched construction of the Quilt; I was now someone affected by AIDS, perhaps not directly in the medical sense, but in the aftermath of its devastation left upon the lives of families, friends, and loved ones. Critic and life scholar bell hooks reminds us that "our collective fear of death is a dis-ease of the heart."[28] For many years and through many medical waves of better to worse health, I feared Stephen's death. When his death came, so did devastation, followed by an overwhelming sense of anger, melancholia for a future with(out) him, and a strongly destabilizing dis-ease that comes with the heartbreak of someone you love and have lost to AIDS. Only now, almost six years later, have I finally appeared to catch my breath. For many years I have been functional and even successful in life and career while slowly yet increasingly working to find a new stride; the loss of Stephen, however, has always been on my mind and in my heart, every step of the way. These days, however, I catch myself smiling when elements of my life with him surface. I laugh at the thought of how funny he was and how unconventionally we lived. Yet even with all this betterment in the recovery from his loss, in an effort to respect his wishes, I have never constructed a panel in his memory.

As noted on the AIDSQuilt.org Web site, "The mission of The NAMES Project Foundation" is "to preserve, care for, and use the AIDS Memorial Quilt to foster healing, heighten awareness, and inspire action in the struggle against HIV and AIDS." Additionally, the Web site reads, "The goals of The AIDS Memorial Quilt" are "to provide a creative means for remembrance and healing, to effectively illustrate the enormity of the AIDS pandemic, to increase awareness of HIV and AIDS throughout the general public, to assist others in providing education on the prevention of HIV infection, and to raise funds for community-based AIDS Service Organizations (ASO's)."[29] I find it disorienting to have connection to some of the elements in the mission and goals of the project yet know that my connection is not a direct one of participation in the construction of the Quilt.

Sometime after Stephen passed on, I took one of his rugby jerseys and handed the worn *material* over to a friend of mine. She knew how to sew well, and I asked her if she would mind sewing his jersey into a pillow for me. I wanted to keep the pillow as something embedded with the personal but also which held a sense of utility. I had given away most of Stephen's clothes, but I had kept selected garments and ball caps to wear, or to simply have near me. For awhile, his clothes smelled like him. When his scent dissipated, I knew it would be time to transform his jersey into something *new*—a stylish pillow to decorate the sofa in my painting studio. But, by the time I was ready to request this transformation of my sewing-skilled friend, too many years had passed on, and I began to feel concerned about asking her if she still had Stephen's jersey. Since the time that she and I had initially spoken about it, and having once spoken about me helping her with the stitching and the stuffing, she had only mentioned that she was ready to work once, but the topic had become one that had gone unaddressed by me for far too long. Today, although

I would like to see his old jersey (the one I most saw and remember him in), I do not want to ask about it, particularly in case my friend has lost the material after so many years. Only now, due to this essay, have I again begun to think about such elements as the *material preservation* of Stephen's memory, his old rugby shirt, and a panel of a quilt that I will not contribute; his rugby shirt is what I would likely put on the Quilt panel if I could. The connection between quilts and loss are long established. As Janet Catherine Berlo writes,

> Looking at my quilt books some months ago, I was moved to tears by a quilt made in 1839 by Elizabeth Roseberry Mitchell of Kentucky. It is a repeating Lemoyne Star pattern, but it has a central square that is a graveyard with a gate. . . . If my mate should die before me, I will make a mourning quilt. Like Elizabeth Mitchell's quilt, mine will be elaborate and detailed, not one that can be completed in a week or month. . . . This will be my path out of sorrow.[30]

Having never made a panel in Stephen's memory (or a homemade pillow either), yet aware of the reasons why one would likely contribute a panel, I have wondered if perhaps my own personal and sociocultural healing had been delayed. Some individuals told me it would be "a couple of years" before I felt present in my life again, but I have taken at least six years to realize that I cannot and do not want to carry the weight of his loss so closely to my heart anymore. Just recently, I breathed differently and let it go. Emotionally and physiologically, I feel different. I believe even in my walk I carry myself differently.

In addition to Stephen's own wishes, I know that there is something overwhelmingly powerful in the symbolism and purpose of the Quilt that steered me away from participating in its construction and away from trying to access his *lost* jersey—the Quilt makes too clear his name, his life, and Stephen, even with all his progressiveness and advocacy, did not want to be remembered for dying of AIDS. I understand the conflict this raises with claims of an individual's progressiveness while simultane-ously opening up criticisms on the politics of shame. But, I know there is no logic sometimes with how one lived his life while living and how he wished to be remembered. With Stephen's death, his own wishes have been the strongest factor in directing me away from completing a panel in his memory. Again, the representational absence of his life within the fabric of the Quilt was his wish, not my need; over time, I have had a strong need to see his life and name as part of the Quilt. I believed that participating in the Quilt would be about healing. Again, for Stephen, the Quilt was different than being embedded into my art or my own academic scholarship. In the end, I have never made sense of his logic and wishes; I suppose I do not need to.

With regard to the never-made pillow, despite its utilitarian function (or perhaps even, *utilitarian masking*), Stephen's rugby jersey reminds me of his body, a body that I held onto in my lifetime and a body that I no longer hold. Although his scent is gone from the fabric of the jersey, it seems easier on my heart to remember him for what he *did* in his lifetime and also for his *advocacy* and strength in *living* rather than for a piece of cloth that rested perhaps too closely to his physical form. Although I can re-create a connection to the good spirit of all he did, I can no longer be in his physical presence, and for me that is where the hardness resided for so many years. As I have thought about the Quilt and how important it became for me to want to participate in it, I am left wondering how the Quilt is fortunately yet complexly not only about *memory* and *remembrance* but also about the *wishes* of those lost, and the *healing* of those left behind.

As a supplement to respecting his memory, I volunteered my voice and skills by serving on the board of directors at the Northern Colorado AIDS Project (NCAP) in Fort Collins for two years. Serving on the board was more challenging than I ever imagined, but it also became a way to engage a different and much needed type of healing, both personally and socioculturally. Important to my love and remembrance of him, it happens to be the manner of social response that most mimics Stephen's way.

Although I undoubtedly choose to respect Stephen's wishes in how he would be remembered, visibly or not in name, materially or not in a most eloquent of quilts, I have wondered if a piece of my healing is lost to the collective stitch of the Quilt. It is clear to me that I will not have participated with so many others whose lives have been affected and whose lives are being remembered and preserved for the generations to come in the Quilt.[31] The spirit and important teachings of the Quilt will have a life beyond our own, a life beyond my ability to participate in community service and advocacy on behalf of Stephen's memory. I continue to think about the fact that his life struggle with AIDS, his identity, his humanity, and his name will not be among those unified and stitched into the collective fabric for the future. So, in the meantime, I celebrate the beauty of community, remembrance, and healing that so many others have engaged in, in meaningful and eclectic ways.

Perhaps Stephen's own remembrance in this world will be revealed through other mediums, perhaps with other important implications, perhaps less material in size, perhaps less visible, perhaps less symbolic in social magnitude, but perhaps just as essential to understanding all that we might come to know about how we remember and heal after losing a loved one to the tragedy of AIDS. This way is what I choose to believe and do, for today, in his memory.

Panel Two: Movement, Materiality, and Memory

Greg Dickinson

In the middle years of the NAMES Project AIDS Memorial Quilt, I was—like the Quilt—moving through. I was moving through graduate school, but I was also moving through the moral, social, and geographic landscapes memorialized in the Quilt. Shifting south from Berkeley and Oakland to Los Angeles and San Diego, my path and the path of the Quilt kept intersecting. Displays of the Quilt in my neighborhoods, participation in HIV/AIDS walks and rallies, and discussions of memory and memorialization punctuated my life as a scholar, community member, and individual. I come to this writing about the Quilt at another particular moment—years into a career of writing about space and place, materiality, and memory. I am struck by the profound (im)materiality of the Quilt and of the relations among the Quilt's materiality, the memories the Quilt encodes, and the theories of memory the Quilt embodies.

It is worth remembering the earliest mnemonic systems of the rhetorical tradition. Young orators in Greece and Rome were advised to memorize an abandoned and striking temple filled with ruined statues and empty rooms. Into this memorized space, orators could place materials to be remembered: the first part of a speech in the entrance of the temple, the conclusion in some backroom, so that by walking through the temple, the orator could also walk through the speech. But, tellingly, behind this architectural mnemonic lies the mythic story of the poet Simonides of Ceos.

Simonides was invited, one day, to present a poem in honor of a rich ruler. But the ruler refused to pay Simonides for services rendered. The gods, desiring to punish the ruler, called Simonides from the banquet hall and then ruined the hall, killing the celebrants inside. The bodies of the dead were so destroyed that their relatives could not identify them. Simonides, remembering where each attendee was sitting, identified each body, making possible a proper burial. Western mnemonics arises out of the ruins of a banquet hall and out of a need to remember the dead. Within this story, remembrance, materiality, and place are interconnected.

And so they are in the Quilt. Here too we see the deep need to memorialize the dead and to do so in ways that connect remembrance with materiality and place. And yet the Quilt offers very particular performances of the connections among remembrance, materiality, and place. The particularities of these relations can be read as generated out of the particular needs to which the Quilt and the Quilt's quilting responds.

FLUID

So many other memorials are made of bricks and mortar, of hard, seemingly permanent materials. The concreteness of these memorials situate them in particular places—the Vietnam Veterans Memorial's materiality is deeply connected to the ground into which it is built.[32] Understanding the material of these built memorials depends not only on taking the granite, stone, or wood of the memorial seriously, but also on attending to the memorial's surrounding landscape.[33]

The Quilt's materiality and spatiality functions differently than we have come to expect from built memorials. Made of cloth and produced by many hands, the Quilt's material marks it as distinctive from other built memorials. The Quilt's softness, composed as it is from cloth,

opposes the hardness of built environments. More, the multiplicity of authors and the variety of designs within each quilt panel sharply contrasts
with the professional designs and relative univocality of more traditional
memorials. Though these differences are often noted, the understandings
of these differences are read primarily as metaphors (the Quilt as comfort
and warmth, for example). But, what of the material itself within the
experience of the Quilt on the Mall or in Cheesman Park in downtown
Denver, where I spent a few hours in September 2007 with the Quilt?

Rather than solidity or permanence, it seems as fruitful to think of
the Quilt's materiality and spatiality as a form of fluidity or nomadism.
In a most literal sense, the Quilt is nomadic. It travels from site to site,
available for display across the country and across the globe. Like the
global economy (or a virus), the Quilt circulates, moves, shifts, changes.
It is global and local. As such, the Quilt is a way of thinking about HIV
and AIDS. It is also a powerful mode of thinking about the contradictions
of family, health, communication, and communicable disease, faith and
faithlessness. It is, in short, a material instantiation of late-twentieth and
early twenty-first-century thinking. Rosi Braidotti writes: "Thinking is a
nomadic activity, which takes place in the transitions between potentially
contradictory positions. It is not topologically bound, especially in the age
of the global economy and telematic networks, but this does not make it
ungrounded, like a view from nowhere."[34] The Quilt, as a particular form
of nomadic thinking, specifies the contradictions. It is not topologically
bound; it is inserted into particular landscapes at particular moments—as
the punctuation of an AIDS walk in Denver, for example. The Quilt—
or pieces of the Quilt—could be anywhere and at any time. But this
"anywhere" and "any time" ought not to be confused with "nowhere" and
"no time." Instead, there is a radical specificity to the Quilt, a radical
materiality and spatiality.

This specificity relies absolutely on the material conditions of the
Quilt. From the very smallest material detail—the broken vinyl record
sewn onto cotton cloth, the leather jacket turned into the backdrop of
one square—to the immensity of displaying even a small portion of the
Quilt panels, the Quilt as experience is always *here*. And, of course, it
is always somewhere/sometime else. The names and the dates, the pictures and detritus sewn into the Quilt trace lines (topoi) to people and

moments gone by. They trace a *passing* (and, sometimes, a passing in too many senses) of a life, of a moment; a passing of a virus, of a word, of communication, of a time. Thus, the Quilt is local and locatable; it offers a material rhetoric of locality: "here lies . . . ," "here are the lies. . . ." or, "come and lie down"—the Quilt can beckon, like a picnic blanket in a park under the sun of a late summer's afternoon.

But the materiality of the Quilt's here and now does not rely only on the Quilt's material. The Quilt demands and constitutes its own audiences and its own authors (and, indeed, the Quilt assiduously works against this authorizing distinction between audiences and authors). The here and now of the Quilt is also, and at the same time, the here and now of the Quilt's visitors. The Quilt invites—no, it demands—the active participation of the viewer. This participation is fully and completely embodied. To see the Quilt is to walk through the Quilt, to stop, move, twist, kneel (as if in prayer, as if in mourning), stand, stroll, sob, cry, laugh, look up, look away, look over, gaze, glance, take in the whole, study the part: synecdoche and metonymy. To visit the Quilt is also, always, a social event. Visitors stand next to each other, look around each other, and look at each other. From across the vast distances of the globe, the Quilt becomes a nodal point of looking and walking, talking and silence.

> To be in process or transition does not place the thinking subject outside history or time: postmodernity as a specific moment of our historicity is a major location that needs to be accounted for. A location is an embedded and embodied memory: it is a set of counter-memories, which are activated by the resisting thinker against the grain of the dominant representations of subjectivity. A location is a materialist temporal and spatial site of co-production of the subject, and thus anything but an instance of relativism. The politics of location, or situated knowledges, rests on process ontology to posit the primacy of relations over substances.[35]

Braidotti here shifts—willy-nilly, it seems—between time and space, here and now. "Historicity," she writes, "is a major location that needs to be accounted for." The Quilt is just this sort of (ac)counting. Visiting the

Quilt and thinking with the Quilt is a powerful reminder of embedded and embodied memory. As we left the Quilt, Eric and I talked of how the losses of our life are most powerfully felt in the loss of a body; the body's smell, feel, warmth, *presence*. This is not only a loss of a body but an embodied loss. The absent body returns as a kind of muscle memory, a memory of the curving of one body into another. The loss of the other's body is the loss of a fluidity of connection where skin seems less like a boundary and more like conduit. And so the loss commemorated and remembered is also radically local—localized in the body of the mourner.

WALKING

"Walking affirms, suspects, tries out, transgresses, respects, etc., the trajectories it 'speaks,'" writes Michel de Certeau. "All the modalities sing a part in this chorus, changing from step to step, stepping in through propositions, sequences, and intensities which vary according to the time, the path taking and the walker."[36] This localizing (and, thus, performing and realizing) of the Quilt depends on walking, on, what Certeau calls the "pedestrian speech act." "If it is true," Certeau writes, "that a spatial order organizes an ensemble of possibilities (e.g., by a place in which one can move) and interdictions (e.g., by a wall that prevents one from going further), then the walker actualizes some of these possibilities. In that way, he makes them exist as well as emerge."[37] The Quilt exists and emerges quite precisely in the walking through the panels. It is easy to think this existing and emerging metaphorically. The visitors quilt the panels together in their walking through the panels. The steps are the stitches, the memories the thread.

While productive, the metaphor of quilting the Quilt with steps may urge us to avoid the materiality of the act. Walking is not so much symbolic (*like* stitching); it is the thing itself. The Quilt's meaning is made not so much in the past or for the future, but in the productivity and performativity of this moment. This performativity of walking in, among, through, by the Quilt creates "a discreteness" of the Quilt and of the Quilt experience. The experience, without a doubt, may be lodged in the memory and may inspire action, but in the first instance walking and the choices created by the walker *is* the Quilt's meaning. Crucially, this walking of the Quilt creates relations: "both a near and a far, a here and a there." These relations are at once relations of connection and disconnection, of saying and silence, of performing and ignoring. This near and far, here and there, produces the Quilt and produces the walker. And so the Quilt and the walker become sutured. The Quilt depends on the walker for its enunciation (just as the structure of the language depends on the speaker for its utterance). The Quilt shifts and sorts the possibilities for the walker but does not determine the walker's path. "These enunciatory operations are of unlimited diversity."[38]

But in moving through the Quilt together, in watching others mourn losses, the Quilt becomes located in the body public. One of the key characteristics of built memorials is that visitors share the memorial with others. Not only does each visitor construct the Quilt out of a walking rhetoric, but the visitors, together, construct the Quilt. This body politic is not a generalized public sphere but is a publicness that occurs in this particular place at this particular time and with these particular people. Further, the publicness of the Quilt does not have as its major rhetorical mode argument or reasoned discourse. Instead, it is a public and embodied sharing of the loss of bodies. In a most fundamental sense, then, the Quilt is co-constructed, made of the materials of the Quilt, the grass on which it lays, the people who wander through, the memories triggered and repressed. The public experience of the Quilt is performed through conversations among the participants, the panels, and the moment. The walking rhetoric of the Quilt, then, is individual and collective, private and public.

MEMORY

What does it *mean,* then, to walk in the Quilt, to walk in the memory/present of HIV/AIDS? And what does it mean to walk in the Quilt with and not with two of my closest friends and writing partners? In part, it means to share with Simonides the duty of remembering the dead, of remembering embodied and emplaced lives. If the mythic story of Siminodes the poet is told as a way to inaugurate an ancient mnemonic system useful for the shift from orality to literacy, perhaps the Quilt is a founding mnemonic of late modernity. In the late modern world, gods no longer kill for retribution (reactionary preachers not withstanding). Instead, viruses circulating among bodies (politic) damage, destroy, and kill. In response to this biologized, depersonalized, globalized, mutating, microscopic danger, a new mnemonic is needed. This new mnemonic has no founding story; it is not located in a single banquet hall, nor locatable on a modernist map, nor woven into a compelling metanarrative. Instead, this new mnemonic is nodal, networked, nomadic, embodied, and performative. This new memory system is not so devoted to *laying to rest* the dead or our fears. Instead, this memory system is about *walking on* in the face of an increasingly inscrutable world. This mnemonic can give shape to the shapeless, location to the placeless, specificity to the abstract. The Quilt materializes and performs memories and theories of memory for and of our time.

Panel Three: Pleasures of the "Text"

Brian L. Ott

On Sunday, September 9, 2007, I made the short jaunt from Fort Collins, Colorado, to Denver to view the NAMES Project AIDS Memorial Quilt.[39] This was only my second time seeing the Quilt and my first in more than ten years. On both occasions, my experience was profoundly moving; indeed, it lies beyond words—exceeds the very limits of language. This failure of language was particularly troubling to me during the more recent visit, as I was there as a critic and scholar. But as I later reflected on my experience, my mind kept returning to Roland Barthes's famous and oft-cited "Theory of the Text" from the *Encyclopaedia Universalis*.[40] Barthes's short, thirty-eight-year-old essay—which begins rather inauspiciously with the question "What is a text?"—remains one of the most noteworthy articulations of poststructuralist theory. As I read and reread the piece, I realized that while I was still unable to discursively capture (to utter) my experience, Barthes's "Theory of the Text" supplied a critical discourse or metalanguage for speaking *about* my experience. My aim in this panel, then, is to employ that language to give an account of viewing, or as Barthes might say, "writing" (*écriture*), the Quilt. But before doing so, I would like to reflect briefly on what can be gained by such an undertaking.

As a cultural critic, I have over the years analyzed a wide assortment of "texts," from films and television shows to rave culture and museums. In one way or another, my interest in each of these cultural artifacts has been animated by questions of identity and ideology, and more specifically by whom the "text" invites me and others to be. The assumption behind these questions is that texts (or textual structures)—while potentially polysemic—are unified, stable, and closed *enough* to make similar demands on readers or viewers. But the Quilt—as a text—is fascinating precisely because it challenges and undermines this assumption. More than any other public memorial, the Quilt is infinitely diffuse, variable, and open. Like Barthes's "writerly" text,[41] the Quilt "answers not to an interpretation, even a liberal one, but to an explosion, a dissemination."[42] The rhetorical force of the Quilt, I contend, lies not in its interpellation of subjects or construction of a preferred subject position, but in its deconstruction of subjectivity itself. One cannot uncover the meaning of the Quilt, for the Quilt abolishes the very possibility of a reading/interpreting subject. To experience the Quilt is, if only temporarily, to unravel—to come undone. Or seen from another angle, the Quilt is living theory, a material instantiation of Barthes's "Theory of the Text." To illustrate this claim, I approach the Quilt via Barthes's five theoretical concepts for defining the Text.

SIGNIFYING PRACTICES

For Barthes, the Text is a signifying practice because signification is generated not at the abstract level of system or structure (*langue*) as Ferdinand de Saussure proposed, but at the level of individual utterance or practice (*parole*).[43] By the late 1960s, Barthes had realized that there were no universal, discursive structures that could function as the ultimate grounds for a text or subject, and he renounced his structuralist past. The insight that accompanies this shift in thinking is that neither text nor subject is ever stable. In rejecting the notion of the Cartesian subject and the supposed unity of the cogito, Barthes had, in effect, sketched a postmodern, antiessentialist view of the self in which subjectivity is itself a discursive performance. Drawing upon experience and available cultural resources, the self is always in a process of becoming and is thus fluid, constructed, and contingent. Consequently, one can never read the same book twice, for one can never return as the same reader. Similarly, one never returns to the Quilt unchanged. Though this is true of other texts and not just of the Quilt, the Quilt destabilizes our sense of self even as we experience it. The Quilt confronts subjects with such a plentitude of deeply personal, yet distinctive images, stories, and memories that responding in a singular, unified way is all but impossible. The multiplicitous voice(s) of the Quilt multiplies responses and splinters subjects, denying would-be visitors any coherent narrative of AIDS, its victims, or its consequences. One loses one's sense of self in the presence of the Quilt.

PRODUCTIVITY

The Quilt, like the Text, is a productivity, for it is a *production,* not a product.[44] It does not generate *a* meaning or even several meanings, for it is never finished; it proliferates meaning endlessly, not just by the constant addition of new panels, but by the never-ending performances it stages. The Quilt, as with the Text, is "the very theater of a production where producer and reader of the text meet."[45] It is a live performance of grief, love, celebration, and remembrance. And, like theater, each performance is unique—an irreducible and irreproducible interplay and exchange between performers, visitors, and venue. As the Quilt, or more accurately as a small selection of its diverse and ever-increasing number of panels, moves from town to town, city park to college gymnasium, a new performance is staged. During my most recent experience of the Quilt, some panels were displayed on a grassy hill overlooking a reflecting pool at Denver's Cheesman Park, while other panels hung like tapestries in a classically Greek-styled pavilion. The day was sunny and warm, and bright colors and metal objects reflecting the sun were the first to capture my gaze. This was a very different performance than the one I had experienced during graduate school, in which the Quilt was displayed on the freshly waxed wood floor of the artificially lit gymnasium at Rec Hall on Penn State University's main campus. The panels and the audience had changed too. The steady stream of college students that had marked my experience more than ten years ago had been replaced by families, couples, and professionals. Part of the power of the Quilt is that one can never see the same Quilt twice. Each performance is fleeting, a singular and never-to-be-repeated experience.

SIGNIFIANCE

Having been trained as a rhetorical critic, I sought to understand the meaning of the Quilt as I walked among its many panels in Cheesman Park. "But once the text is conceived as production (and no longer as product)," Barthes argued, "'signification' is no longer an adequate concept." Indeed, the harder I searched for one or several fixed signifieds in the Quilt, the more they eluded me. In place of canonical signification, which suggests "that the text possesses a total and secret signified" that can be revealed through interpretative criticism, Barthes proposed the notion of 'signifiance' (not to be confused with significance) in which the text is read/written as a mobile play of signifiers. Though I had not set out to play with the Quilt, each question I posed to it returned three, eight, a dozen more. Soon, I was thinking not of the Quilt (at least not in any limited or limiting sense) but of flowers, relationships, mortality, and my own life. My thoughts continuously generated new connections and dis/associations, but never answers. At one point, I was so overcome by a sense of spinning that I stumbled and nearly fell on/into the Quilt. "'Signifiance' is a process," observed Barthes, "in the course of which the 'subject' of the text, escaping the logic of the ego-cogito and engaging other logics (that of the signifier and that of contradiction) struggles with meaning and is deconstructed ('is lost')."[46] As I tried to reorient myself, I caught a glimpse of my friend and colleague Greg. Still feeling light-headed, I made my way over to Greg and told him that I needed to sit down and rest for awhile. Slumped over on the concrete bench/retaining wall of the reflecting pool, I slowly began to regain my sense (of logic, balance, and wholeness). In stepping out of or departing from the Quilt, I reentered a world of boundaries, categories, and classifications.

GENOTEXT

The notion of the *genotext* comes from one of Roland Barthes's students, Julia Kristeva, who contrasts it with the *phenotext*. For Kristeva, the phenotext denotes "language that serves to communicate"; the genotext, alternatively, "is not linguistic" and entails presymbolic processes such as psychological "drives, their disposition, and their division of the body."[47] Adopting the vocabulary of rhetorical scholars, the phenotext might be thought of as the symbolic inducements of a text and the genotext its material inducements. The Quilt, I argue, offers a particularly clear instance of how texts operate on a material, bodily, and affective level, as well as on a symbolic, linguistic, and rational level. The Quilt, for instance, literally engages the bodies of its visitors, who, on perhaps the most obvious level, move between and through its many panels. Movement involves time and space, pace and direction, and, consequently, is primary (not secondary) to the experience of the Quilt, for its many symbols are framed by the velocity and vector of its visitors. Vision is central too, not just as a mechanism for processing signs and symbols, but also as a tool that allows the body to pursue its own drives and desires. "The pleasure of the text," commented Barthes, "is that moment when my body pursues its own ideas—for my body does not have the same ideas I do."[48] The Quilt entails so many signs, so many personal objects and belongings that the body (not the mind) chooses what to see; it selects a jean jacket over a teddy bear, not because the former is more significant, but because it activates signifiance, which derives from a pulsional resonance.

INTERTEXT

According to Barthes, "any text is an intertext; other texts are present in it, at varying levels, in more or less recognizable forms: the texts of the previous and surrounding culture. Any text is a new tissue of past citations."[49] Though I certainly concur with Barthes that any text is an intertext, I would note that the intertext is often not readily apparent. Many texts *appear to be* the original work of an autonomous author. The Quilt, however, explicitly exposes this authorial illusion, as it is comprised of nearly 6,000 blocks, each of which consists of eight "individual" memorial panels, many of which were themselves collaboratively created. The more than 44,000 panels that are recognized as the NAMES Project AIDS Memorial Quilt so fragment and disperse the notion of the Author as to render it obsolete. One cannot interpret the Quilt, not simply because the interpreting subject is mutable, the object is fluid, the signifying process is boundless, and the body is primary, but also because "it reads without the inscription of the Father."[50] It is for this reason that the reader comes to occupy the space of the author—that he or she produces rather than consumes the Text, and that writing is opened up rather than closed down.[51] The two occasions on which I have written (perhaps *sewn* is the better metaphor here) the Quilt lie beyond words, not because of a lack of language, but because of an overflowing of it. Barthes could just as easily have been describing the Quilt when he wrote, "the current theory of the text turns away from the text as veil and tries to perceive the *fabric* in its texture, in the interlacing of codes, formulae and signifiers, in the midst of which the subject places himself and is undone, like a spider that comes to dissolve itself into its own web."[52]

REFLECTIONS AND REVERBERATIONS

In this brief essay fragment, I have attempted to illustrate how the Quilt, like the Text, "is that which goes to the limit of the rules of enunciation (rationality, readability, etc.)."[53] I do not mean to suggest that the Quilt is meaningless. On the contrary, the Quilt is so meaningful—so full of meanings—that my experience cannot be yours and vice versa. One's experience of the Quilt is not, I maintain, the result of idiosyncratic impressions of its plentiful signs. It is, at least to the extent it is experienced as Text, a singular and momentary deconstruction of the self. As the Text "is bound to *jouissance*,"[54] so the Quilt is necessarily an ecstatic experience in the manner that Judith Butler understood it: "To be ec-static means, literally, to be outside oneself, and this can have several meanings: to be transported beyond oneself by passion, but also to be *beside* oneself with rage or grief. . . . I am speaking to those of us who are living in certain ways *beside ourselves*, whether it is in sexual passion, or emotional grief, or political rage."[55] The Quilt, then, is an intensely political memorial, not in the traditional sense of a carefully constructed rhetorical message designed to persuade its audience of a particular point of view, but in its affective ability to foster a moment, a flash of experience, outside the confines of ideology. The Quilt temporarily frees us from a world of prejudice, injustice, and inequality. And therein lies not its meaning, but its power.

On *"Quilting"/Reading the Quilt*

"What," queries one of this chapter's authors in another context, "is the role and function of the critic when confronted with postmodern textuality?"[56] It is the same question that plagued us as we began to think, talk, and write about the Quilt as a postmodern text(ile). In the course of this essay, we have suggested that one possible answer—following the lead of critics such as Gregory Ulmer and Susan Sontag—is to practice an erotics of art in place of a hermeneutics of art. In temper and disposition, such an approach is immersive, embodied, and sensual rather than distant, rational, and objectivist. In style and execution, such an approach favors collage/montage rather than mimesis. Though such an approach is well suited for engaging the Quilt, we wonder along with Ulmer, "Will the collage/montage revolution in representation be admitted into the academic essay, into the discourse of knowledge, replacing the 'realist' criticism based on the notions of 'truth' as correspondence to or correct reproduction of a referent object of study?"[57] In closing, we make a case for why collage/montage, as well as other nontraditional critical forms and practices, ought to be admitted into academic discourse by reflecting on its productive and interventionist dimensions.

First, as a device for criticism, collage/montage is *productive,* for it "invent(s) social knowledge rather than discovering it."[58] Unlike more traditional critical modes, which attempt to accurately reflect or re-present the object of study, collage/montage utilizes Derrida's principles of grafting and textual miming to create something more (and other). *Grafting* is the process of writing "on" not just "about" an object; it adds to the object, builds upon and is superimposed on it, combines, joins, and assembles with it.[59] Just as visitors add their own voices to the Quilt, grafting adds the (voice/body of) the critic (as text) to the text. Grafting can be enacted in a wide variety of ways. But when the technique is specifically one of collage/montage, what is grafted onto the text is a *textual mime* or a "compositional structuration of the referent, resulting in another text of the same 'kind.'"[60] In other words, the critical text (criticism) mimes (formally imitates) its object of study (the text).[61] In the case of the AIDS Quilt, the practice of collage/montage necessarily grafts "a quilt" upon the Quilt. This secondary "critical quilt" produces knowledge of the Quilt through performance rather than explanation. With Eric, it produces knowledge of mourning and healing; with Greg, movement, materiality, and memory; and with Brian, pleasure and critical theory.

Second, collage/montage as critical practice is *interventionist*. Since this practice writes on, adds to the text, it therefore transforms the text (and the critic). The "procedure of montage" is governed, according to Walter Benjamin, by "the principle of interruption," for it "disrupts the context in which it is inserted."[62] Elaborating on this perspective, Ulmer explains that "montage does not reproduce the real, but constructs an object . . . or rather, mounts a process . . . in order to intervene in the world, not to reflect but to change reality."[63] To understand how our critical quilt intervenes in the world, it is useful to recall the chief functions of quilting—historical, practical, aesthetic, and political—discussed earlier in this essay, and to view our essay through them. In "quilting"/reading the Quilt, we have recorded our own stories and voices, and we have done so in a manner—namely, academic writing—that preserves something of our unique (professional) traditions. Moreover, as we wrote (that is, grafted our voices onto the Quilt), the Quilt aided each of us in confronting struggles of our own, be they highly personal ones like Eric's struggle with loss or highly abstract ones, like Brian's struggle with language. That is to say, "quilting"/reading the Quilt had (practical) consequences. It also allowed us to express ourselves creatively (and aesthetically) through writing—a writing whose very form functions (politically) to challenge the dominant mode of criticism.[64] And if these interventions seem insignificant, we would simply remind readers that the Quilt activates and multiples them infinitely.

NOTES

1. James Davison Hunter, *Culture Wars: The Struggle to Define America* (New York: Basic Books, 1992).

2. Edwin Black, "Gettysburg and Silence," *Quarterly Journal of Speech* 80 (1994): 22.

3. Gregory L. Ulmer, "The Object of Post-Criticism," in *Anti-Aesthetic: Essays on Postmodern Culture,* ed. Hal Foster (New York: New Press, 1998), 93–125.

4. Susan Sontag, *Against Interpretation and Other Essays* (New York: Picador USA, 2001), 14.

5. Ulmer, "The Object of Post-Criticism," 94.

6. Catherine Amoroso Leslie, *Needlework through History: An Encyclopedia* (Santa Barbara, CA: Greenwood Publishing Group, 2007), 170.

7. Karen J. Warren, *Ecofeminist Philosophy: A Western Perspective on What It Is and Why It Matters* (Lanham, MD: Rowman and Littlefield Publishers, 2000), 68.

8. Joan Mulholland, "Patchwork: The Evolution of a Women's Genre," *Journal of American Culture* 19 (1996): 57.

9. Judy Elsley, "The Rhetoric of the NAMES Project AIDS Quilt: Reading the Text(ile)," in *AIDS: The Literary Response,* ed. Emmanuel S. Nelson (New York: Twayne Publishers, 1992), 188.

10. Charlotte Pierce-Baker, "A Quilting of Voices: Diversifying the Curriculum/Cannon in the Traditional Humanities," *College Literature* 17 (1990): 152.

11. Elsley, "The Rhetoric of the NAMES Project AIDS Quilt," 188.

12. Warren, *Ecofeminist Philosophy,* 68.

13. Jill Schachner Chanen, "Stitchin' Time: Quilting Helps Lawyers to Uncover Their Own Creative Patterns," *ABA Journal* (March 1998): 88.

14. Leslie, *Needlework through History,* 169.

15. Peter S. Hawkins, "Confronting AIDS: The NAMES Project Quilt," *AIDS Patient Care and STDs* 12 (1998): 745.

16. Van E. Hillard, "Census, Consensus, and the Commodification of Form: *The NAMES Project Quilt,*" in *Quilt Culture: Tracing the Pattern,* ed. Cheryl B. Torsney and Judy Elsley (Columbia: University of Missouri Press, 1994), 118.

17. Hillard, "Census, Consensus, and the Commodification of Form," 115–116.

18. Christopher Capozzola, "A Very American Epidemic: Memory Politics and Identity Politics in the AIDS Memorial Quilt, 1985–1993," *Radical History Review* 82 (2002): 96; Jacquiline L. Tobin and Raymond G. Dobard, *Hidden in Plain View: A Secret History of Quilts and the Underground Railroad* (New York: Doubleday, 1999), 35.

19. We are using "tactics" here in de Certeau's sense of "a maneuver 'within the enemy's field of vision'" and "the art of the weak" (Michel de Certeau, *The Practice of Everyday Life,* trans. Steven Rendall [Berkeley: University of California Press, 1984], 37). On the transgressive and tactical potential of quilts, see Linda Pershing, "'She Really Wanted to Be Her Own Woman': Scandalous Sunbonnet Sue," in *Feminist Messages: Coding in Women's Folk Culture,* ed. Joan Newlon Radner (Chicago: University of Illinois Press, 1993), 98–125.

20. Capozzola, "A Very American Epidemic," 95, 98.

21. Hawkins, "Confronting AIDS," 744, 745.

22. Capozzola, "A Very American Epidemic," 92.

23. Hawkins, "Confronting AIDS," 745.

24. Capozzola, "A Very American Epidemic," 104.

25. Dwight Conquergood, "Rethinking Ethnography: Towards a Critical Cultural Politics," *Communication Monographs* 58 (1991): 180.

26. Ibid. The distinction we are making here resonates with McKerrow's distinction between "rhetorical criticism" and "critical rhetoric." Our own practice is much closer to the latter, which "is a performance played out in and among the discursive practices it enjoins in critique" (Raymie E. McKerrow, "Space and Time in the Postmodern Polity," *Western Journal of Communication* 63 [1999]: 274).

27. See, for example, Eric Aoki, "An Interpersonal and Intercultural Embrace: A Letter of Reflection on My Gay Male Relational Connections," *Journal of Couple and Relationship Therapy* 3 (2004): 111–121.

28. bell hooks, *all about love: New Visions* (New York: William Morrow and Co., 2000), 198.

29. The NAMES Project Foundation, "The AIDS Memorial Quilt," http://www.aids-quilt.org.

30. Janet Catherine Berlo, *Quilting Lessons: Notes for the Scrap Bag of a Writer and Quilter* (Lincoln: University of Nebraska Press, 2001), 11–12.

31. Seeing and experiencing the Quilt at the public park in Denver with my colleagues Brian and Greg was an emotional journey. I had spent that morning walking AIDS Walk Colorado in silence mostly and in high reflection on my life with Stephen, knowing that I would engage the Quilt at the walk's end. Brian and Greg know that I have decided to keep this experience with the Quilt mostly to myself.

32. Of course, as Carole Blair points out, the seeming permanence of built memorials can, in fact, mark their impermanence. If the stone is destroyed or the building neglected, the memorial can eventually disappear. Carol Blair, "Contemporary U.S.

Memorial Sites as Exemplars of Rhetoric's Materiality," in *Rhetorical Bodies,* ed. Jack Selzer and Sharon Crowley (Madison: University of Wisconsin Press, 1999), 37–38.

33. Greg Dickinson, Brian L. Ott, and Eric Aoki, "Spaces of Remembering and Forgetting: The Reverent Eye/I at the Plains Indian Museum," *Communication and Critical/Cultural Studies* 3 (2006): 27–47.

34. Rosi Braidotti, "Posthuman, All Too Human: Towards a New Process Ontology," *Theory, Culture and Society* 23 (2006): 199.

35. Braidotti, "Posthuman, All Too Human," 199.

36. de Certeau, *The Practice of Everyday Life,* 100.

37. Ibid., 99.

38. Ibid., 100.

39. I, of course, viewed only a small portion (or fragment) of the Quilt. It has not been displayed "in full" since October 1996, when it was shown on the Mall in Washington, D.C. Given its size today, it is unlikely that the Quilt will ever be displayed again in its entirety.

40. Originally published in 1973, the essay was later reprinted as Roland Barthes, "Theory of the Text," in *Untying the Text: A Post-Structuralist Reader,* ed. Robert Young (Boston: Routledge and Kegan Paul, 1981), 31–47.

41. In *S/Z,* Barthes contrasts "writerly" or producerly texts with "readerly" or consumerly texts. Roland Barthes, *S/Z: An Essay,* trans. Richard Miller (New York: Hill and Wang, 1974), 5.

42. "The Text is plural," added Barthes, "which is not to say that it has several meanings, but that it accomplishes the very plural of meaning: an *irreducible* (and not merely an acceptable) plural" (Roland Barthes, *Image, Music, Text,* trans. Stephen Heath [New York: Hill and Wang, 1977], 159). I specifically wish to distinguish Barthes's point as well as my argument from what I regard as the limited plural of a postmodern "multivocal rhetoric." See Carole Blair, Marsha S. Jeppeson, and Enrico Pucci Jr., "Public Memorializing in Postmodernity: The Vietnam Veterans Memorial as Prototype," *Quarterly Journal of Speech* 77 (1991): 289–308.

43. Barthes, "Theory," 36.

44. Indeed, Barthes argued that *"the Text is experienced only in an activity of production"* (*Image,* 157).

45. Barthes, "Theory," 36.

46. Barthes, "Theory," 37, 38. "The Text," wrote Barthes, "practises the infinite deferment of the signified, is dilatory; its field is that of the signifier. . . . the *infinity* of

the signifier refers not to some idea of the ineffable (the un-nameable signified) but to that of *playing;* the generation of the perpetual signifier" (*Image,* 158).

47. Julia Kristeva, *Revolution in Poetic Language,* trans. Margaret Walker (New York: Columbia University Press, 1984), 86–87.

48. Roland Barthes, *The Pleasure of the Text,* trans. Richard Miller (New York: Hill and Wang, 1975), 17.

49. Barthes, "Theory," 39. Elsewhere, Barthes explained, "The intertextual in which every text is held, it itself being the text-between of another text, is not to be confused with some origin of the text: to try to find the 'sources,' the 'influences' of a work, is to fall in with the myth of filiation; the citations which go to make up a text are anonymous, untraceable" (*Image,* 160).

50. Barthes, *Image,* 161.

51. On this point, see Barthes, *Image,* 147.

52. Barthes, "Theory," 39 (emphasis added).

53. Barthes, *Image,* 157.

54. Ibid., 164.

55. Judith Butler, *Undoing Gender* (New York: Routledge, 2004), 20.

56. Brian L. Ott, "The Pleasures of *South Park* (An Experiment in Media Erotics)," in *Taking* South Park *Seriously,* ed. Jeffrey Andrew Weinstock (Albany: State University of New York Press, 2008), 39.

57. Ulmer, "The Object of Post-Criticism," 97.

58. Robert L. Ivie, "Productive Criticism," *Quarterly Journal of Speech* 81 (1995): editor's introduction.

59. See Jacques Derrida, *Dissemination,* trans. Barbara Johnson (Chicago: University of Chicago Press, 1981), 355.

60. Ulmer, "The Object of Post-Criticism," 107.

61. Derrida, *Dissemination,* 206, 294.

62. Walter Benjamin, "The Author as Producer," in *Reflections: Essays, Aphorisms, Autobiographical Writings,* trans. Edmund Jephcott, ed. Peter Demetz (New York: Schocken Books, 1978), 234.

63. Ulmer, "The Object of Post-Criticism," 97.

64. Given our (visually) playful use of language, this is an essay that must be seen and not simply heard to be fully appreciated.

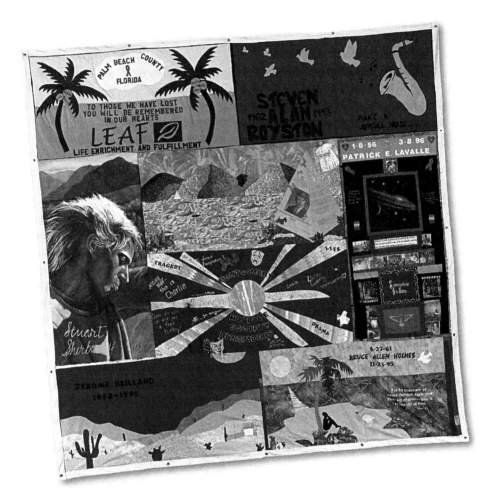

A Stitch in Time: Public Emotionality and the Repertoire of Citizenship

Jeffrey A. Bennett

The narratives resonating from the AIDS Memorial Quilt speak to its power as a cultural text. The snapshots of lives lost to government neglect and incurable disease spark feelings of rage and sentimentality, generating both alienation and bonds of stranger-relationality.[1] If AIDS represents a "crisis of signification," the incomplete narratives of the Quilt are an embodiment of that calamity.[2] It gains its emotive force not from a unified message, but from a series of incommensurable tensions: it is both utopian and apocalyptic; therapeutic and traumatic; speaks to the universal limits of the body and to individual demise; transcends time but alters the spaces in which it is situated; it is oddly normative even as it is discerningly queer. The fragmentary narratives of those lost to AIDS necessitate onlookers to negotiate these complications, navigating the discursive gaps of this anomalous memorial.[3]

Many of the Quilt's panels could speak to the multifarious implications stemming from these tensions. One panel elucidating this rhetorical quagmire was unveiled as the memorial was displayed on the Washington Mall for the third of its five complete showings. The *Washington Post* featured the story of a man named "Robert W." At the time, Robert was one of the latest people to have his name added to the vastly expanding Quilt. Though the country was eight years into the epidemic, the atmosphere for people living with HIV/AIDS remained volatile. Out of concern for their safety and his legacy, Robert's family stitched a strip of blue cloth across his last name. On it, they embroidered a message: "Family fear removed this name. Love can remove this patch."[4] The anxiety expressed by his family was exceeded only by the profound hope they embraced for the capacity of others to love. Fear and hope, remembrance and evolution, immobilization and exigency all radiate from the family's emotive call for action. Imploring participants to transform their attitudes, this single panel illustrated that the love of one family was insufficient for reconstituting debilitating prejudices in the polity. To be public required a wider disposition toward kinship and identification. The collective effort to eliminate that swatch would alter the meaning of Robert's panel, the composition of the Quilt, and the performances it enabled. Of course, love alone could not promise transformation—this was a faith in strangers that held no guarantees.

This moving, though little noticed, act draws attention to the memorial's unusual aptitude for constituting publics and civic identities. The Quilt is a peripatetic site of public emotionality that engenders repertoires of public citizenship. It embodies the emotive aspects of citizenship typically shunned in democratic practice, including normative rhetorics that have been privileged in AIDS discourse, such as science and public health. The emotive quality of the Quilt has played a central role in both resisting dominant cultural discourses and conforming to neo-liberal narratives highlighting individualism and equality. However, the Quilt complicates the process of entextualization because the narratives it perpetuates are continually unfolding, always being stitched together, even as they appear to stabilize over time. In short, the Quilt has adopted an itinerant peculiarity not only in space, but in time, allowing it to act as a site where narrative understandings of AIDS and stranger-relationality can be constantly reimagined. Though the Quilt's purpose and visibility are seemingly diminishing in the public sphere, its potential as a mobile scene of public emotionality remains a powerful conduit for addressing the challenges of HIV/AIDS.

For the purposes of this essay, the Quilt is conceptualized not as an archive, but a performative repertoire of civic belonging.[5] Diana Taylor notes that the repertoire "enacts embodied memory: performance, gestures, orality, movement, dance, singing—in short all those acts usually thought of as ephemeral, nonreproducible knowledge."[6] People do not simply recount history when they are immersed in the Quilt's miles of fabric. In their encounters with this unusual memorial, people become active participants in the creation of knowledge about the impact of AIDS and its circulation in the polity. Displayed in spaces generally associated with public life (churches, schools, rallies), the Quilt gives presence to the mediation of public emotionality and its centrality in the polis. Unlike the archive, which works to stabilize texts, signifiers, and practices, the repertoire is exacted in scenarios forged in cultural fantasies and executed in the performances of everyday life.[7] These performances edify enigmatic histories "always in situ, every particular instantiation marked by the confluence of traditions in a particular scenario."[8] The Quilt was conceived at the juncture of neglect, absence, and betrayal, instigating a host of passions at a time when rituals of public mourning for AIDS-related deaths were limited. The hope projected by the Quilt and the indictment it symbolically conveys allowed loss to be publicly communicated in ways not previously imagined. Indeed, even as the meaning of AIDS continues to shift, and the Quilt rapidly disappears from view, the emotive repertoires it enables still have the potential to resist normative conceptions of disease and citizenship. The Quilt itself is empty without the meanings generated by our practices. Like Robert W.'s family, the Quilt's burden is not to reconstitute the norms of the polity: it is but one panel that can move us closer to the goals of motivating government agencies, educating publics, and bringing strangers closer together, knowing all the while that identification never assures action.

This essay unfolds in four segments. First, rational appeals used to explain the epidemic are briefly reviewed to illustrate how the official discourses of science and government gave rise to the emotive necessity of the Quilt. Second, having evolved into a national memorial, the public emotionality engendered by the Quilt is explored for both its peculiar embodiment and its role in cultural memory. The complications of public emotionality in the entextualization process are probed in the third section. Finally, the ways in which these repertoires of civic performance both limit AIDS activism and expand the potential for stranger-relationality are revisited.

AIDS *and the Limits of Reasoned Mourning*

The devastation of AIDS is perhaps the greatest tragedy of Ronald Reagan's administration. The common refrain that Reagan refused to utter the word "AIDS" publicly for seven years speaks to the monstrous political environment that confronted people with HIV/AIDS and their loved ones. This carefully planned public relations campaign, one that perpetuated negligence and paranoia, positioning people with HIV/AIDS as dangerous creatures lurking in the shadows of American life, continues to wreak havoc.[9] Thomas Yingling rightfully contended that "the benign neglect of government agencies makes the epidemic a passive-aggressive act on the part of rational society."[10] It is too easy to assert that high-ranking government officials such as the president feared "the Other." The White House's overt silence and refusal to combat fears about people living with HIV/AIDS illuminates the political rationalism that allowed erratic information to disseminate throughout the polity and advance the careers of politicians, demagogues, and bigots.[11]

While the administration seemed content with its silence on AIDS, medical officials and scientists (who were usually connected to government institutions) addressed the epidemic in both productive and harmful ways. The development of a language to signify the many facets of HIV/AIDS created opportunities for sparking initiatives to combat ignorance, but it also gave rise to a classification system that (further) stigmatized various communities, including gay men, sex workers, and Haitians.[12] Paula Treichler explains, "the construction of scientific facts, the existence of a name plays a crucial role in providing a coherent and unified signifier—a shorthand way of signifying what may be a complex, inchoate, or little-understood concept." Unfortunately, the practice of creating a signifier for what is a bewildering syndrome is often lost in translation when relocated to the public sphere. The original signification of AIDS as GRID (Gay Related Immunodeficiency), for example, left many people believing they were insulated from the reach of AIDS. When individual cases materialized outside of the aforementioned classification systems, scientists often assumed those aberrations would simply fall into place.[13]

The reliance on medicine and science allowed for the constitution and perpetuation of several partial truths about AIDS. While science rightfully told the world HIV could be prevented by using condoms, could not be spread by casual contact, and made no distinctions among human bodies, it also erroneously asserted that AIDS originated in Africa, that health-conscious gay men should not be allowed to give blood, and that testing drugs on impoverished populations in non-Western countries was in the best interest of the people being exploited.[14] Cindy Patton observes that any "cultural stereotype or political idea that could be recirculated or challenged by this association with science had far greater power than a stereotype that stood on its own."[15] Narratives supported by science generally play a critical role in the acceptance of public health policies, and in AIDS rhetoric the most egregious of stereotypes could be advanced with the help of science. These negative associations did not exclusively infringe on gay men or drug users. They also explain why many people believed they were immune to HIV: they were never a component of cultural narratives grounded in "empirical fact."[16]

As AIDS continued to march resolutely toward the homes of people around the globe, the epidemic quickly became articulated with notions of liberal democracy in America. Across the country a campaign was under way that asserted "we're all equally at risk" and "we're all in this together."[17] This attitude, which democratized disease, fabricated a false notion of unity by allowing all to mourn, even when losses were categorically unequivocal. Themes of individual responsibility, the destruction of the nuclear family, and protecting the borders had become fixtures in the media.[18] The year the Quilt had its debut the government began prohibiting people who were HIV-positive from entering the country.[19] Flowing throughout official discourses was a simultaneous essentialism and segmentation of identities, borders, and sex practices. In the wake of these isolating practices, the Quilt provided an emotional outlet for scores of people who knew little of science or public health, but everything about the loved ones they were consecrating.

The rational narratives guiding AIDS discourse did not provide a cathartic forum for people coming to grips with the impact of the epidemic in their everyday lives. Government silence left a void, and scientific "discoveries" offered little comfort. The rational discourses being disseminated left a conspicuous absence. Shifting the focus from statistical oneness to political wholeness, the Quilt became a site of "popular civil religion."[20] It made AIDS "meaningful in a way that allows those affected and infected by it to secure it as an experience and not merely as information."[21] Even if we accept this claim, the panels on the Quilt provide remarkably little information about the people it enshrines. We know almost nothing of people like Robert W. (and sometimes no name is embroidered at all). Those narrative features the Quilt fails to express leave a space where humanity's capacity for ingenuity beams bright. At the heart of that inventive spirit is emotion.

Pubic Emotion and the Repertoire of Citizenship

While science and public health were (and continue to be) a guiding force of the crisis, few outlets for publicly channeling the emotive impact of AIDS existed. The partners, parents, friends, and children of people grappling with AIDS were still developing and learning a language that captured the enormity of the epidemic and the rapid pace at which the syndrome's tentacles were spreading. The Quilt was certainly not the *only* outlet that people embraced in their effort to understand the devastation of AIDS, but it offered communal spaces for working through the syndrome's perplexities. The Quilt propagated an emotive quality that allowed publics to be constituted around reflection, loss, despair, anger, and hope. For some the Quilt was public acknowledgment of queer lives lost, for others a space where loved ones who did not "belong" to the classification schemes of official discourses could be recognized. One visit to the Quilt illustrates easily enough that these losses are neither equivalent nor hierarchical in their emotive expression. Contra "rational" understandings of AIDS, the Quilt did the important work of suturing voids left by lives impossible to signify. Public emotion seems especially crucial for the performance of citizenship in relation to this crisis for two reasons: it initiates change and constitutes particular embodiments of cultural memory. Each of these alters the repertoires of civic life reflected in the Quilt.

Exploring the emotive features of the Quilt does not suggest an absolute division between reason and emotion. The two are not only interdependent but also often indistinguishable from one another. Reason, as is increasingly transparent in much academic research, is not possible without emotion. Reason is not thought or deliberation free of emotion; nor is emotion an excessive remainder that distorts the reasoning process. Reason is built on a foundation of situated and practiced emotion, some of which is conscious, but much of which is not. George Marcus argues that "emotion talk has explanatory power because embedded in it are some central metaphors that do the actual explaining. And, as often happens with good metaphors, their use becomes invisible to those who use them and their presumptions remain hidden."[22] Emotion in the public sphere is often castigated as "getting in the way," even when it is acknowledged that emotion is foundational to being reasonable.

The driving force of emotion in public life continues to influence theories of citizenship. Similarly, ideals of citizenship "deeply engage our received conceptions of reason and emotion."[23] Writing against models of citizenship privileging reason over emotion, several scholars have refuted claims that emotion disrupts reasonable decision making.[24] In these works, as in the philosophical writings of Aristotle, emotion is central for the rise of moral action and political participation. In Marcus's view, reason is "a set of conscious skills that are recruited by emotion systems for just those occasions when we wish them to be available and applied, situations that compel explicit consideration and judgment."[25] In fact, emotion enhances a citizen's ability to be reasonable because it affords a flexibility to make political judgments in particular situations.[26]

Nonetheless, even compelling works on public emotion have difficulty breaking with the reason/emotion binary. For example, Barbara Koziak's excellent text on the subject sometimes retreats into the realm of duality. Koziak asserts "although emotions may involve thought, in the sense of a background belief or judgment, emotional capacity is not thought or reason itself." Concepts such as loss and grief clearly complicate this frame. Attempting to capture the pain of loss without emotion is at best melancholia, but certainly not a form of "reason." Despite this, Koziak rightfully contends there is a "governing scenario of emotion," and particular situations (such as traumas) incite "emotional repertoires" because there are no historical events to aid in molding public decorum.[27] AIDS was one such trauma when public emotionality needed to be discursively defined for the purposes of coping and meaning production.

The power of public emotion to initiate change is especially pertinent for eras afflicted by trauma. The complicated relationship between loss and signification—of recognizing the limits of words to capture that which is absent—is mitigated by emotion, even as emotions themselves are impossible to encapsulate with words. The enigmatic qualities of the scenario are managed by emotion, forging new pillars of tradition and novel forms of decorum. Personal pain can be an instigator of change, and public emotion provides the catalyst for stimulating action in the public sphere. Cautiously avoiding direct causality, Taylor recognizes such potential, remarking that "performances enter into dialogue with a history of trauma without themselves being traumatic. These are carefully crafted works that create a critical distance for 'claiming' experience and enabling, as opposed to 'collapsing,' witnessing."[28] The Quilt facilitates such experiences, allowing actors to express feelings of loss and anguish in ways that are both cathartic and plausibly empowering. Rather than be stunted by narratives that long for explanation or conclusion, these embodied practices engender repertoires of citizenship steeped in emotion. Here it is not the "authenticity" of the experience transpiring that is important. It is the repertoire of emotion that produces experience to energize meaning for unfathomable events.[29] Perhaps because the trauma of AIDS is no longer central to contemporary public discussions (though assuredly AIDS still traumatizes plenty of people), public emotionality has taken on a different form.

The emotive healing generated by the Quilt can be found in various cultural artifacts that eschew the rational narratives associated with AIDS. One writer noted, "The Quilt is certainly not a pure monument of the twilight of the Age of Reason, like the obelisk to George Washington; nor is it a brilliant work of poetic minimalism, like Maya Lin's Vietnam

Memorial. Unlike a monument built of stone, it is mutable, capable of—and encouraging—growth and replication."[30] Perhaps the most recurring way the Quilt reworks the rational impetus of public institutions is in the preoccupation people place on breaking down the statistical obsession of the sciences. A quick glance at popular press coverage of the Quilt highlights this subtle renegotiation. In 1989 a reporter contended the Quilt provided a space for "focusing on the lives and faces and names behind the statistics."[31] Three years later, a woman told the *St. Louis Post-Dispatch* that the panels "prove that no one is a statistic, every life has its own fabric and its own colors—no two are alike."[32] Gwenn Barteld, who lost her twenty-five-year-old brother to AIDS said the Quilt, "tells a story and personalizes it for people. . . . Now he is not just another statistic. He is a person."[33] The final time the Quilt was displayed on the National Mall, Anthony Turney, executive director of the NAMES Project, commented, "What it has done always in the past, and will continue to, is put a face on this epidemic. It makes this epidemic human."[34] As comforting as this may seem, these statistics also represent absence. At one point organizers estimated that roughly 10 percent of the panels did not include full names.[35]

The relationship between social change and emotionality is even more significant when one considers the ways embodiment is central to cultural memory. Memory is itself a practice that cannot be understood separate from the body, always being wrapped up in the ideas and experiences of the person remembering. Attempting to come to terms with the diffuse performances that transpire when people come into contact (or not) with the Quilt is itself an insurmountable task.[36] Peggy Phelan has noted that attempting "to write about the undocumentable event of performance is to invoke the rules of the written document and thereby alter the event itself." Technologies privileging the archive (such as writing) can never capture the performative nature of identity creation forged in the realm of the lived practices to which emotive response is central. The failure to capture ontological essences—those incomplete narratives one is exposed to when in contact with the Quilt—is the void where identity emerges. Phelan advocates writing toward disappearance rather than preservation (the archive), arguing the "after-effect of disappearance is the experience of subjectivity itself."[37]

The idea that moving toward disappearance affords a space for producing personal or political empowerment is captured by the idea of the repertoire and its relationship to emotionality. Although absence has mainly been conceived in the form of death when deciphering the Quilt, the erasure of particular identities also necessitates attention. The Quilt has been criticized because it severely lacks panels featuring women and minorities, two populations now disproportionately affected by HIV/AIDS. A mere 616 blocks of the memorial include women, and only 260 represent African Americans. These are massively uneven figures when compared to both new infection and mortality rates, not to mention the 91,000 names affixed to the Quilt. However, pushing the Quilt into arguments about statistical representation does little more than reproduce the logic of empiricism it resists. These unaccounted representations provide an opportunity for rethinking the Quilt's purpose and the epidemic's changing nature.[38] Bringing this discomforting oversight into public view, contrasting these absences to the immensity of the Quilt itself, could further highlight the enormity of the epidemic that is not only seen—but unseen. The Quilt has long been regarded as a memorial that is malleable and changing. Altering the mode of performance to stress absence could serve a useful function, but humans must alter the repertoire of the Quilt—the Quilt itself does little. The NAMES Project has provided some workshops in minority communities about Quilting, and while such spaces can be empowering, the absences are equally significant and have been since the start of the pandemic. Public emotionality is not always inherently inclusive, but it can be discursively transformed. There is a struggle in negotiating repertoires of emotion, of anger, and of absence, but without these forms, no body of reason for grappling with the epidemic can emerge. The ability to produce identifications among members of a community is dependent on these shared understandings of emotionality and what remains unseen could provide new avenues of activism.[39]

Of course, not all cultural fantasies, even in the most hegemonic of states, are ever fully shared. The sphere of fantasy requires memory and knowledge common among a people to constitute the fabric of community. With the partiality of fantasy, its wholeness never being fully captured, people forge identifications, suturing voids and creating meaning from the incompleteness. The repertoire of performance and the emotions on which it is built will never be consistent among all people. This schism in signification can be both enabling and debilitating. While writing this essay I was discussing the Quilt with an acquaintance whose former partner died of AIDS complications. I relayed the experience of walking around the Quilt at Atlanta Pride and the distinct differences among those who clearly had loved ones who had died from AIDS and those who had not. Most noteworthy were the contrasts among the generations. While most people were undeniably solemn, younger people were not as visibly impacted by the devastation of the epidemic. Without missing a beat, the man sadly retorted, "I don't want them to get it." The relationship between knowledge, memory, and embodied performance was transparent for this man. It is common to argue that young queers are in a compromised position because they do not understand the devastation of AIDS. But this altered sensibility affords them an understanding of the epidemic that engenders a particular freedom in their everyday lives. At the same time, the identity of young queers has been conceived and continues to be transformed by AIDS. They are the product of PSAs, of health education, of popular representations, and of rising infection rates. These interpenetrating discourses of naivety and interpellation incite emotive responses that shape repertories of public performance, highlighting new challenges for those memorializing and fighting against HIV/AIDS.

The heterogeneous qualities of the Quilt make it difficult to assert anything regarding emotional response with certainty. But this fleeting attribute is a positive characterization, allowing the Quilt to act as a peripatetic site that fosters public emotionality appropriate to specific eras and generations. So, when Marita Sturken pondered if the Quilt takes away a sense of anger that should be expressed over the deaths of people who battled AIDS, it is difficult to surmise an answer.[40] Certainly, some will approach the Quilt with an overwhelming sense of loss where the potential to exert anger is not possible. But that same loss renders others devastated by the impact of AIDS, inciting anger. This conflict was captured well by Eve Sedgwick, who describes being furious at a viewing of the Quilt while her friend Michael Lynch was dying. She was enraged by the Quilt's "nostalgic ideology and no politics, with its big, ever-growing, and sometimes obstructive niche in the ecology of gay organizing and self-formation." She describes the mixed emotions of seeing the panel of a man that read "HE HATED THE QUILT."[41] This incongruent perspective magnifies an explicit rift between the need to mourn and the desire to take vengeance on a world that did (and still does) little for people living with HIV/AIDS. That collusion of feelings illustrates what is at stake in the performative repertoire of the Quilt itself. Moving from panel to panel provokes more than a singular feeling. Nonetheless, this puzzling crash of meanings can be a productive site of stranger-relationality.

Entextualization and the Problems of Neoliberalism

The artificial divide between reason and emotion has generated a number of cultural associations about each concept. Reason, with its supposed well-plotted path toward discovery, is often conceived linearly. Both inductive and deductive reasoning, for example, follow a course that un-folds over time with calculated precision. Emotion, conversely, is rarely envisioned with such exactness. More often than not, emotion is seen as interference or explosion, being couched in metaphors of containment and risk. The ephemeral quality of emotion provides novel avenues for exploring the process of entextualization and artifacts such as the Quilt. As the years have gone by, the performances enabled by the Quilt have changed. Decades have passed since the memorial's unfolding, and while pain and grief linger, that anguish has taken on new forms of mourning. Likewise, for those coping with recent losses, the lack of commemoration for people with AIDS might produce melancholia difficult to verbalize. Although these practices have changed largely because of cultural at-titudes about HIV/AIDS, community awareness, and a lack of media coverage, the Quilt's participation in these forms of mourning highlights a transformation in the repertoires of performance mediated by the memo-rial. While this reifies elements of neoliberalism, the memorial's flexibility provides resistive spaces for constituting civic identities.[42]

Entextualization is "the process through which narratives are made stable and crafted into tangible texts and other material expressions" to constitute discursivity.[43] While materializing standardized scenarios for consumption, these narratives also empower some to speak at the expense of others. Inherent in these practices are attempts to manipulate, recuperate, and generate cultural and ideological meanings.[44] Emotion is central to this process because the constitutive features of memory invigorate feelings privileged among a people, guiding their actions and their capacity to induce change. The ways we entextualize the dead, and performatively engage with them, solidifies foundations of memory and tradition, even if this condensation is illusory.[45] Reason is dependent on emotion for defining that which is essential to a people, in large part because memory is situated entirely on emotive energies.[46]

The problems of entextualizing performances facilitated by the Quilt are evident in the efforts to clinch the magnitude of the epidemic in the archive. People often attempt to empirically comprehend the emotive power of the Quilt and the enormity of the epidemic it represents. One of the first stories featuring the Quilt in the *New York Times* observed that the Quilt measured 150 feet by 470 feet. Just a year later it was "the size of seven football fields," or five times bigger than the year before. In 1989 the Quilt expanded to fourteen acres, or forty-nine collective miles. In 1992, just a month before Bill Clinton was voted into office, the Quilt had grown tenfold from its initial viewing. It was up to twelve and a half football fields, with one new panel being added every two hours. By 1996 it included twenty-three miles of walkways alone and was now twenty-four football fields.[47] During the final viewing in D.C., the Quilt "was so large that visitors were directed to five different subway stations, depending on which panels they wished to see."[48] Repeatedly readers have been told the Quilt was composed of 1,920 panels in 1987; 8,000 in 1988; 10,000 in 1989; 20,000 in 1992. In 1996 it doubled to 40,000. Surprisingly, these empirical facts serve an important emotive function. They attempt to constitutively alter people's thinking about AIDS as it is mediated by the Quilt. But again, efforts to capture the magnitude of the epidemic can never be attained. The Quilt features a miniscule percentage of American deaths from AIDS and an even smaller amount of the deceased globally.[49]

The most frequently reoccurring statistics involve not only the Quilt's size, but, interestingly, its weight. This is a feature of media reports and academic scholarship alike. The burden of dealing with AIDS was clearly growing heavier with each passing year. In 1987 the Quilt already weighed three-and-a-half tons. Two years later it had substantially grown to thirteen tons. By 1992 it weighed twenty-six tons without walkways and almost thirty-one tons with them. And in 1996 it was composed of forty tons of fabric.[50]

The statistics that frequently surface in the media are undoubtedly the work of press releases composed by the NAMES Project. Equally important are the connotations of public emotionality underlying these facts. Note the obsession with "football fields." The image of the football field conveys more than mere magnitude. It offers explicit encapsulation of cultural measurement, alluding to a specifically American identity, and an identification that transcends the realm of gender typically associated with the queer bodies on the Quilt.[51] Likewise, the idea of "weight" is more than statistical. It signifies an emotive sense of burden and immobility. Despite these cultural inferences, the Quilt will never foster the emotive feelings people have with the layers of fabric that constitute a transient hallowed ground.

As an experiential artifact of profound emotive magnitude, the Quilt instigates disparate performances. But simply because the repertoire initiated by the Quilt can never be fully captured does not mean it is free of ideological discourses guiding understandings. In many ways, the Quilt does conform to discourses of neoliberalism that prize individuality and reify multiculturalism. Being prominently displayed on the National Mall, in the halls of educational institutions, and during gay pride parades and festivals, the Quilt has secured a place for public expression that is prey to hegemonic forces. Sometimes it is articulated with progressive social causes; at other times it is joined with discourses seemingly counterproductive in the fight against HIV/AIDS. The democratization of the Quilt, for instance, is apparent in the description of the panels themselves. While all are equal in size, they carry their own characteristics that emphasize individual personalities. As one reporter noted, by "including details about those who have died—hobbies, birth dates, favorite songs and photographs—Quilt organizers hope to emphasize that people who die of AIDS are as diverse in philosophy and background as the general population."[52] Queers have long been excluded from conceptions of the "general population" in AIDS discourse and the process of entextualization may do little more than move them toward erasure.

Indeed, some have argued that the Quilt is marred by the larger heterosexist culture that concocts diabolical images of queer men. Speaking to the NAMES project, Jeff Nunokawa writes:

> If a homophobic reticence helped to prompt the Names Project in the first place, a different homophobia has contributed to its canonization in the dominant media; if the majority culture is not inclined to recognize the death of the male homosexual, it is also not inclined to recognize anything else about him; if the majority culture grants no notice to his death, it also inters him from the start. The gay community is thus taxed during its sad time by a double burden: the variegated regime of heterosexism not only inhibits the work of acknowledging the loss of a gay man, it also exacts the incessant reproduction of this labor, by casting his death as his definition.[53]

Although some have accused Nunokawa of being "paranoid" in his reading of the Quilt, a more vexing question involves the context in which he was writing.[54] At the time, there was indeed a troubling way in which death and queerness were intimately linked (a connection that lives on today). But equally significant is the modernist (and almost overly rational) ways in which Nunokawa plots the ideas of death and queerness. Nunokawa longs for the idea of the individual. He is steeped in understandings of the Quilt that prohibit the inventive possibilities that it yields. For him, the Quilt has been "canonized," there is a "reproduction of labor," and queer men are transparently defined by their death. The Quilt for him is not a scenario that sparks emotive repertoires of civic identity and memorializing. In his account queer men can never win because the entextualization process condemns them from the start. This overlooks a number of practices that might otherwise run contrary to his thesis, not the least of which is the way many queer men living with HIV/AIDS have produced their own panels.

The memories cultivated by the entextualization process offer clues into the ideological position adopted by a polis. Similarly, the emotive features of memory always mirror the cultural norms in which they are situated. In American culture, the outlook is perpetually toward the future. Unlike many societies, Americans are predisposed to a discourse that pushes us forward at all costs. Progress remains our most valued God-term, and the Quilt is consistent with a therapeutic ideology that literally allows participants to "move on." Progress is the instigator of science and public health, and the Quilt's "healing" capacity shares the forward moving impulse of these fields. However, just as emotion and citizenship fundamentally alter one another, so too does the Quilt hold some promise—even if minute—to transform the ideas of stranger-relationality circulating in the polity.

The Quilt is unique in its situatedness, in its use of both time and space. The protean relationship between the past and the present is one example of its unusualness. Walking through the aisles of the Quilt, one quickly learns that time is a labyrinth with no clear exit. Participants can never escape the blurry line between past and present. It is difficult to situate AIDS firmly in the past when panels featuring present day are easily observed. Memories are always filtered through the lens of the present, and the Quilt is fast to remind those who come into contact with it that the epidemic lives on. There are no official starting points when immersing oneself into the fabrics, no chronological beginning that travels a straight line to a conclusion. The memorial's long stream of panels, each covered with touchstones to various moments of the past, is somewhat disorienting, as citizens do not simply reflect on the slow creep of change, but leapfrog from date to date. The Quilt constantly reminds us that everything has changed, but nothing has.

Just as the Quilt alters time through repertoires of public emotionality, so too does it change the spaces it occupies. The Quilt has a peripatetic quality, meaning it teaches as it moves among locations. Like Aristotle's method, in which movement is central to learning, the Quilt travels to spaces and transforms them as it unfolds and new bodies (both living and dead) flow through its aisles. Usually displayed in small segments, the Quilt reconstitutes public spaces like gymnasiums and university ballrooms. It has no center, being constrained only by the area where it is exhibited.[55] Silence is manufactured by the Quilt, disrupted only by the sounds of names being read and the occasional emotive responses of those in contact with the memorial.[56] Adapting to local communities and appealing to regional identifications, it materializes bonds between participants. For example, in the state of Indiana there are often several panels dedicated to Ryan White on display in schools where the Quilt makes appearances. This is coordinated not only because White was a student who was cast aside by educators, but because his hometown is Kokomo, Indiana. Participants enter these spaces, filling in the narrative details and allowing the dead to speak to them in ways that will and will not forge identifications.

The heterogeneous qualities of the Quilt make it at least partially resistive to the discourses that so often move us forward at the expense of remembering those who have been lost to devastating afflictions. This resistance to the progressive narrative is especially significant when contemplating the unity denied by the Quilt. Despite the impulse to articulate the Quilt in relation to national identity, it remains conspicuously fractured. In Yingling's words, the Quilt "seems to successfully resist the last move of the sublime (reincorporation) precisely because the unity it allows and constructs, the identity it offers through its collective scope, remains outside all of our corporate structures of knowledge."[57] The cloudy arrangement of time and its role in the performative repertoire perpetuates an anxiety that is profoundly perplexing. Its incomplete narrative structures the voids that those engaged with the Quilt must fill and prohibits the therapeutic qualities of the Quilt from eliminating possibilities for change.

A Stitch in Time: Narratives of Stranger-Relationality Reimagined

At a time when our understanding of HIV/AIDS has changed dramatically and our performances with the Quilt have largely moved into the realm of memory, one of the more pressing questions to ask is how the Quilt maintains its relevance in the fight against HIV/AIDS. Certainly the NAMES Project continues with its goals of educating publics and attempting to provide spaces of remembrance for those who have lost loved ones. However, the spaces available for communal reflection and the desire to do so are taking on different meanings. What happens now that the Quilt cannot be displayed in its entirety? Does its incompleteness alter cultural performances? In truth, the Quilt has made thousands of appearances, and only five of them have been collective. Perhaps the fantasy of wholeness is itself a suspicious claim.[58] What emotions are now provoked by the Quilt? Which can be made public? Who do they memorialize? How has the sedimentation of contemporary history altered the scenarios of performance?

At the beginning of this fight, NAMES Project founder Cleve Jones said, "part of making an event real is just saying it, over and over."[59] Continuing these reiterations, making these discourses more secured over time, eventually alters the message. Now that the signifying process of HIV/AIDS has transformed from a rhetoric of death and disaster into a rhetoric of management and control, it would seem that the emotive possibilities associated with the Quilt have fluctuated as well. Much like the discourse surrounding diseases like diabetes, AIDS is endemic, but no longer positioned as the public health threat it once was. The Quilt's occupation of small spaces in gymnasiums and lobbies may reflect the changing nature of the epidemic itself—powerfully emotive, but ultimately contained. HIV/AIDS is always ubiquitous, but its enormity is increasingly difficult to accentuate. Yet the changing nature of public emotionality from something discrepant than it was in 1987 need not be apocalyptic. Some element of public emotionality will always be present in this struggle. What should be feared is the waning anxiety some people have about AIDS and its debilitating consequences. The bigger question becomes, how do strangers ensure the Quilt continues to generate a sense of anxiousness necessary for keeping people alive? Should this be done through the creation of more panels, or perhaps the recognition of those panels not present? Theories of public emotion have been instrumental in advancing the idea that anxiety is a productive emotion for initiating change. Anxiety not only generates immediate learning, it also interrupts habits that have been previously learned. Emotions motivate people to alter their lives.[60] But the rhetoric of control—no doubt a rational and well-plotted schema if ever there was one—threatens this potential for action by justifying the capacity for containing HIV and relinquishing the anxiety that has propelled change.

Emotion continues to be a guiding force of political change in a culture where we are still largely strangers to one another, where AIDS continues to be whispered and the lives of millions continue to be lost.

Robert Hariman and John Lucaites remind us that "in a world lived among strangers, emotional resonance becomes an important measure of connection."[61] Just as the characters of Greek tragedy make their gravest mistakes when they do not recognize the stranger as kin (think Oedipus), so must we remember the connections to others propagated by the Quilt.[62] We need not see bodies to be reminded that our capacities for humaneness continue to be a necessary force in public life. Anxiety, anger, and sentimentality remain an imperative part of the fight against HIV/AIDS. Meaning can still be generated through the medium of the Quilt, but it requires a public that wishes to remain engaged. This need not happen through a unified public response. A multitude of responses, Peter Hawkins reminds us, is best for addressing the complicated scenarios generated by HIV/AIDS.

There remains hope that the Quilt can engender performances of citizenship that alter understandings of AIDS, even as the project for combating AIDS evolves. A group of high school students who saw the Quilt the final time it appeared in Washington, D.C., shows the continued value of the memorial. One of the students reflected, "I know all the technical stuff—how its transmitted, how not to get it, how many people are dying—but to come here and actually see all the lives it's touched, how many people have died, it's like reality hitting you in the face. This makes it real." Central to their newfound understanding was not what they were reading in their textbooks—a powerful tool in the archive of public life. The reporter following the story noted that "some of the students seemed surprised at the opportunity of emotion they saw—people crying, embracing and offering each other support. Several students said they were surprised at their own feelings of sadness and pain for people they didn't know, and many left messages and tributes on sections of the Quilt."[63] It was the repertoire of emotive citizenship playing a central role in these people's lives—and the quotes above are insufficient for capturing what was moved (or not) in their souls.

The Quilt can have an effect on the quotidian performances of people looking to impel change in a world where AIDS continues to devastate millions. But the idea of moving the Quilt into a San Francisco museum should make us shudder.[64] The Quilt's emotive power has always best exerted itself in public spaces that can be transformed, where the repertoires of citizenship can unfold in innovative ways. Absences can be a powerful source of motivation, and the changing face of the epidemic must be aggressively addressed. Though somewhat different from the losses the Quilt once sanctified, these tragic deaths can be combated in numerous forms, those that are material and those that remain unmarked. The Quilt may instigate a scenario of mourning that radiates privilege. But it can be more if the desire to recreate the fabric of our world is pursued and the cultural narratives surrounding the Quilt continue to be reconstituted among strangers in the polity.

At a moment of intense pain and reflection, a family stitched a blue swatch across their loved one's name to protect themselves from the harsh response of a malicious public who justified their hate through every avenue possible. People were told God demanded the sacrifice of young men because their sexual practices defied nature. Religious fundamentalists suddenly embraced survival of the fittest. We even convinced ourselves that everything happens for a reason. As the decades passed and as emotions made room for change, the opportunities for living in this world have became more bearable. But comfort has not come for all, much suffering remains, and much action is left to be taken. The world continues to change. And love can still remove that patch.

NOTES

1. For more on stranger-relationality, see Danielle Allen, *Talking to Strangers: Anxieties of Citizenship since Brown v. Board of Education* (Chicago: University of Chicago Press, 2004); Michael Warner, *Publics and Counterpublics* (New York: Zone Books, 2002).

2. Paula Treichler, *How to Have Theory in an Epidemic: Cultural Chronicles of AIDS* (Durham, NC: Duke University Press, 1999), 19.

3. John Durham Peters reminds us that gaps may be the most fundamental unit of communication. See Peters, "The Gaps of Which Communication Is Made," *Critical Studies in Mass Communication* 11 (1994): 117–140.

4. Brooke Masters, "AIDS Quilt Captures the Fear Behind the Loss," *Washington Post*, October 8, 1989, D3.

5. For more on performative repertoires, see Isaac West, "Debbie Mayne's Trans/scripts: Performative Repertoires in Law and Everyday Life," *Communication and*

Critical/Cultural Studies 5 (2008): 245–263.

6. Diana Taylor, *The Archive and the Repertoire: Performing Cultural Memory in the Americas* (Durham, NC: Duke University Press, 2003), 20.

7. Taylor makes an important distinction between *scenario* and *trope.* Scenarios "exist as culturally specific imaginaries—sets of possibilities, ways of conceiving conflict, crisis, or resolution—activated with more or less theatricality." Unlike tropes, scenarios are not constrained by language to transmit a set pattern of behavior or action. See Taylor, *The Archive and the Repertoire,* 13.

8. Taylor, *The Archive and the Repertoire,* 272.

9. There is little denying that the Reagan administration systematically annihilated gay people in the early years of the AIDS epidemic (the countless dead are proof enough). Writing of the White House's attempts to squander AIDS research through budget restrictions, Randy Shilts noted: "Even the most cynical critics of the Reagan administration were staggered when the Office of Management and Budget released its proposed AIDS budget for the 1986 fiscal year. Not only had the administration *not* increased AIDS funding but the budget called for reducing AIDS spending from the current level of $96 million to $85.5 million in the next fiscal year. The 10 percent reduction would be felt across the board in AIDS research but most heavily at the CDC, where funds would be cut back 20 percent to just $18.7 million. The government's planned appropriation for education aimed specifically at the gay community was $250,000, which, again, was to be channeled through the U.S. Conference of Mayors in an effort to ensure that no federal agency was in the business of telling gays how to perform sodomy safely."

These lethal actions are documented throughout *And the Band Played On,* and it is especially disturbing to see how these measures were put into place so late in the epidemic's scourge. As Shilts reflects, "by early 1987, the only major Western industrialized nation that had not launched a coordinated education campaign was the United States." Shilts is not alone in the clear documentation of Reagan's malcontent. Cleve Jones points out that even after Reagan finally uttered the word "AIDS" in public, he never did say the word "gay." Steve Epstein writes of Reagan officials who admitted discussions of quarantining entire populations. Reagan's White House AIDS adviser Gary Bauer penned callous editorials against safe-sex education. The executive branch was so overtly hostile toward pouring resources into combating AIDS that the surgeon general of the United States at the time, C. Everett Koop, developed educational materials without the administration knowing, so as to avoid the ideological censorship threatened by the White House. But perhaps Larry Kramer put it best: "Year after year of his hateful and endless reign we knew we were not a part of the American People he was President of. He would never talk about us, of course, or do anything for us except murder us. There were no social services for us. There was no research into our health. Even as we were dying like flies. How could he not have seen us dying? The answer is he did see us dying and he chose to do nothing. There was no representation in his government of us. There was never anything for us but his ignoble dismissal of us. All of Washington, indeed the world, knew that Reagan hated us."

See Randy Shilts, *And the Band Played On: Politics, People, and the AIDS Epidemic* (New York: St. Martin's Press, 1987), 525, 589; Cleve Jones, *Stitching a Revolution: The Making of an Activist* (San Francisco: HarperCollins Publishers, 2000), 188; Steve Epstein, *Impure Science: AIDS, Activism, and the Politics of Knowledge* (Berkeley: University of California Press, 1996), 95–96; Douglas Crimp, *Melancholia and Mourning: Essays on AIDS and Queer Politics* (Cambridge, MA: MIT Press, 2002), 189; Treichler, *How to Have Theory in an Epidemic*, 57; Larry Kramer, "Adolph Reagan," *Advocate*, July 6, 2004, 32–33.

10. Thomas Yingling, *AIDS and the National Body* (Durham, NC: Duke University Press, 1997), 53.

11. Douglas Crimp, *Melancholia and Moralism: Essays on AIDS and Queer Politics* (Cambridge, MA: MIT Press, 2002), 69.

12. The U.S. government was not the only one to advance problematic responses to AIDS. The British, for example, also developed reactionary policies and educational initiatives that were sometimes unintentionally stigmatizing and at other times overtly murderous. In 1986 a Tory leader announced, "As a cure I would put 90% of the queers in the ruddy gas chamber . . . We must find a way of stopping these gays going round." See Colin Chuter and Gill Seidel, "The AIDS Campaign in Britain: A Heterosexist Disease," *Text* 7 (1987): 347–361.

13. Treichler, *How to Have Theory in an Epidemic*, 20, 28.

14. Cindy Patton, *Inventing AIDS* (New York: Routledge, 1990), 77–97.

15. Cindy Patton, *Globalizing AIDS* (Minneapolis: University of Minnesota, 2002), 50.

16. See, for example, Cathy Cohen, "Contested Membership: Black Gay Identities and the Politics of AIDS," in *Creating Change: Sexuality, Public Policy, and Civil Rights*, ed. William B. Tuner, John D'Emilio, and Urvashi Vaid (New York: St. Martin's Press, 2000).

17. Cohen, "Contested Membership," 76.

18. The press largely stopped covering the AIDS crisis after 1987 because they worried

about oversaturation and public disinterest. See Edward Alwood, *Straight News: Gays, Lesbians, and the News Media* (New York: Columbia University Press, 1996), 235.

19. This is no small irony considering the rest of the world largely viewed AIDS as an American disease. The emergence of AIDS in American communities such as San Francisco, Los Angeles, and New York supported the widely held belief that AIDS was a U.S. affliction.

20. Peter S. Hawkins, "Naming Names: The Art of Memory and the NAMES Project AIDS Quilt," *Critical Inquiry* 19 (1993): 760–762.

21. Yingling, *National Body,* 54.

22. George Marcus, *The Sentimental Citizen* (University Park: Pennsylvania State University Press, 2002), 9.

23. Marcus, *The Sentimental Citizen,* 12.

24. Marcus, *The Sentimental Citizen,* 19; See also Barbara Koziak, *Retrieving Political Emotion: Thumos, Aristotle, and Gender* (University Park: Pennsylvania State University Press, 2000); Martha C. Nussbaum, *Upheavals of Thought: The Intelligence of Emotions* (New York: Cambridge University Press, 2001).

25. Marcus, *Sentimental Citizen,* 28, 49.

26. George Marcus, W. Russell Neuman, and Michael MacKuen, *Affective Intelligence and Political Judgment* (Chicago: University of Chicago Press, 2000), 124.

27. Koziak, *Political Emotion,* 27–28, 95.

28. Taylor, *The Archive and the Repertoire,* 210.

29. In making this claim, I am not assuming direct causality between making a panel and global awareness of AIDS. However, the feminist movement reminds us that consciousness-raising is an imperative element of social change. Some studies have already alluded to the potential action that can be forged between the AIDS Quilt and action. See Jacqueline Lewis and Michael R. Fraser, "Patches of Grief and Rage: Visitor Responses to the NAMES Project and AIDS Memorial Quilt," *Qualitative Sociology* 19 (1996): 433–451.

30. George Shakelford, "Fabric of Remembrance," *Washington Post,* October 4, 1992, C5.

31. Jeff McLaughlin, "AIDS Quilt Becomes Symbol of Caring," *Boston Globe,* October 5, 1988, 89.

32. Helen Gregory Affton, "AIDS Quilt Has Healing Spirit," *St. Louis Post-Dispatch,* October 3, 1992, 2B.

33. Howard Schneider, "Acres of Anguish and Healing," *Washington Post,* October 11, 1992, A1.

34. Marc Sandalow, "AIDS Quilt Covers National Mall," *San Francisco Chronicle,* October 11, 1996, A1.

35. Masters, "AIDS Quilt," D3.

36. In the words of Diana Taylor, "The bodies participating in the transmission of knowledge and memory are themselves a product of certain taxonomic, disciplinary, and mnemonic systems" (*The Archive and the Repertoire*, 86).

37. Peggy Phelan, *Unmarked: The Politics of Performance* (London: Routledge, 1993), 148.

38. Alan Zarembo, "The Quilt Fades to Obscurity," *Los Angeles Times,* June 4, 2006, A1; Jesse McKinley, "Fight Over Quilt Reflects Changing Times in Battle Against AIDS," *New York Times,* January 31, 2007, 16.

39. I recognize this is a difficult task since the NAMES Project claims not to be an author and would therefore be hesitant to draw attention to the absences of the Quilt. At the same time, the organization has taken efforts to do outreach in African American and Latino communities and might push for such efforts.

40. Marita Sturken, *Tangled Memories: The Vietnam War, the AIDS Epidemic, and the Politics of Remembering* (Berkeley: University of California Press, 1997), 200.

41. Eve Sedgwick, *Tendencies* (Durham, NC: Duke University Press, 1993), 265.

42. There are many ways to define "neoliberalism." Lisa Duggan notes that neoliberals "advocate privatization of economic enterprises, which they consider fundamentally 'private' and inappropriately placed in any 'public' arena. They go further than this, though, in advocating that many ostensibly public services and functions also be placed in private profit making hands," including cultural production. She continues, this "rhetoric promotes the *privatization* of the costs of social reproduction, along with the care of human dependency needs, through *personal responsibility* exercised in the family and in civil society—thus shifting costs from state agencies to individuals and households." See *The Twilight of Equality? Neoliberalism, Cultural Politics, and the Attack on Democracy* (Boston: Beacon Press Books, 2003). For other works on neoliberalism, see especially David Harvey, *A Brief History of Neoliberalism* (Oxford: Oxford University Press, 2005); Aihwa Ong, *Neoliberalism as Exception: Mutations in Citizenship and Sovereignty* (Durham: Duke University Press, 2006); Wendy Brown, "Neo-liberalism and the End of Liberal Democracy," *Theory and Event* 7 (2003).

43. Stephen Olbrys, "Disciplining the Carnivalesque: Chris Farley's Exotic Dance," *Communication and Critical/Cultural Studies* 3 (2006): 253.

44. Eileen Moore Quinn, "Entextualizing Famine, Reconstituting Self: Testimonial

Narratives from Ireland," *Anthropological Quarterly* 74 (2001): 72.

45. Olbrys, "Disciplining the Carnivalesque," 253.

46. Marcus, *Sentimental Citizen,* 76–78.

47. *New York Times,* "Memorial Quilt Rolls Out," October 12, 1987, 11; McLaughlin, "AIDS Quilt," 89; Lynne Duke, "D.C. Crowds Recall AIDS Victims through a Common Thread," *Washington Post,* October 9, 1988, B1; Masters, "AIDS Quilt," D3; Shackelford, "Fabric of Remembrance," C5; Sandalow, "AIDS Quilt," A1.

48. David Dunlap, "AIDS Quilt Grief on Capital Mall," *New York Times,* October 13, 1996, 22.

49. *St. Louis Post-Dispatch,* "AIDS Quilt Carpets National Mall," October 13, 1996, 18A; Craig Wilson, "AIDS Quilt: Patchwork Memories," *USA Today,* October 5, 1992, 4D.

50. Judy Elsley, "The Rhetoric of the NAMES Project AIDS Quilt: Reading the Text(ile)," in *AIDS: The Literary Response,* ed. Emmanuel S. Nelson (New York: Twayne Publishers, 1992), 187; Marcia Stepanek, "AIDS Quilt: A Work of Love, Protest," *Houston Chronicle,* October 9, 1992, A12; *New York Times,* "Grown Too Large, Full AIDS Quilt Is Displayed for the Last Time," October 7, 1989, 1; Wilson, "Patchwork Memories," 4D; Sandalow, "AIDS Quilt," A1.

51. For more on the relationship between gender norms and the Quilt, see Hawkins, "Naming Names," 765; Lawrence Howe, "The AIDS Quilt and Its Traditions," *College Literature* 24 (1997): 114.

52. Stepanek, "A Work of Love," A12.

53. Jeff Nunokawa, "'All the Sad Young Men': AIDS and the Work of Mourning," in *Inside/Out: Lesbian Theories, Gay Theories,* ed. Diana Fuss (New York: Routledge, 1991), 319.

54. Sarah Brophy, *Witnessing AIDS: Writing, Testimony, and the Work of Mourning* (Toronto: University of Toronto Press, 2004), 46.

55. Hawkins, "Naming Names," 764.

56. Peter S. Hawkins, "Confronting AIDS: The NAMES Project Quilt," *AIDS Patient Care and STDs* 12 (1998): 746.

57. Yingling, *National Body,* 53–54.

58. Hawkins makes the important point that without an "official" space, the overall impact of a traveling memorial might be lessened. Hawkins, "Naming Names," 762.

59. Elsley, "The Rhetoric of the NAMES Project AIDS Quilt," 190.

60. Ibid., 102; Marcus, Neuman, and Mackuen, *Affective Intelligence and Political Judgment,* 95.

61. Robert Hariman and John Lucaites, "Public Identity and Collective Memory in U.S. Iconic Photography: The Image of 'Accidental Napalm,'" *Critical Studies in Media Communication* 20 (2003): 61.

62. Koziak, *Political Emotion*, 139.

63. Benning, "AIDS Quilt's Moving Message," B01.

64. McKinley, "Fight Over Quilt," 16.

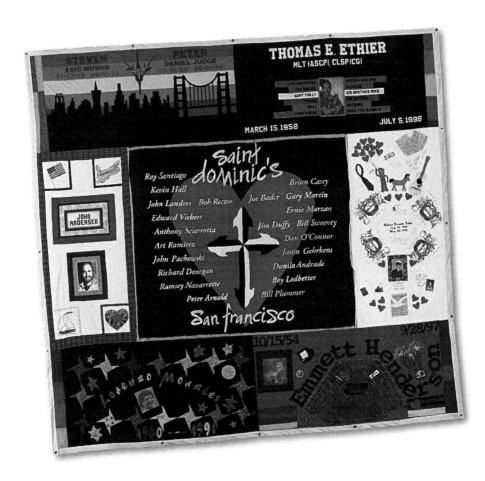

From San Francisco to Atlanta and Back Again: Ideologies of Mobility in the AIDS Quilt's Search for a Homeland

Daniel C. Brouwer

H*aving been approved to teach an undergraduate special topics course on "Rhetorics of HIV/AIDS" during the Spring 2006 semester, I programmed readings about the AIDS Quilt for a unit on ritual. Midway through the semester, I invited students to design, as one of two options for a formal, graded assignment, a panel for someone they knew who had died from AIDS-related complications and defend why they chose to memorialize the person in that particular way. To craft this assignment, I visited the NAMES Project AIDS Memorial Quilt Web site for the first time in many years. Although my main task of finding the organization's instructions for making panels was highly instrumental, I was struck by the very first image that greeted me at the site and returned to it after finding the information I was seeking. In the image, nine women of color, one sitting and eight standing, appear behind a long table upon which a panel rests. The intricate patterns and stitching evidence great skill. A textual fragment*

on the panel reading "Lord Remem" is visible. The image seemingly captures a communal effort to complete a new panel for a loved one.

The image both made perfect sense and startled me. Sensibly, the image articulated important intersections among women, race, and HIV/AIDS. I have long essayed to attend to these intersections in my service, pedagogy, and politics. Indeed, in 2000 I taught a class titled "Women and AIDS: Rhetorical Investigations," and in preparation for and conjunction with that course I volunteered for nearly eight months at the Chicago Women's AIDS Project, where on a weekly basis I invested in learning more about and helping to respond to the urgent needs of women, particularly women of color. Further, across the span of a decade, my curricula for that and three similar courses have reflected my desire to learn and teach about intersections of race, sex, and infection and changing demographics of HIV/AIDS nationally and internationally. More, I have been generally cognizant of the histories of quilting among African American women. For these reasons, the AIDS Quilt Web site image made perfect sense. But still, even as the Quilt has always described itself as an artifact for the full variety of people who die from AIDS-related complications, and even as I have always known and believed this, my startled response to the NAMES Project image revealed to me my habitualized thinking of the Quilt as an artifact especially significant to gay men. The image reminded me that the NAMES Project had relocated from San Francisco—its queer birthplace—to Atlanta—a center of New South black politics—in part to be closer to and better serve communities of color, specifically African Americans. I wondered further about the dynamics of its travels—where it had gone geographically, politically, pedagogically, and in the social imaginary—since I had been away from it for so long.

Two key controversies about the AIDS Quilt span the years 2001–2007. Specifically, these controversies are the relocation of the Quilt from San Francisco to Atlanta in 2001 and the firing of NAMES Project founder and spokesperson Cleve Jones in 2003, a dispute that prompted a number of lawsuits and settlements between Jones and the national organization. These controversies bring to the forefront the importance of ideologies about place and movement. Embedded in these controversies is an assumption about the nature of the Quilt—that it does its work best when it engages in "promiscuous mobility." Yet this assumption stands along-side an equally strong assumption about the Quilt's need to rest in an appropriate homeland. Thus, these controversies nominate *mobility* as both a key topic for analysis and a conceptual resource.

I employ *mobility* as a conceptual framework for exploring themes of movement, space, place, homeland, and ownership in these two contro-versies and for exploring the intersections of these themes with sexuality and race.[1] The key mobilities in these controversies include the invocation of homelands, shifting commitments to mobility, and competing notions about the proper relationship among texts, people, and places. Further, while especially the Quilt's relocation from San Francisco to Atlanta pivots on sexuality and race, these controversies are not easily reducible to or fundamentally attributable to eruptions of racism in the queer com-munity or homophobia in communities of color. Instead, variegated lines of identification demonstrate the provisional and constructed nature of home, homeland, and travel.

Ideologies of Mobility

Studies in mobility make movement the figure instead of the ground of critical analysis.[2] Such studies typically couple the fact of movement—whether grand (as in an "exodus") or mundane (as in a "stroll around the block")—with exploration of ideologies about place, space, home, homeland, travel, tourism, and other variations of movement. Describing mobility as "socially produced motion," Tim Cresswell invites analysis of mobility at three related levels: the plain fact, or empirical reality, of mobility; representations of mobility; and embodied experiences of mo-bility. A critical approach to the study of mobility, in his view, invests in adding "power, politics, and ideology" to its lexicon.[3] Attending to power, politics, and ideology, Mimi Sheller and John Urry nominate "questions of exclusion, disconnection, bypassing and differentiation . . . [as] . . . central to thinking about mobilities and their implications."[4] Mobility is rarely unfettered, for example, and mobility is best recognized as a disparately available symbolic resource or material possibility. Mobility is also best understood as a historical production, its meanings having been as strongly associated with freedom, opportunity, and progress as with deviance, danger, and "social pathology."[5] Whether mobility takes the form of tourism, diasporic dispersal, or other sorts of travel, whether it is chosen or coerced or forced, joyful or reluctant, critical studies of mobility attend to the facts of movement, representations of movement, and embodied experiences of movement.[6] More, mobility studies attend to reticence or intransigence toward movement, or the value of staying still and defending place, home, and homeland.

Ideologies of Mobility in HIV/AIDS

AIDS is both an epidemic and an "epidemic of signification."[7] When AIDS is understood as an epidemic, mobility emerges as "a key issue in understanding patterns of HIV infection."[8] Charting how HIV moves from cell to cell, person to person, population to population, and nation to nation have long been interests of virologists and epidemiologists. Notably, in epidemiology mobility has largely been understood as a problem or detriment. Indeed, epidemiologists have long addressed the seeming threat posed by the unchecked circulation of HIV-infected people (as immigrants, sex workers, or agriculture laborers, for example), and nations have frequently crafted legislation to regulate the flows of HIV-infected people within and across their borders.[9] When AIDS is understood as an epidemic of signification, or a proliferation of meanings, mobility emerges as a recurrent theme shaping the meanings of representations of HIV/AIDS. In that spirit, Meredith Raimondo's analysis of HIV/AIDS mobilities in U.S. media representations explores "the ideologies of race, gender, sexuality, class, and nation" and "the relationship of identity and place."[10] Raimondo argues that mobility occurs and is conceptualized at various "scales" (such as the cellular, the individual, the community, and the national) and that conceptualizations of HIV at one scale often inform conceptualizations of HIV at other scales. Further, Raimondo's analysis illustrates that when we study AIDS as an epidemic of signification, meanings of mobility also tend toward the detrimental. As an illustration, people who are imagined to practice excessive or clandestine mobility, such as wealthy and jet-setting gay white men, sex (and other) tourists, flight attendants, philandering spouses, bisexuals, and men on the down low, have appeared as insidious characters in representations of HIV/AIDS.

Key features of the AIDS Quilt interrupt the tendency to think of HIV/AIDS mobilities as detrimental. Attending to the manner by which single panels make their way into the larger U.S. AIDS Quilt, for example, foregrounds mobility as participatory and communal. Makers of single panels (which, at three-by-six feet, approximate the size of a grave) transport the panel either to a local NAMES Project chapter or directly to the national NAMES Project office. Local chapters perform a number of functions, including the integration of new panels into the national artifact and a national community of people with HIV/AIDS. Importantly, for those who choose to transport their panel to a local chapter in person or by mail, doing so may allow those vernacular memorializers to ritualize the letting go of their panel and the addition of the loved one's name to the national artifact in a place that is close to home. After the national office receives a panel, the office processes the panel, notifies the sender of receipt, and sews the panel into a twelve-by-twelve-foot block with other panels. When a block is complete, it becomes available for travel and display.

From its inception the Quilt has been assumed to function best under conditions of "promiscuous mobility," or unfettered circulation.[11] As a key feature of the AIDS Quilt, promiscuous mobility describes the need for the panels that compose the Quilt to circulate vigorously and endlessly so that they can perform their political and pedagogical functions of naming the dead, raising visibility, informing and inspiring people, and promoting solidarity and collective memory. At different moments during the controversies that I am studying, for example, eventual adversaries Cleve Jones and Julie Rhoad agree that, as Rhoad affirms, the "Quilt is always on the road."[12] In addition to traditional local site displays and occasional national and international tours of the U.S. Quilt, the NAMES Project facilitates the Quilt's promiscuous mobility through creation and support of more than forty international affiliate chapters (in Guam, Guatemala, Romania, Taiwan, Uganda, Northern Ireland, Japan, Argentina, Suriname, Cuba, and elsewhere) and through online image display of all received and processed panels. Yet the announcement of the Quilt's relocation from San Francisco to Atlanta animated a different version of mobility that affirmed ideologies of home and homeland; these affirmations of home and homeland were not entirely consonant with the principle of promiscuous mobility. Its move from San Francisco to Atlanta represented a significant and controversial rerouting of the Quilt, crafting new combinations of memory, fantasy, people, and place as it unsettled long-standing combinations of those elements.

From San Francisco . . .

Michael Lee Tiffany—son, brother, partner, artist, paleontologist, and more—died of AIDS-related causes in San Francisco in December 1998. In December 2005 family and friends completed a Quilt panel for him. To Eddie, who moved to San Francisco in 1988, Michael was an unrequited love whose affective policy of not falling in love with seronegative partners cast Eddie into the bittersweet realm of friendship.[13] Michael's mother and several of his friends engaged in conversations about how to memorialize Michael. With another friend designing the panel and a second friend performing most of the initial labor, Eddie received the work-in-progress, labored on three smaller portions, and made the final hand stitches to complete the panel.

Eddie's labors on the textile fragments dramatize the Quilt's potential mobilities. In San Francisco parks, at softball games, on airplanes, on camping trips, and elsewhere, Eddie worked on panel fragments, publicly performing the act of memorializing and testifying. In ways mundane and profound, this public labor engendered queries about Michael, the challenges of quilting, and the process of remembering. A worker at a fabric store donated twenty dollars after learning about Michael and the effort to create a panel for him. A UPS employee who asked Eddie if the package, on its way to Michael's mother in Montana, contained anything fragile or of value listened to the story. Well-traveled in San Francisco, the completed panel then traveled to Bozeman, Montana, for a temporary stay with Michael's mother, Irma. Restless in Montana, the panel traveled with Irma as she visited with her other children. Four months later, the panel returned to Eddie in San Francisco, where, for about two months, he displayed the panel in his office in the

U.S. Court of Appeals for the Ninth Circuit, thereby creating a temporary, unofficial home for the panel in the city that was the former homeland of the AIDS Quilt in toto. Finally, on June 30, 2006, Eddie sent the panel via UPS to its ultimate destination of the NAMES Project warehouse in Atlanta.[14]

San Francisco's status as a national and international queer homeland barely seems to need elaboration. Historian Nan Boyd observes, "the strength of the city's queer communities is world renowned."[15] Boyd historicizes the emergence of publicly visible queer politics and socializing in San Francisco by historicizing the city itself. She starts with the commonly used expression that San Francisco has long been a "wide open town" and strives to elaborate the specific policies and practices that confirm, in important ways, that perception. While queer practices were long a part of this wide-open city, in Boyd's assessment publicly visible queer mobilizing (political and social) emerge after 1933. In more recent times, Andrea Howe observes "guidebooks that routinely boast that San Francisco is 'the gayest city in the United States' and 'gay central USA.'"[16] The Castro neighborhood in Eureka Valley, in fact, typically stands in as queer "ground zero"—the gayest part of the gayest city.

Complicating the meaning of San Francisco, Howe advances an important argument about the difference between the frequently invoked descriptor of "queer capital" and her preferred conceptualization of "queer homeland." She explains, "while capitals are the legislative nexuses of states, homelands offer a symbolic refuge for believers who make the pilgrimage." In that sense, "San Francisco . . . serve[s] as an imagined homeland for queers . . . who often experience exile from, and ostracism living in, their places of origin (nation-state, community, family, and so on) . . . [and who in San Francisco] find their 'return' in a pilgrimage to a homeland."[17] In his memoir, *Stitching a Revolution: The Making of an Activist,* Cleve Jones narrates his own arrival to San Francisco in terms of a pilgrimage from small-town Indiana through Phoenix, Arizona, and on to "my home, its natives my people."[18]

The power of a homeland to inspire and unite is substantial, but as Howe and others caution, uncritical embrace of this queer homeland elides the significant differences that distinguish individuals' and collectives' participation in and attachment to that homeland. Marlon Riggs's poignant critique of the toxic, racist dimensions of the Castro neighborhood in *Tongues Untied* (1989) still stands as painful testimony to this fact.[19] Further, sitings of the Castro neighborhood as ground zero of queer San Francisco figuratively and ideologically displace lesbians of myriad races and ethnicities, as well as people of color of myriad sexualities who physically settled and congregated in other neighborhoods of the city, such as the Tenderloin District and Forbidden City.[20] Just as important, recognition of other collectives' (including people of Chinese, Japanese, Filipina/o, Latina/o, and African ancestries) variegated and complex histories with and within San Francisco tempers overcoding the city as queer or assuming that the city is singularly or primarily a queer site.

The Quilt's connections to San Francisco are extensive and varied. The story of Cleve Jones's inspiration for the Quilt arriving while attending a commemoration in San Francisco of Harvey Milk's assassination is well known and often told. Incorporating and opening its first office in San Francisco in 1987, the NAMES Project tapped into and was galvanized by the half century of visible queer activism that had occurred in the city. In 1987, as AIDS disproportionately appeared in gay men and warranted intensification of already existing homophobic ideologies, one can hardly imagine a more appropriate place for the Quilt to emerge and grow. Indeed, the first two panels memorialized Marvin Feldman and Ed Mock, a Jewish man and an African American man, and both gay residents of San Francisco, a fact that simultaneously indexes sexuality's participation in complex intersections of social identities and articulates gay, AIDS, and San Francisco to each other. In sum, San Francisco has become in the popular imaginary the Quilt's place of origin and its original homeland.

Despite a *Sacramento Bee* journalist's claim that the Quilt was born in Sacramento because Jones sewed the first panel there in 1987, counternarratives about the Quilt's origin gain little traction.[21] Still, this journalist's boosterism demonstrates the important fact that claims about homelands are disputable and plural. Recognizing this, I invest in exploring, not defending, the presumption of San Francisco as the Quilt's proper homeland. That presumption is forceful: even though the NAMES Project has always invited and accepted panels for any sort of person, the Quilt has been repeatedly associated with queer activism. For some, that strong and enduring association renders the Quilt's move to Atlanta unsettling and controversial.

To Atlanta . . .

For both "economic and strategic reasons," the NAMES Project relocated the Quilt to Atlanta, thereby newly inflecting W. E .B. DuBois's century-old heralding of Atlanta as "the new Lachesis, spinner of web and woof for the world."[22] The board of directors sought someplace other than San Francisco to find more affordable rental prices and thus reduce its debt. Economically, the move to Atlanta allowed the NAMES Project to increase its storage space, improve its space-to-cost ratio, and create a climate-controlled environment to aid the preservation of the Quilt. As someplace else, Atlanta was additionally appealing because it would place the Project in close proximity to the Centers for Disease Control and Prevention and in proximity to an African American community especially beleaguered by AIDS in a city with a visible and political African American community and a history of civil rights and human rights activism. Endorsing "strategy above sentiment," Cleve Jones argued that relocating to Atlanta would help to render the Quilt "as useful and as powerful and as important to the African American community and its struggle against this terrible disease" as the Quilt was to the gay community of the San Francisco Bay area in earlier years.[23] Conspicuously, across the decades of the Quilt's existence, scholars and activists, including members of ACT UP / New York, have endorsed the remarkable artifact while condemning the organization and/or its leaders for failing to materialize its rhetorics of inclusion and diversity.[24] Thus, Jones's forceful and careful endorsement of the relocation and retooling of the Quilt seems to function as a compelling rejoinder to years of criticism about the Quilt's overriding status as a chronicle of the deaths of gay white men.

Atlanta's emergence as a center of New South black politics significantly inflects the meanings of the Quilt's relocation there. Allison Dorsey describes Atlanta as "the preeminent city of the New South in the first generation after the end of slavery," rising from post–Civil War ashes "like a phoenix from the flames."[25] African Americans striving to make a home and a life in Atlanta created various social organizations and mobilized through black churches, whose legacy as "centers of education, social services, and political activism" continues today.[26] Experiencing an economic boom throughout the twentieth century, Atlanta emerged as a center of black politics, especially in the 1970s.[27] Atlanta's status as a center of New South black politics is not uncomplicated, of course. Karen Ferguson argues that the significant class and status differences that divided black communities after the Civil War, when conservative elites and a more radicalized working class benefited disparately from Atlanta's energetic rise, persist today.[28] Such variation in blacks' experiences of Atlanta undermines the ability of the city to function as an equally available material or symbolic resource.

Atlanta's complexity as a homeland is heightened when it is recognized as a southern gay capital. Galvanized by the Stonewall riots in New York City, gay and lesbian people in Atlanta began formally organizing in 1969.[29] In time, Atlanta gave rise to a visible and powerful LGBTQ movement, whose success was dependent upon an economically and politically progressive climate, diminishing religious opposition, recognition as a significant voting bloc, and a conscious effort to build on the city's black civil rights legacy.[30] Mayor Shirley Franklin and revered civil rights leader Coretta Scott King famously expressed support for local and national LGBTQ rights. Indeed, for LGBTQ African Americans, Atlanta is recognized as a "black gay capital."[31]

Despite Atlanta and San Francisco's complexities as homes and homelands for a variety of collectives, in the controversy about the AIDS Quilt's relocation the cities overwhelmingly represent, respectively, a black homeland and a queer homeland. What the basic fact of the Quilt's relocation mobilizes are particular ideologies about San Francisco and Atlanta that shape the meanings of relocation.

According to the NAMES Project Web site, the national board of directors decided in 1997 to relocate the Quilt from San Francisco to Atlanta and Washington, D.C.[32] According to Edward Gatta, then-president of the NAMES Project board of directors, the national office informed the forty-six local chapters about its decision to move the Quilt in March 2000.[33] The actual transport of the Quilt did not occur until March 2001.[34]

Despite one account that the Quilt "moved without much fanfare from its former home of San Francisco," the move occasioned significant consternation and opposition.[35] Even as she chose to move with the Quilt to Atlanta, devoted Quilt activist and long-term Quilt sewer Gert McMullin proclaimed, "we know San Francisco is the city that made the quilt, loved it, supported it during the hard times. The quilt should be there." Further, Felicia Elizondo threatened legal action to retain and thus keep in San Francisco the over fifty panels that she had sewn and noted that some activists considered "stealing" panels to prevent their move to Atlanta.[36] Additional newspaper accounts report somber crowds and the refusal by some Quilt supporters to attend the unbearable farewell ceremony.

As a member of the NAMES Project board of directors and an official spokesperson for the Quilt, Cleve Jones managed a complicated set of values, emotions, and goals by endorsing a retooling of the Quilt based on epidemiological shifts and by attenuating the link between the Quilt and its San Francisco homeland. At the time of the move, Jones affirmed that "the Quilt will always be remembered as a gift from the people of San Francisco," even as he endorsed its journey to Atlanta.[37] Capitalizing on the quality of promiscuous mobility, Jones also noted that because portions of the Quilt are always in circulation, even internationally, the national office in San Francisco was best understood as a way station rather than a resting place.[38] That is, the very nature of the Quilt prevents its sedimented, sacred linkage to any home or homeland. Two years later, Jones emphasized pedagogical and political efficacy as a valuable reason for the move: "Let's face it. The world identifies San Francisco with white gay men, but AIDS is doing its worst in women of color. The directors decided, correctly, that Atlanta would be the proper place from which to continue to get the word out."[39] Recognizing the reductive significations of places, Jones nevertheless affirms the value of place and the value of thinking in terms of the careful integration of people, texts, and places. This affirmation of the pedagogical and political significance of Atlanta to women of color seems to run counter to his earlier effort to attenuate the link among San Francisco, gay men, and the Quilt, but these claims do not rise to the level of contradiction. That is, a claim about the Quilt's inability to settle definitively into a specific homeland because of its promiscuous mobility does not contradict a call for rhetorical sensitivity.

Especially notable here is Jones's unequivocal recognition of women of color as the most vulnerable population for HIV transmission. This is not just an epidemiological claim; it is also a political claim in that it warrants a targeted investment of resources.

And Back Again?

As a second and related controversy involving mobilities, the firing of Cleve Jones from his paid role as spokesperson for the Quilt took a decidedly more circuitous route. Twisting and turning from a denied request to a call for firing to a lawsuit, and through several settlements, each of which unsettled the previous, this controversy was decidedly complicated. In this controversy, mobility figured in two important ways: the need for Quilt panels to circulate promiscuously in order to optimize their good works, and the effort to return the Quilt to its San Francisco place of origin.

In anticipation of the November 2004 national elections, Cleve Jones hoped to conduct a voter registration drive for people who are HIV-positive and to underscore gay rights issues by launching a national tour that would culminate in a display of the full Quilt on the National Mall, a display last accomplished in 1996. Jones shared his plan with the board of directors in the summer of 2003, and by several accounts he was told that by November 15, 2003, he would have to raise $2 million to fund the display. Perceiving such a task as unnecessarily cumbersome, Jones submitted a letter to the fifteen-member board of directors in which he outlined complaints against board president Julia Rhoad and board member Edward Gatta and requested greater decision-making authority in his role as spokesperson. Jones failed to raise $2 million by the deadline, and the board of directors decided not to support the national display.[40] More, on December 31, 2003, the board fired Jones for insubordination.[41]

Jones responded vigorously, filing a lawsuit on January 20, 2004, in which he claimed wrongful firing, breach of contract, and intentional emotional distress and asked for financial compensation, retention of his health benefits, which for years had made his expensive anti-HIV medications affordable, and, perhaps most dramatically, the return of the entire Quilt (with its more than 44,000 panels at the time) to San Francisco. In the spring of 2005, Superior Court judges in California permitted only the mental distress charge to move forward in the lawsuit. By September 2005, the litigants' lawyers proposed a settlement that would grant Jones the freedom to create a nonprofit "friends of the Quilt" organization affiliated with the NAMES Project, the opportunity to forward four nominations for NAMES Project board members, and receipt of thirty-five blocks of panels to be returned to San Francisco and governed by Jones's organization in exchange for Jones's willingness to drop the lawsuit. The next month, the settlement was derailed. In December 2005, a new settlement was proposed, only to be derailed over one year later.[42]

Given his conscientious defense of the Quilt's move to Atlanta in 2001 and given the economic, symbolic, and emotional immensity of that move, it is perhaps startling to hear Jones demand the full return of the Quilt to San Francisco. Although Jones eventually agreed to settle for the return of thirty-five of the over 5,700 blocks of panels, this significant reduction does not similarly diminish the significance of his call for the return of the Quilt to its birthplace. In Jones's view, because the NAMES Project abdicated its responsibility to optimally circulate the Quilt (in the form of, for example, his proposed 2004 national display), it abdicated the privilege of shepherding the Quilt. Further, this abdication reactivated San Francisco's special link to the Quilt and nominated San Francisco as the proper (re)new(ed) homeland. In December 2005, Jones contended "the Names Project continues to keep the quilt locked up in a warehouse in Atlanta where no one from San Francisco has any access to it at all," a boldly hyperbolic claim that nevertheless indicts the national office for breaking an implied promise to the previous keepers of the Quilt. In the midst of his lawsuit and settlements, Jones revised his gentle disavowal of a sacred connection between the Quilt and San Francisco into a commitment to his queer homeland, noting, for example, the disproportionate contributions of "thousands and thousands of quilt panels . . . from San Francisco made by San Franciscans," and explaining, "I fought hard to get the entire quilt back because I believe strongly that the quilt, like the rainbow flag, like the Gay Games, could only have started in San Francisco."[43]

Jones's mission statement for his new organization offered a vigorously partisan account of his relations with the NAMES Project and featured particular qualities of mobility. Accusing the national office of "years [of] neglect . . . to support the education and activist activities associated with the original mission of the Quilt when it began in San Francisco" and declaring that he was victorious in his lawsuit against the NAMES Project, Jones hailed the work to be done: "to begin anew the educational and memorial mission of the Quilt in the San Francisco Bay Area." Framed as a recovery of the original mission of the Quilt as conceived in San Francisco, Jones's new mission was "to demonstrate the continuing need for AIDS education and awareness by means of displaying memorial panels of persons who have died of HIV."[44] Astute observers will recognize in Jones's call to recover the original mission of the Quilt a tension that seems to rise to the level of contradiction: why condemn straying too far from original commitments after endorsing in 2001 the need to retool the Quilt to meet the needs of the newest disproportionately affected populations? Jones mitigated this seeming contradiction by affirming the premise that disparately affected populations need to be targeted through the Quilt but devoting himself to youth and young people as the constituency to which the Quilt most needs to be retooled.

While Jones did not name young people in the San Francisco Bay Area Friends mission statement, he frequently discussed the needs of young people in his 2000 memoir, emphasized youth in January 2004 as soon as he announced his lawsuit, and iterated youth in September 2005: "if you look at new infection rates, you see a vast majority of newly infected are young people."[45] Keenly, Jones did not argue that educators and activists should shift their focus away from the needs of women of color. Indeed, many of the young who are newly infected are people of color, so a retooling of the Quilt to focus on youth would ostensibly serve communities of color. Instead, with the return of the Quilt to San Francisco as his starting point, Jones fulfilled his rhetorical precedent of naming a population other than gay men to maintain the coherence of his endorsement of retooling the Quilt. Yet in his public statements, Jones failed to distinguish San Francisco as an exceptional site of youth populations; that is, he did not argue that San Francisco had a significantly higher population of youth than Atlanta or other cities in the United States or that San Francisco had recently experienced a significant rise in the numbers of its youth population, nor did he argue that San Francisco was a recognized homeland for youth politics. As such, Jones abstained from the earlier rhetorical precedent of expressing a unique linkage between place and people to defend moving the Quilt.

More, Jones's advocacy on behalf of youth simply iterated the NAMES Project's ongoing focus on youth through its National Youth Education Program. Beginning in the late 1990s, this program's description named young people as "the fastest growing group in the United States to be infected with HIV" and dedicated itself particularly to "youth of color, young women, and GLBT youth in under-served urban and rural communities."[46] For the NAMES Project, then, youth was not a desperate, disparately infected population that the organization had neglected. While Jones did not accuse the organization of such neglect, his own post–2004 lawsuit emphasis on youth startled with its redundancy.

Conclusions

Thus far, I have interrogated the various ideologies of mobility at play in the controversies over the Quilt's move to Atlanta and Cleve Jones's dismissal from the NAMES Project. I have affirmed the value of thinking through these controversies with special attention to themes of home and homeland and to relations between place and movement. In doing so, I have also affirmed that claims about home and homelands are both powerful and complicated. Specifically, I have attended to the challenges of endorsing both promiscuous mobility and habitation in a proper homeland. I have argued that Jones successfully negotiated this challenge in his defense of the Quilt's move from San Francisco to Atlanta, but that after his dismissal he abstained from his rhetorical precedent in failing to articulate a unique relationship between youth and San Francisco. Following are some of the implications of my choices and findings.

First, my choice to characterize the AIDS Quilt through the concept of "promiscuous mobility" should make sense on two levels. On one hand, I advance the concept earnestly as an especially apt way of expressing how the Quilt's advocates think about its ends and means. On the other hand, I advance the concept with some irony, heartened and inspired by its erotic and immodest dimensions. In his original vision of the Quilt,

Cleve Jones was explicit about his desire to capitalize on the presumed capacity of the medium of quilting to dismantle the stigma of gay male promiscuity: "That it was women who did the sewing was an important element. At the time, HIV was seen as the product of aggressive gay male sexuality, and it seemed that the homey image and familial associations of a warm quilt would counter that."[47] Douglas Crimp and others have famously criticized this temperate motivation given that sex—indeed, promiscuity—occupied a key material and symbolic place for some in the process of queer "liberation."[48] My choice, then, should be read as an expression of agreement with Crimp's and others' critiques.

Second, I want to insist on the value of imagining that a San Francisco homeland for the Quilt was neither inevitable nor necessary and that San Francisco was not a singularly appropriate place for the Quilt to have domestically emerged. Indeed, if we consider other constituencies disproportionately affected by HIV in the earliest years of the U.S. epidemic—hemophiliacs, female sex workers, and intravenous drug users, for example—we might profitably wonder where the Quilt might have originated had those constituencies created it—Peoria? Nevada? New York City? My point here is to note that while the Quilt's emergence in San Francisco was not random, neither was it inevitable.

Third, in terms of explicit multiplication and targeting of audiences, the "retooling" or "reinvention" of the Quilt preceded by several years its relocation. By the mid-1990s, for example, the NAMES Foundation had, with Cleve Jones's enthusiastic endorsement, established its National Interfaith Program and National High School Quilt Program. Further, in 1999 the organization created the Historically Black Colleges and Universities Initiative to target young people of color. Thus, the Quilt's relocation to Atlanta did not occasion a sudden or unprecedented rethinking of its potential good works. Still, for someone who views the relocation of the Quilt from its ostensible queer homeland as an index of a related reconfiguration or detachment of the Quilt from queer histories and queer politics, the following NAMES Project description of its ongoing efforts to archive each of its panels might evoke anxiety about the ideological distance traveled in the Quilt's relocation: once archiving is completed, "a student in the rural South exploring her heritage might search for all the panels that contain kente cloth, read about the memorialized persons' lives, and access video interviews with the panel makers to learn about the significance of the African patterns."[49] To turn a ghastly phrase, the artifact imagined here is not your dead gay white uncle's Quilt.

Fourth (and related), strange fears about being shut out from the Quilt upon its move to Atlanta express an underlying commitment to homeland and betray anxiety about the loss of one of its artifacts. Upon announcement of the relocation, one activist wondered: "The majority of the panels were made here in San Francisco. How am I going to be able to go and view the panels I have made?"[50] As I noted above, in 2005 Jones claimed that the NAMES Project had "locked up" the Quilt in a warehouse, where "no one from San Francisco has any access to it at all."[51] In a similar vein, a June 2006 *Los Angeles Times* article bookends its discussion of the Quilt's obscurity with evocations of the quiet, cold, secluded warehouse in Atlanta.[52] Factually, the relocation of Quilt panels to Atlanta does not make them unavailable to residents of San Francisco. At various levels of financial ability, those residents can travel to Atlanta to see panels, travel to nearby local displays, or request panels (indeed, very specific panels) for their own local displays. Certainly, those who fear being shut out from the Quilt know this. Yet anxious expressions like these perform the work of affirming the value of the mundane—of the value of being able to encounter a revered artifact on a daily, local, and embodied basis.

Fifth, even as we affirm the special significance of specific places to specific constituencies, we must attend to plurality within those places. Places are inhabited by more than one type of person, and individuals' claims of identity and place affiliations are rarely singular. This complicated fact should, I hope, temper efforts to claim ownership of the Quilt and its meanings. This fact thus suggests that it is worth the effort to imagine the Quilt's openness to multiple constituencies and its ability to foster coalitional politics. The "painful progress" of building coalitions sometimes requires a willingness to countenance or create a "revision in the text," a willingness to recognize seemingly enduring and intractable stories about origins and trajectories as stories that are subject to change.[53] In that spirit, I end with two evocations.

*From San Francisco to Atlanta traveled the Quilt panel that Eddie and oth-
ers crafted for Michael Lee Tiffany. Eddie's description of his experiences
and emotions helping to create the panel and directing its various travels
bear witness to the complicated and contradictory pulls of home, homeland,
travel, and textual transformation. Expressing a strong sense of connection
between the AIDS Quilt and San Francisco as its queer homeland, Eddie
laments the NAMES Project's departure: "It's unfortunate. Given the devastation in this region, it seems appropriate for the Quilt to be here, even a
few panels." Further, Eddie fondly remembers the days when one could walk
down Market Street to the Bay Area chapter office, where newly completed
panels were taken in and processed, opining about this ritual that he "would
prefer to do it here where [Michael's panel] could have been in communion
with other panels" crafted for and by members of the local San Francisco
community. Yet despite voicing these keenly felt emotions about the Quilt
and its home(land), Eddie was prepared to relinquish complete ownership of
Michael's panel to Irma ("I was prepared for her to want to keep the panel"),
an act that, while honoring the wishes of a biological family member, would
have chastened the panel's promiscuous circulation back to Michael's chosen
home and fictive kin, back to the nation's ostensible queer homeland, on
to the Quilt's new home, and to not-yet-determined destinations beyond.[54]
More, in settling upon the sentiment "as long as it has a home," Eddie expresses willingness to relinquish the Quilt in toto to a new home.*

*In the fall of 2006, a sabbatical leave afforded me the opportunity to
drive across much of the United States. Curious about potential conver-
gences between my travels and the AIDS Quilt's mobilities, I discovered via
the NAMES Project online display schedule that two blocks of the Quilt
would appear at the annual gospel brunch fund-raiser for the Women at
Risk (WAR) organization, held at the House of Blues in Los Angeles during
my planned stay there. In 1991 Ann Copeland and Linda Luschei founded
WAR after being diagnosed with HIV and discovering meager and alienating
services for seropositive women in the LA area. During an interview with
WAR event coordinator Suzy Herbert before the gospel brunch fund-raiser,
she clarified that the Quilt blocks would appear not as the event centerpiece
but as a literal "backdrop," to be hung at the back of the stage, for the day's
events.[55] In Suzy's description, the Quilt blocks would offer constant, quiet
commentary—a reminder of the purpose of the fund-raiser, a reminder that*

lives are still being lost, a reminder of the people who have come before us, a public voicing of the people named in the panels on display, a symbol of the need to create safe spaces for seropositive women—as speakers declared and musicians performed on stage. Poignantly, while both cofounders have Quilt panels made in their names, and while Suzy Herbert requested both panels for the fund-raiser event, only the block containing Linda Luschei's panel was available. This point underscores the fact that the Quilt's circulation is chastened by a variety of factors, including the possibility that a block containing a desired panel for display might already be temporarily routed elsewhere.

After the event, I essayed to get a closer look at Linda Luschei's panel. Warned by House of Blues technicians to be careful about the electrical cords, I was permitted onto the stage. At this range and in a particular sense, I met Linda Luschei, my understanding of her significance to the organization animating the memory enacted by her panel. "It's amazing to think about the fact that the Quilt travels all around the world," Suzy said. There on the stage, I considered the domestic but no less evocative voyage of Linda's panel from a storage warehouse in Atlanta to her LA-area community in the service of the organization that she cofounded.

NOTES

The author wishes to thank Brandon B. Ferderer for his invaluable work as both a research assistant and a scholarly interlocutor for this project, Kenneth Morrison for his generous and thoughtful commentary about homelands and artifacts, and Suzy Herbert and Eddie Hosey for sharing their narratives and insights about the AIDS Quilt. Thanks also to Erin Rand and Charles E. Morris III for their insightful commentary on earlier versions of this essay. Portions of this essay were presented in February 2007 as a guest lecture sponsored by the Honors Tutorial College and the School of Communication Studies at Ohio University in Athens.

1. Mimi Sheller and John Urry interrogate the ideological in mobility and representations of mobility in their "Introduction: Mobile Cities, Urban Mobilities," in *Mobile Technologies of the City*, ed. Mimi Sheller and John Urry (London: Routledge, 2006), 1–17. In thinking about HIV/AIDS mobilities, Meredith Raimondo calls for "mapping representations of mobility," with the goal of "unpacking the ideological

implications of some of the conventional terms for talking about the epidemic" (Raimondo, "'Corralling the Virus': Migratory Sexualities and the 'Spread of AIDS' in the US Media," *Environment and Planning D: Society and Space* 21 [2003]: 389–390).

2. Tim Cresswell describes an interdisciplinary "mobility turn," or "new mobilities paradigm," gaining momentum in 1996. Tim Cresswell, *On the Move: Mobility in the Modern Western World* (New York: Routledge, 2006), ix.

3. Cresswell, *On the Move,* 3–4, 55.

4. Sheller and Urry, "Introduction," 8.

5. Cresswell, *On the Move,* 1–2, 15, 31, 39.

6. In their theorizing of tourism as a particular type of mobility, Sheller and Urry foreground the "relational mobilizations of memories and performances, gendered and racialized bodies, emotions and atmospheres" that constitute tourism practices and experiences. Further, they note, "tourism mobilities involve complex combinations of movement and stillness, realities and fantasies, play and work." See Mimi Sheller and John Urry, "Places to Play, Places in Play," in *Tourism Mobilities: Places to Play, Places in Play,* ed. Mimi Sheller and John Urry (London: Routledge, 2004), 1. Cresswell, *On the Move,* 3–4.

7. Paula A. Treichler, *How to Have Theory in an Epidemic: Cultural Chronicles of AIDS* (Durham, NC: Duke University Press, 1999), 11.

8. Raimondo, "Corralling the Virus," 389.

9. From 1987 to 2010, the United States banned the entry of people who declared themselves to be HIV-positive. Such travelers to the United States could apply for waivers, but the application process was typically cumbersome. This restriction on mobility inspired a boycott against the 1990 International AIDS Conference held in San Francisco and led the international AIDS community to discontinue choosing locations in the United States as host sites for annual international AIDS conferences. In 2009, the U.S. Department of Health and Human Sciences removed HIV from the list of infections and diseases that disqualify people from entering or migrating to the United States. That policy took formal effect on January 4, 2010.

10. Raimondo, "Corralling the Virus," 391, 403.

11. Scientific and humanistic scholars alike employ the phrase "promiscuous mobility" to denote unfettered or unregulated circulation. In the biological sciences, the phrase refers to the circulation of molecular elements at a cellular level. In the humanities, scholars employ the phrase variously—to denote, for example, the circulation of historical images and citations or the diffusion of queer sexual pleasure.

See, respectively, Geoff Eley and Atina Grossman, "Watching *Schindler's List:* Not the Last Word," *New German Critique* 71 (1997): 41–62, and Christopher Nagle, "Sterne, Shelley, and Sensibility's Pleasures of Proximity," *ELH* 70 (2003): 813–845.

12. Avram Goldstein, "Region's AIDS Quilt Group Disbands," *Washington Post*, March 23, 2002, http://web.lexis-nexis.com (accessed August 26, 2006).

13. I met Eddie Hosey, a self-identified gay man and nearly twenty-year resident of San Francisco, through a mutual friend, John Milton Hendricks. John explained Eddie's participation in the creation of a Quilt panel and his display of the panel at their shared workplace of the library of the U.S. Court of Appeals for the Ninth Circuit. In San Francisco, I interviewed Eddie on September 21, 2006, and engaged in several follow-up e-mail exchanges with him about his relationship to the panel and its honoree, Michael Lee Tiffany.

14. Throughout, I vary (and by varying, play with) attributions of agency to the Quilt. That is, I have the Quilt searching for a homeland, traveling, and exhibiting restlessness, as well as being sent, being relocated, and being displayed. I mean for this ambivalence to be productive by capturing the Quilt's dual status as an object and subject of ideology and by demonstrating that mobility, while it can mean many different things, rarely means just one of them. I thank Erin Rand for drawing attention to the productive possibilities of ambivalent attributions of agency.

15. Nan A. Boyd, *Wide-Open Town: A History of Queer San Francisco to 1965* (Berkeley: University of California Press, 2003), 1.

16. Andrea C. Howe, "Queer Pilgrimage: The San Francisco Homeland and Identity Tourism," *Cultural Anthropology* 16 (2001): 52.

17. Howe, "Queer Pilgrimage," 36, 44, 53.

18. Cleve Jones (with Jeff Dawson), *Stitching a Revolution: The Making of an Activist* (New York: HarperCollins, 2000), 93.

19. Marlon Riggs, *Tongues Untied* (San Francisco: Frameline, 1989).

20. Boyd, *Wide-Open Town*, 79, 135. Boyd importantly notes conscious acts of queer divestment from political coalition-building with communities of color. Boyd, *Wide-Open Town*, 179–180, 185–186.

21. Walt Wiley, "AIDS Quilt Out of Spotlight, but Big Plans Are in the Works," *Sacramento Bee*, January 10, 2003, http://web.lexis-nexis.com (accessed August 26, 2006).

22. Gracie Bonds Staples, "AIDS Quilt Preparing to Find Home in Atlanta," *Atlanta Journal and Constitution*, February 9, 2001, http://www.lexis-nexis.com (accessed August 26, 2006); W. E. B. DuBois, "Of the Wings of Atalanta," *The Souls of Black Folk* (Chicago: A. C. McClurg and Co., 1903; repr., New York: Penguin Books,

1989), 64. Citations are to the Penguin edition.

23. Staples, "AIDS Quilt Preparing to Find Home in Atlanta"; Katie Szymanski, "SF Bids Farewell to AIDS Quilt," *Bay Area Reporter,* April 6, 2001, http://ww2.aegis. com/news/bar/2001/BR010401.html (accessed August 26, 2006); Margie Mason, "AIDS Quilt Readied for Move," *Associated Press,* March 30, 2001, http://www. aegis.com/news/ap/2001/AP010339.html (accessed August 26, 2006).

24. See, for example, the anonymously authored "The NAMES Project Exposed: What Cleve Jones Doesn't Want You to Know," available in the Northern California GLBT Historical Society's AIDS History Research Project archive or in Wendell Ricketts Papers (1961–2004), Cornell University, Collection Number 7681 (box 5, folder 4), n.d.; Peter S. Hawkins, "Naming Names: The Art of Memory and the NAMES Project AIDS Quilt," *Critical Inquiry* 19 (1993): 752–779; and ACT UP / New York, Letter to the Names Project Foundation, September 16, 1996, http:// www.actupny.org/campaign96/NAMESltr.html (accessed December 6, 2006).

25. Allison Dorsey, *To Build Our Lives Together: Community Formation in Black Atlanta, 1875–1906* (Athens: University of Georgia Press, 2004), 2, 30.

26. Dorsey, *To Build Our Lives Together,* 2.

27. See Ronald H. Bayor, "A Voteless People Is a Helpless People: Politics and Race," *Race and the Shaping of Twentieth-Century Atlanta* (Chapel Hill: University of North Carolina Press, 1996), 15–52.

28. See Karen Ferguson, "The Politics of Inclusion," in *Black Politics in New Deal Atlanta* (Chapel Hill: University of North Carolina Press, 2002), 253–268.

29. Arnold Fleischmann and Jason Hardman, "Hitting Below the Bible Belt: The Development of the Gay Rights Movement in Atlanta," *Journal of Urban Affairs* 26 (2004): 414. In discussing non-heterosexualities in Atlanta, I have altered my language from "queer people" to "gay and lesbian people" to follow the findings of the Black Pride Survey 2000 of the Policy Institute of the National Gay and Lesbian Task Force, which found "Black GLBT people do not readily, or even remotely, identify as 'queer.'" Indeed, in that survey, which included respondents from the 2000 Atlanta Black Pride event, only 1 percent of the 2,408 respondents to the question of sexual identity labels chose "queer" as their preferred self-identification, while 42 percent of those surveyed identified as "gay" and 24 percent identified as "lesbian." To be sure, the phrase "gay and lesbian people" itself elides other forms of sexual self-identification among black people (e.g., "bisexual" and "same gender loving"). My main point here is to recognize that "queer" does not always function as an umbrella term for all nonnormative sexualities. See Juan Battle, Cathy J.

Cohen, Dorian Warren, Gerard Fergerson, and Suzette Audam, *Say It Loud: I'm Black and I'm Proud; Black Pride Survey* 2000 (New York: Policy Institute of the National Gay and Lesbian Task Force, 2002), 19.

30. Fleischmann and Hardman, "Hitting Below the Bible Belt," 423.

31. Edward Brown, II, "We Wear the Mask: African American Contemporary Gay Male Identities," *Journal of African American Studies* 9 (2005): 31.

32. The NAMES Project Foundation, "Quilt Relocation Facts," http://www.aidsquilt. org/pr/pr_archive/pr_farewell_relocation_fact.htm (accessed August 23, 2006). The Quilt itself traveled to Atlanta, while the administrative office was meant to relocate to Washington, D.C., in order to facilitate relations and collaborations with private and governmental institutions located in the nation's capital. In fact, the administrative office never made it to D.C., instead following the Quilt to Atlanta. Washington, D.C., barely registers as a place or home or potential homeland in the controversies that I examine; thus, I do not address it here.

33. Christopher Heredia, "AIDS Quilt to Be Stored in Atlanta—AIDS Quilt Moving East," *San Francisco Chronicle,* February 6, 2001, http://web.lexis-nexis.com (accessed August 26, 2006).

34. This relocation of the Quilt, its corollary retooling, and the corollary reorganization of formal and financial relations between national and local chapters were followed by the closure of many local chapters. For over a year after the Quilt left San Francisco, the local Bay Area chapter remained open to receive and process new panels created by Bay Area residents and to send those panels to the Atlanta office. Yet in May 2002, the Bay Area chapter announced that it was folding, citing a lack of volunteers, changes in national rules for chapters, and high rents in San Francisco. Before the doors closed in July 2002, Bay Area residents could witness firsthand for the last time panels on local display at an official NAMES Project site. See Christopher Heredia, "Rip in the Quilt—Bay Area Chapter of the NAMES Project Reluctantly Ends an Era of Activism," *San Francisco Chronicle,* July 30, 2002, http://ww4.aegis.org/news/sc/2002/SC020731.html (accessed August 26, 2006). A 2002 *Advocate* article situates the Bay Area chapter closure within a larger trend of chapter closures, allegedly catalyzed by the national organization's newly coercive funding scheme and its apportionment of too many funds for international events. Local chapters of the NAMES Project facilitate memorialization of those proximate to the chapters and facilitate the integration of new, locally produced panels into the larger national artifact and broader HIV/AIDS community. As such, closures of local chapters might profitably be thought of in terms of

the loss of local, microhomelands. See Bob Adams, "A Rip in the Quilt," *Advocate,* June 25, 2002, http://www.findarticles.com/p/articles/mi_m1589/is_2002_June_25/ai_88583368 (accessed August 26, 2006).

35. Patricia Guthrie, "Home of AIDS Quilt: In an Inman Park Warehouse Sits Poignant Reminder of Pandemic," *Atlanta Journal-Constitution,* December 2, 2004, http://web.lexis-nexis.com (accessed August 26, 2006).

36. Heredia, "A Rip in the Quilt" and "AIDS Quilt to be Stored in Atlanta."

37. Cleve Jones, "Power of the AIDS Quilt: Comforting, Consoling and Convincing," *San Francisco Chronicle,* June 1, 2001, http://www.commondreams.org/views01/0601-02.htm (accessed August 26, 2006).

38. Szymanski, "SF Bids Farewell."

39. See Wiley, "AIDS Quilt Out of Spotlight." At about the same time, Mike Smith, a cofounder of the NAMES Project, defends the move in pedagogical and political terms: "The quilt never belonged to any one community. . . . Some chapters have felt like it was owned by the gay and lesbian community, but the quilt needs to be going where the epidemic is going—black communities, black churches." See Heredia, "A Rip in the Quilt."

40. The board of directors named both a lack of funds and discomfort with associating the Quilt with a federal political campaign as reasons for rejecting Cleve Jones's plan. It is unclear if Jones was made aware of the second reason before gaining approval to raise money for the 2004 national display. See Lance Williams, "AIDS Quilt Caught Up in Tempest," *San Francisco Chronicle,* January 21, 2004, http://www.sfgate.com/cgi-bin/article.cgi?f=/c/a/2004/01/21/MNG6Q4EAE51.DTL&hw=aids+quilt&sn=010&sc=382 (accessed August 26, 2006).

41. Cleve Jones was not the executive director of the NAMES Project when he was fired. Jones conceived of the Quilt in 1985, incorporated the NAMES Project in 1987, and served as its founder and director until 1990, when he became very ill from AIDS-related complications and ceded his leadership position. Rejuvenated by favorable reactions to anti-HIV drugs, Jones returned to the organization under the title of "founder." It was from this position that he was fired.

42. Andrew Keegan, "AIDS Quilt Lawsuit Settlement Unravels," *Washington Blade,* November 21, 2005, http://washblade.com/ (accessed December 5, 2006). Under the December 2005 terms, Jones founded and directed the San Francisco Bay Area Friends of the AIDS Memorial Quilt, a nonprofit organization sponsored by the progressive Tides Center in San Francisco. Believing that he had fulfilled the legal stipulation that he secure funds to pay for the Atlanta–San Francisco shipment of

the thirty-five blocks, attain storage for the blocks, and create a 501(c)3 nonprofit organization to steward the blocks by a December 31, 2006, deadline, Jones was dismayed to encounter in early January 2007 the NAMES Project's charge that his nonprofit organization did not technically qualify as an independent 501(c)3 because it benefited from the Tides Center's facilities and financial and managerial support services. Jones's failure, the NAMES Project charged, disobliged the latter from abiding by any of the terms of the settlement, including the return of the thirty-five blocks. After January 2007, there seems to be little media coverage of the conflict between Cleve Jones and the NAMES Project, suggesting that the thirty-five blocks never returned to San Francisco. See Matthew S. Bajko, "Names Project Delivers New Setback to AIDS Quilt Creator," *Bay Area Reporter,* January 4, 2007, http://www.ebar.com/ (accessed April 14, 2009); and Wyatt Buchanan, "AIDS Quilt's Permanent Return to City in Doubt: Portion of Project Destined for S.F. Still Entangled in Legal Battle," *San Francisco Chronicle,* January 4, 2007, http://www.sfgate.com/ (accessed April 14, 2009). Details from these two news stories suggest that while the NAMES Project had legal grounding for its objection, it showed no interest in tempering legal proceduralism with affective substance.

43. Bajko, "AIDS Quilt Settlement Talks Collapse"; Bajko, "AIDS Quilt Panels to Return to San Francisco," *Bay Area Reporter,* September 15, 2005, http://ww5.aegis.org/news/bar/2005/BR050902.html (accessed August 26, 2006).

44. San Francisco Bay Area Friends of the AIDS Memorial Quilt, "Project Detail," *Tides Center,* http://www2.tidescenter.org/directory/project_detail_new.cfm?id=60287.0 (accessed December 5, 2006).

45. Bajko, "AIDS Quilt Panels." See also Williams, "AIDS Quilt Caught up in Tempest," and Lance Williams, "AIDS Quilt Creator Can Keep Benefits," *San Francisco Chronicle,* January 23, 2004, http://web.lexis-nexis.com (Accessed August 26, 2006).

46. The NAMES Project Foundation, "National Youth Education Program": http://www.aidsquilt.org/programsnyep.htm (accessed January 11, 2007).

47. Jones, *Stitching a Revolution,* 108.

48. Douglas Crimp, "The Spectacle of Mourning," *Melancholia and Moralism: Essays on AIDS and Queer Politics* (Cambridge, MA: MIT Press, 2002), 196–200.

49. The NAMES Project Foundation, "The Quilt Archive Project," http://www.asidsquilt.org/archive.htm (accessed December 6, 2006).

50. Terry Beswick, "Names Project Is Moving to Washington, D.C.: Quilt to Be Housed in Atlanta," *Bay Area Reporter,* February 2, 2001, http://www.aegis.com/

news/bar/2001/BR010205 (accessed January 11, 2007).

51. Bajko, "AIDS Quilt Settlement."

52. Alan Zarembo, "The Quilt Fades to Obscurity," *Los Angeles Times,* June 4, 2006, http://www.latimes.com/ (accessed June 6, 2006).

53. Tony Kushner, *Angels in America: A Gay Fantasia on National Themes, Part Two: Perestroika* (New York: Theatre Communications Group, 1992), 46, 144.

54. Kath Weston, *Families We Choose: Lesbians, Gays, Kinship* (New York: Columbia University Press, 1991).

55. With both Suzy Herbert and Eddie Hosey, I shared the portions of this essay in which they appear and invited their critique and requests for revisions.

PART 3

Transformation

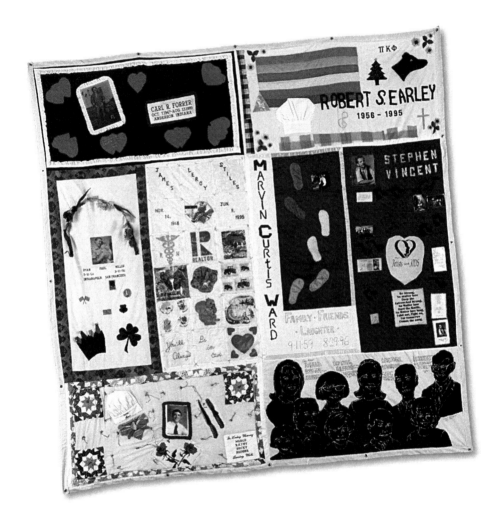

Rhetorics of Loss and Living:
Adding New Panels to the AIDS Quilt
as an Act of Eulogy

Bryant Keith Alexander

My partner and I both love quilts. They adorn every room of our house—draped over chairs, mounded on racks, displayed as slipcovers and wall hangings, and, most important, layered on beds for warmth. And even though we now live at the foothills of the San Gabriel Mountains in sunny Southern California, we both grew up in families, homes, class designations, and regions of the country where quilts had a significant meaning, a necessity. Long before the recent kitsch of nostalgia or the emergence of using quilts as decorating centerpieces—for families in West Virginia and Southwest Louisiana, quilts brought comfort on cold winter nights, and, for me, in a house without central heat and with floor heaters whose mystical fire glow offered close comfort but not sustained warmth from a distance—our quilts were cozy companions. These quilts, made by aunts and grandmothers, individually and in quilting circles with family and friends, were stitched with a particular necessity: patches of layered fabrics, some found, others bartered and bought, but most often reclaimed from garments that had lost their wearable function and drafted into another form of service. These quilts were put to work, washed, worn, and refabricated over and over again.

These quilts, while created for their functionality, were patterned, in the sense of templates, for the ease of creation. With the aesthetic astuteness of care, they were pieced, appliquéd, and sometimes embroidered as a display of pride in workmanship. But their function was clear, and the women in our childhood lives engaged the act of making these quilts for the purpose of use. The thought of quilts as mere adornment would horrify them, and while many of them will now make quilts for pleasure or to sell to local tourists, they understood the intention and process of making quilts as acts of care and necessity. My partner's aunt has now made a quilt for our six-year-old cocker spaniel, a two-by-three-foot quilt that fits into her puppy bed. It has her name on it, PEPPY, with embroidered dog bones as signifiers of her station, sewn in colors and a fabric that does not show dirt and is easily washed. We playfully extend our family heritage into the life of our canine progeny; the creation of the quilt for the dog is a traditional act of love and care to us.

And while most of the quilts from my childhood have disintegrated with time and use, they have painfully been discarded and replaced with newer and easier to care for modern renditions. We have quilts from my partner's life before me. Yet I mourn the comfort of my own older quilts, not just for the warmth but also for the care of intent, the intensity of desire, and the act of love that went into their construction. Each quilt was like a symbolic hug from its creator. And maybe this is the reason that my partner and I are forever purchasing quilts from skilled artisans, mostly from West Virginia and Southwest Louisiana, and ritually giving them as gifts to friends and family, a cloak of care.

The aesthetics of quilts are sometimes trapped not only in the warp and woof of fabrics, but also of and in the rhythms of the effort signifying traditional aesthetic uniformity and desirous intent that is as diverse as those whose lives are enveloped in the social construction of the engagement. In speaking of African American women's quilting, Maude Southwell Wahlman and John Scully suggest the following:

When the colors of the strips are different from the color in the rows of blocks or designs, two distinct movements can be seen: one along the strips and the other within the designs . . . This represents a textile aesthetic which has been passed down from generations among African-American women who were descendants of Africans . . . African-American quilters do not seem interested in a uniform color scheme. They use several methods of playing with colors to create unpredictability and movement.[1]

I use this quote, as does Elsa Barkley Brown, to build a framework for conceptualizing. For her it is a key to building a *framework of conceptualizing and teaching African American women's history.* She writes, "in my course on African-American women's history, I seek to create a polyrhythmic, 'nonsymmetrical,' nonlinear structure in which individual and community are not competing entities."[2] A part of her project is "about coming to believe in the possibility of a variety of experiences, a variety of ways of understanding the world, a variety of frameworks of operation, without imposing consciously or unconsciously a notion of the norm."[3] Quilts, in this sense, become metaphor for social and political constructions of identity made manifest in artifacts of culture.

I also use the quote as a framework of conceptualizing the AIDS Memorial Quilt as a series of individualized panels, individually constructed and aestheticized with personal intentions; isolated panels that are not designed for uniformity outside of the context of its own intent. However, when placed adjacent to other panels embroidered with the same intent, they too formulate *a polyrhythmic, "nonsymmetrical," nonlinear structure in which individual and community are not competing entities,* building an image of collective struggle through buttressing and stitching individual expressions of mourning. It is in the moment of joining the panels that a collective vision is presented and the nonsymmetrical nature of the whole develops its own rhetoric. Yet while the individual panels represent the past (lives lost), the collective Quilt "constitutes a set of practices and cultural negotiations in the present" and becomes a collective narrative *performing presence, absence, and historical memory.*[4]

In presenting this idealistic notion of a collective narrative I also know that the racial representation in the quilt and the politics of the quilt of those non-white victims of AIDS has not always been fully present. Hence a more complex intention in using Brown's quote is to foreground the absence of color, the asymmetries of representation in a project of memorialization; the missing voices of those men of color who have passed from AIDS but also those living with HIV/AIDS—voices that must be heard both to expand the narratives told by the quilt and to invoke the possibility that the quilt as a memorial shrouds. In this light, when as a black gay man I think of the actuality of the NAMES Project as one of the largest community arts projects in the country, I am less taken with the politics of the collective than of the acts of care and compassion that went into constructing the individual panels—self-contained quilts within the larger fabric of the effort.[5] The thought of friends, lovers, and loved ones taking up arms, fabric, and needles, stitching manifestos that are as much political statements as expressions of remembrance and remorse; fabric stitched together with laughter and tears, with memories and dreams; panels offered as arguments and as one last symbolic hug, stretched over the expanse of multiple football fields. This thought gives me comfort in the social politics of love that often run shotgun to governmental politics that link desire and disdain in relation to HIV/AIDS and opens spaces for additional stories.

I am interested in partially reflecting on the historical nature of the AIDS Memorial Quilt, but in a more performative and narrative approach to telling stories of AIDS and HIV-positive status that traverses the boundaries between death and life, between loss and gain, between fear and a powerfully embraced self-determination, between acceptance and regret; and between regret and a righteous transcendence into self-knowing and liberation. And maybe more important, I seek to include voices of black gay men living with HIV/AIDS in the particular discussion of memorializing that the quilt addresses and politicizes.

Critical ethnointerpretive methodology engages a particular focus on critique but uses a highly personalized, reflexive, narrative, and autoethnographic mode of exploring the invested self-implication of the author and those he engages in the telling of the told. This is a form that engages an interpretive ethnography that foregrounds the actual expressions of particular cultural members, while also allowing the researcher the opportunity to illuminate both his self-implication and his broader cultural membership in the community of interest that he investigates.

Here I present a series of autoethnographic narratives that situate me in the story I am telling as a black gay man and the brother of a black gay man who died from HIV/AIDS. There are also brief ethnographic narratives drawn from ten interviews with black gay men living with HIV/ AIDS. Their voices are mournful and hopeful, funny and tragic—yet illustrate the diversity of conditions that inform their situated being. The work of ethnography in this project helps to illuminate the meaningful contributions of these interlocutors. Drawing from D. Soyini Madison's work on critical ethnography:

> As ethnographers, we employ theory at several levels in our analysis: to articulate and identify hidden forces and ambiguities that operate beneath appearances; to guide judgments and evaluations emanating from our discontents; to direct our attention to the critical expressions within different interpretive communities relative to their unique symbol systems, customs, and codes; to demystify the ubiquity and magnitude of power; to provide insight and inspire acts of justice; and to name and analyze what is intuitively felt.[6]

Constructing a Panel for My Brother: Narrating Remembrance and Remorse in a Panel

I saw the AIDS Memorial Quilt in its first display on October 11, 1987. I made the pilgrimage to see for myself the carefully crafted insertions and assertions of lives into three-by-six-foot individual cloth paneled tombs that laid down like recalcitrant lovers as memorials—key phrases, dates of birth and death, and character traits, signifiers of being, pictures, diagrams, messages of personal and political intent; mournful displays of remembrance and remorse laid bare in front of the U.S. Capitol in Washington, D.C.[7] The display was a "performance environment where we are asked to change from spectator/bystander to witness, where we were asked to make our specific memory into historical memory."[8]

Yet the Quilt was only a temporarily placed memorial that through reflection of its social significance and the fragility of its substance became transient as a national marker of dignity, a banner of a war symbolizing urgency and necessity—this in comparison to such fixed memorials as the Lincoln Memorial, the Washington Memorial, and the Vietnam Memorial. Later I saw the Quilt as a display traveling across America, segmented from the whole to politicize its significance as a mobile sideshow of a political cause. The reduced (re)presentation simultaneously exposed a wider population to the aesthetic and performative politics of the Quilt while diminishing the visual magnitude of the epidemic.

In my viewing of the Quilt in its varying constructions, totality and traveling road show—betwixt and between the nonsymmetrical multicultured panels of the Quilt—I always seem to miss the bodies of color. I did not doubt their existence, as much as how a lack of visibility suggests absence and thus a lack of representation. In 1994, when my brother died from HIV/AIDS, I wanted to create a panel for him, but in the midst of loss and remembrance, and the absence of presence, I was stupefied by the process of reducing a life to a panel on a Quilt; the politics of submission and inclusion, and the manner in which the literal gesture would memorialize my brother in the textile narrative and political gestalt of the quilt of AIDS victims. This panel would reduce him to an enshrined corpse in a perpetual wake—like Vladimir Lenin, Eva Peron, or James Brown. Which, while desperately attempting to hold onto a physicality of presence, prolongs the process of witnessing a slow deterioration of departure.

I resisted then, but now I would like to symbolically insert this narrative rendition of his panel, for I believe that his story, that our story as black gay men, have not adequately been represented in the historiography of both the Quilt and the AIDS epidemic.

STANDING AT THE CROSSROADS

I am the fifth of seven children, the fourth of five boys—born into a social experiment that my parents called a family. In spite of the dynamic social interaction that goes on in a large family, I grew up a very private kid, constantly demanding his own space, his own place, his own identity—separate from my brothers (the athletic brother, the talented brother, the handsome brother, the younger brother). I always felt that I was at a crossroads between who I was and wanted to be and who they were and the directions their lives were taking them.

The house that I grew up in was located on a corner lot in the center of our neighborhood—at a crossroad between Simcoe Street and 12th Street. All the local kids flocked over to our house. My mother used to say, "with seven kids you're bound to attract a lot more." Our yard was the place to be. We had pecan trees and fig trees, mulberry trees and a pine tree. We had a big front porch, a field for football and a dirt basketball court. This was the main attraction. Guys from around the neighborhood would come with their attitude and bravado, fighting over who would be shirts or skins. Sporting their new Converse tennis shoes, these guys would walk into our yard talking a whole lot of shit . . . who would win, by how many points, who would make it to the NBA. These guys performed the pageantry of youthful dreaming and the ritual of growing up. I watched these guys from the side window—one of two in the living room of our house. I would watch these guys, young Olympians in the prime of their manhood—calling up the dirt, swirling in a dust cloud of hopes and dreams, their bodies caked with a mixture of sweat, dirt, and tenacity. The basketball court was a crossroads, a passage into another time, another space—a ticket to another place.

The other window in the living room looked out to the front. The house that I grew up in was located across the street from Syrie Funeral Home. During the evening I would often look through it and see the pageantry of death and the ritual of saying good-bye. In the distance I could hear the mournful wails of those feeling grief. I could see the old men sipping from a bottle of courage near the dumpster. I saw children doing what children do—some playing games, others engaged in solemn social banter. I saw people looking silently, longingly into the distance, standing at the crossroads of their memories and their reality.

On September 7, 1994, I drove from Carbondale, Illinois, to Lafayette, Louisiana, to attend the funeral of my brother Nathaniel Patrick Alexander—who died from complications of AIDS three days earlier. Many asked why I didn't fly, but I needed the time. In my informed confusion I thought that if I delayed getting there I could somehow suspend time. During that eleven-hour drive I crossed real and imagined borders—traveling down a road that took me to painfully familiar places. The day he told me he was gay. The day he introduced me to a partner. The day he called me and said, "Are you coming home this summer?" The day I helped him move home. The day I found out he had AIDS. The day he said, "I'm sorry I let you down." The day he said, "I love you." The day he died.

As I pulled into Lafayette I reflected on another special day: after a name-calling episode with some of the local boys in which I was the focus of their pro-masculine anti-sissy juvenile male posturing, my brother sat me down and said, "I see me in you. We are so much alike. There are many versions of being a man. Find the one that is best for you that does not cause harm to others. Be who you are, what you are, and how you are, and to shit with them." I was thirteen. He was seventeen.

I enter my parent's house at 10:30 P.M. and family immediately surrounds me. I navigate myself through childhood memories and put to rest sibling rivalries. I greet my sisters, my older brother, his wife and children. I talk to the other older brother—on the phone—who is incarcerated in the local jail for drug dealing. He is feeling the pain of his absence in that time of family grief. I hold a strained conversation with the younger brother, who, since dropping out of high school, finds it difficult to talk to me, his graduate-student-teacher-older-brother.

The next day my family arrives at the funeral home early for a private viewing of the body. This is the first that I have seen my brother in months. He looks thin and ashy. Surprisingly, I find myself more angered than sad. I am angry at his carelessness. I am angry that as a black man he carried himself recklessly through the world. I am angry because his hair is combed forward instead of backwards. I am angry because he is wearing a plaid jacket that even he would not be caught dead in. His skin is darkened, his eyes are deep, and the clothes are draped over his body like they are hanging on a rack. His eyes are closed; there is a slight smile on his face—a glimmer of recognition, but no real acknowledgment. I miss him. I miss seeing me in him. This is not the brother that I fought with for years, the brother who helped me to cross over into being.

Later that evening I see faces from my past, all older and a little grizzled. I have not seen many of these faces in years. As the resident family recluse and all-around shy guy, I retreated from the neighborhood years before and busied myself with high school, then college, then graduate school, and then teaching. Many of them hesitate when they see me, an adult version of the child memory; the face in the window. Then almost predictably, they comment: "You look like him. You sound like him. You act like him." It is an attempt to re-create him—it's a form of celebration and renewal. I smile uncomfortably and welcome them. I see a number of my brother's friends, gay men who float in on a trail of tears. I know many of them. We greet. We hug. We kiss. And as gay men we stand at the crossroads of our lives. We look at each other searching our faces for some sign, for some assurance—for denial, for escape.

During a novena, a repetitive chanting of prayers, I step out. While standing outside of the funeral home I realize that I am engaged in the pageantry of death and the ritual of saying good-bye. In the distance I can hear the mournful wails of those feeling grief. I could see the old men sipping on a bottle of courage near the dumpster. I can see children doing what children do—some playing games, others engaged in solemn social banter. I am looking silently, longingly into the distance, standing at the crossroads of my memories and my reality.

I look across the street at an empty lot where my childhood house used to stand, long removed. I hear the faint sounds of brothers and sisters fighting and laughing. The trees are still there, but the grass has long grown, covering the arena of boyish dreams—where guys performed the pageantry of youthful dreaming and the ritual of growing up—in the swirl of dust and clouds of dreams. In the distance, leaning against the pecan tree, I see a figure. Standing there is the memory of a boy named Donald, one of my childhood friends, a basketball player—a titan of the court. Now he is a shadow of a man, frail from drug and alcohol abuse. The tree holds him up as he sips a bit of courage before he begins to cross the road to pay his respects. As he approaches me, I see that his skin is darkened, his eyes are deep, the clothes are draped over his body like they are hanging on a rack. He conceals his bottle as he pulls up his pants. I stand there dressed in a tailored suit, manicured fingernails, and designer glasses. When he crosses my path he hesitates. Our eyes meet. There is a glimmer of recognition but no real acknowledgment. I mourn the loss of Donald. I mourn the loss of my brother. I mourn the loss of young black men and youth-filled dreams.

I am standing. I am standing at a crossroads between my brothers (the married brother, the dead brother, the jailed brother, the dropout brother). I am standing at the crossroads of my life looking through a window to another time—onto a dusty basketball court—seeing young black Olympians in the prime of their manhood performing the pageantry of youthful dreaming and the ritual of growing up. I am standing at a crossroads of my life as a gay man living in the age of AIDS. I am standing at a crossroads looking through the window, seeing myself engaged in the pageantry of death and the ritual of saying good-bye. I am standing at the crossroads between Simcoe Street and 12th Street, between my childhood home and the funeral home, between boyish dreams and adult realities. I am at a crossroads—looking, reflecting, remembering, moving and being moved, but standing still at an intersection in space and a breach in time.

Each panel of the AIDS Memorial Quilt, like the narrative I just told, tells a story, a story often pictorially presented: *epitaphs*, panels as tombstones; *epithets*, panels as substitutes for names and lives; *effigies*, panels as substitutes for bodies; *eulogies,* panels as remembrance and celebration. Each panel is a narrative of a life in a restricted space allocated by the conventions of time and location. Each panel seeks, like my own more explicit narrative, to tell a story of a life and relationship that has ended in death; a death particularized by the implications of a disease; a disease reductively associated with the politics of gender and sexuality; a disease often relegated to the politics of negligence and self-gratification; a social condition that implicates the politics of medical research and the politics of a community and culture to witness and mourn. The politics of HIV/AIDS are always situated, situated in family, culture, class and society—politics that implicate our sense of knowing ourselves and encountering others in the face of threat and the vulnerability of desire. And while a particular expression of remembrance and remorse, my narrative seeks to illuminate these qualities that are stitched between the fabrics, seams, and emblems of the panels as larger rhetorics of loss and commemorations of life on the quilt. The following ethnoperformative narratives, like my own, offer the particularity of experience in the face of loss; but unlike in my narrative, the men whose voices are presented speak from a space of affective knowing as they negotiate their own HIV-positive status, constructing and offering counternarratives to the situated panels on the AIDS Memorial Quilt.

Ethnoperformative Narratives: Living in the Face of Diagnosis

The ethnoperformative narrative is, for me, a narrative drawn from ethnographic interviews, a personal narrative that stands on its own as a performative expression of desire. It stands as a counternarrative, a self-expression that disrupts and disturbs public discourses or master narratives from the dominate culture by exposing the complexities and contradictions of the unspoken and the cloistered lives that public discourses do not include, revealing nuanced differences in which private lives, usually minority lives, respond to the situatedness of living.⁹ In a series of ethnographic interviews with ten black gay men self-identified as either HIV-positive or living with AIDS, I draw the following thematically linked and stitched narrative responses back to the overarching notions of building *rhetorics of loss and living.* While the AIDS Memorial Quilt documents and concretizes a particular history of death, and a political medium of marking such deaths, "the voices [that echo within the Quilt] are full of the weight of a history that cannot be absorbed, full of sorrow that cannot be managed, full of absences that never can be filled, full of contradictions that never can be resolved."¹⁰ And thus the Quilt makes a resolute contribution to the historiography of HIV/AIDS, but not always to all of the lives affected by the disease, or at least not in equal measure.

Within the following brief and singular utterances from these ten men, my attempt is to offer *counternarratives,* "short stories" that offer individualized perspectives of experience that are sometimes cloaked and silenced within the official narrative of HIV/AIDS that the AIDS Memorial Quilt seems to signify, pervading social consciousness. I believe that these short stories as ethnoperformative narratives, presented in the active voice of men living with HIV/AIDS, resist the finality of closures in the moment of their utterance. They may even serve as *disidentifications,* as practiced positionalities within a lived circumstance that critiques from within, and as a method that seeks to subvert mainstream constructions of queer identities in the particularity of the AIDS Memorial Quilt.[11]

These stories reveal the limits of manageability. Like the disease with which these men are infected, there is a careful selection of memory, a liberal dosage of invective, and linguistic excess that is palpable within the social economy of their expressions. But the reader and audience of these short stories also can see the fixity of particular features of the disease (psychological, physiological, and sociological) that demands accountability. These expressions do not bear the same *weight of a history that cannot be absorbed* or *a sorrow that cannot be managed* in the Quilt. They only offer perspectives on living with the disease and open new spaces of possibility in the ever-present specter of probability.

These are a series of vulnerable stories and subjectivities. They are not vulnerable because they demand empathy or sympathy from the reader. They are vulnerable because they expose that which is always being concealed in the discourse of the AIDS Memorial Quilt—and maybe more important in HIV/AIDS discourse, the positionality of the dead in relation to those living with HIV/AIDS, as well as a particular admission of self-implication in the context of suffering, death, and mourning. As an organizational and interpretative mechanism, a series of themes with brief framing logics emerged in the ethnographic interviews. The themes and the accompanying analytical frames are not meant to override or dominate the voices featured; they are to help the reader contextualize the offerings of the narrative in the larger context of this project and reveal the ways in which the narratives *defy and demystify the ubiquity and magnitude* of the AIDS Memorial Quilt, while contributing new insights to its continued power as a trope of HIV/AIDS. The first theme deals with the relationships between individuals, the cultural communities in which they claim membership, and the pressure of being cultural members in the face of HIV/AIDS. The second theme addresses the conundrum of living and dying at the same time. Men infected with HIV/AIDS articulate a sense of living not in the margins but in spaces of liminality, betwixt and between. The third theme provides a brief glimpse of black gay men who use their HIV/AIDS disposition as an opportunity for public information and activism.

Stitching Notions of the Individual, Community, and AIDS

AIDS has its own stigma, both for the particularity of the individual and for the community to which the victim holds membership. Whether through the stigma of the disease or the manner of assumed contraction, sex or intravenous drug use, both the private and the public becomes implicated in the statistical chronicling and the categories of designation that are part of the disease and the marked lives of those infected. I use the preceding heading as a thematic precursor to utterances made by these black gay men as an immediate response and reflection on their HIV-positive diagnosis.

Black gay men's awareness of the growing number of AIDS cases in the black community, and the still-contested nature of the black community's orientation to "gayness," places a particular racial and cultural burden on their self-realization, forestalling their moments of personal grief in the alchemy of race, sexuality, and the mediated space of home.[12] In the interview protocol the question framing this response was "What was your immediate response to receiving the news of your HIV-positive status?"

> JAMES: The first thing I said when I got my test results was, "I am a God Damn Statistic!" How many times have I heard the growing statistics of black gay men contracting HIV/AIDS? How many fucking times had I thought of black friends and Black people that I know who got the bug? How many fucking times had I thought about how stupid they must be—don't fuck without a condom, don't rim, don't swallow, don't share needles, don't fucking share bodily fluids! And here I am . . . I sat there for a while, in the waiting room of that free clinic and just thought *What the fuck?* . . . Really as a question, not a statement of fact . . . and because I was sitting in this public space reading something so private and personal . . . made to be so clinical . . . I was also trying to control or maybe contain my response . . . but I saw other stunned, blank, and

worried faces looking down on test results or looking into space waiting for test results and thought . . . how in the fuck did I get here?

. . . And then I began to think about my mother, and my family. I began thinking about how disappointed they would be in me . . . and that somehow they would do what everybody does with this disease . . . just think that it is the ultimate cost of being gay, the payback, the punishment, GOD's wrath . . . and they are being punished too . . . being shamed. I knew that people would be disappointed in me for somehow voluntarily throwing away my life . . . me the former altar boy, . . . the first-generation college boy who should know better, . . . the one who presumably made "a choice" to be gay, . . . the one who did something nasty, and now I had to pay the price. For black people AIDS was a white man's disease . . . hell, being gay was for white boys . . . And here I am another black boy with a white man's disease . . . another black boy lost.

DARRYL: I didn't know what to say . . . I didn't know who to tell . . . For the first time I didn't think that I could go home . . . it was bad enough that I was a black fag, but now to be a black fag with AIDS just seemed like I was a random statistic . . . it was almost laughable . . . Years before, I remember attending the funeral of this older black guy in the community. Nobody ever really talked about Mr. Clyde. My Clyde was never married and had no children—in that way in my community, in which signs of being straight was either being seen in the company of women or having children, as the evidence of being with women. No one really talked about him, he did work in the church and in the community and for those reasons people didn't talk about his personal life . . . But as a little black gay boy I remember looking at Mr. Clyde and seeing how he looked at me . . . it was that gay look that people sometime called the gaydar. It was a way of looking that suggested interest, but not in that lecherous old man look, but a way of seeing me and letting me know that he really saw me . . . until Mr. Clyde, I didn't think that anyone saw me as gay. And in some ways I liked that, but I didn't really want to be seen by others because being seen and being known in this way in the black community was dangerous . . . at his funeral people said nice things about him, but no one broached the subject that he might have died from AIDS . . . I had seen him in my years of going back and forth . . . and in his face I saw that face of some of my gay friends who had died or were dying with AIDS . . . partially gaunt and hollowed but overly muscular, eyes bulging, and a body trapped somewhere between wasting and gaining . . . I saw it in his eyes and he would see me seeing it in his eyes . . . and I said nothing and he said nothing. Mr. Clyde is like so many black gay men in my childhood—their gayness was markedly real for other black gay men, but somehow invisible to others in the community . . .

When I came out people immediately called me fag, black fag, bitch . . . and I could not go unnoticed and uncritiqued . . . maybe like Mr. Clyde . . . I could have been tolerated, if I just didn't talk about it . . . then I had to tell my parents I was HIV-positive . . . because I just didn't want to disappear . . . but when I told them I really became invisible . . . I could see the shame and embarrassment . . . I saw them staring at me and then not seeing me at all. So I left.

Maybe I am just a statistic, not really from AIDS but of the homophobes in the black community . . . I think about Mr. Clyde's funeral a lot and wonder about the consequences of being out . . . the only difference is that my parents attended Mr. Clyde's funeral.

The narratives of James and Darryl move me, and I am not surprised by the nature of their talk, which is not exclusively of their own mortality but about the social and cultural implications of their diagnosis. Each addresses the issues of family, culture, and community as key elements in responding to their diagnosis. Each invokes issues of stigmatization, alienation, and the silence in the black community on issues of HIV/AIDS, but they clearly signal the racial expectedness of heterosexuality as a performance of masculinity and of being a black man.

The politics of the AIDS Memorial Quilt invokes the rhetoric of loss, the rhetoric of memorials, and the rhetoric of activism. The sheer expanse of the original display of the quilt was in many ways a piece of visual rhetoric, a political statement on the magnitude of the epidemic and a call for more federal funding for research.[13] But what I am particularly interested in is the potentially unspoken narratives that are also written in the Quilt; narratives of gay men living cloistered lives; narratives of boys and men being ostracized from their families at the knowledge of them being gay; narratives of family shame and embarrassment at their diseased child that forestalls the immediacy of embrace, leaving men like James and Darryl isolated from family and community at a time when such support might inform the care that they need.

My mother was a nurse's aid, often caring for sick and dying children on a pediatric ward at a state run hospital in Lafayette, Louisiana. While my brother was not quickly forthcoming with the news of his diagnosis, my mother detected his symptoms. It was she who recommended that he move from his apartment in New Orleans back home to Lafayette. It was she who cared for him in the last year and a half of his life as the disease quickly progressed. It was she who initially called me at graduate school in Southern Illinois and told me of his illness, and, knowing that I too was gay, she told me to practice safe sex. It was she who told me that she was taking an early retirement to care for him and that she did not want me to come until it was over. This was an act of care; this was a precaution to keep from seeing me in the company of him—(like James) her two gay college boys. After my brother's death my mother began to speak at local churches and town meetings about HIV/AIDS. She spoke to mostly black audiences about the disease, explaining the links between caution, care, community, and culture. I assisted her with her speaking notes and sat once in the back of a partially filled cafeteria as she spoke. These are experiences of HIV/AIDS that are not narrated on the current Quilt but could serve as powerful expressions—those *living with* HIV/AIDS and negotiating the boundaries between culture and mortality, between compromised health and cultural compromise, and between loss and renewed conviction of possibility.

RESISTING FORECLOSURE: CONSCIOUS AWARENESS OF LIVING AND DYING AT THE SAME TIME

Performance theorist Richard Schechner wrote, "performance is not a passive mirror of . . . social changes but a part of the complicated feedback process that creates change."[14] In the stories in this set, the act of telling is an act of resisting the foreclosure of the told and the actuality of living. The act of telling is a resistance to the limited narrative of HIV/AIDS that says *you contract it and you die*. The stories told by Jason and Thomas are whimsical and painful resistance to this reductive aphorism in ways that acknowledge the perils of diagnosis buttressed against the reality of being. The oral presentations of thought serve as moments of *therapy discourse*—outing concerns of self and building a "mutating, transitory cultural intelligibility of agency, within the frame of social temporality that renders the . . . self culturally 'coherent.'"[15]

And while I am using Judith Butler's construction in this moment, I am less interested in the ways in which such *coherence* is a reference to some link between sex, gender, sexuality, and sexual practice. In these short stories these men are establishing coherence between the reality of illness and the sustainability of their unbroken spirits, who they were and continue to be in the face of the intervening complications of HIV/AIDS. Within these stories, their performance and presentation of self is part of a feedback loop of sustainability that is not just about living, but also about thriving in shifting conditions of being. In the interview protocol the question framing this response was "What is your general outlook on life or living with HIV/AIDS?"

JASON: I have good days and bad days, count up/count down, strong and looking healthy/weak and looking sick . . . In some ways I don't mind being sick. After 10 years of being diagnosed, I've come to grips with my situation . . . I just don't like looking sick . . . you know? The precarious nature of this disease is that it takes over and while I have the choice to care for myself and keep up on my meds—there are things going on in me that are beyond my control—so I am *kinda living and dying at the same time* and each day tells the tale of which side is winning . . . but I am not dead yet. I have a lot of things that I need to accomplish . . . I want to finish my Master's degree. I want to realize my dream of teaching in a Community College, I want to really fall in love . . . you know . . . to find someone that really loves me and me him . . . not just somebody to fuck—that's easy, and I think that is what got me like this . . . just fucking.

You know I was one of those rare kids that my parents actually had the "birds and the bees" talk with . . . well it was actually my grand-mother . . . The only thing I really remember her saying was something about sex and marriage, but she said sex in love is the best . . . and the fruits of that love would flourish . . . that's how I remember that . . . She was probably talking about children—even though I thought that she was the only one that really got me . . . So when I was told that I was HIV-positive I thought that *that* sex wasn't love, and if I was in love then, I wouldn't be sick now . . . I know that's silly . . . but I ain't dead yet—so I am still looking for love, and maybe that will make this living hell better.

THOMAS: I went to a party last week and there was this guy that I dated . . . well I just fucked him regularly . . . but I hadn't seen him in years. He knew that I had AIDS, and I knew that he had AIDS, but we had eliminated the possibility of co-infecting each other . . . he was years ago . . . And when he saw me he said, "You're still alive?" And I said, "I'm not dead yet!" and we both laughed. It was a funny moment . . . I guess someone hearing that story might think "how sick!" But it was damn funny. We weren't really laughing at AIDS or being sick—because we've lost a lot of friends . . . We weren't really laughing at being still alive because that would be looking a gifted horse in the mouth . . . I think that we were laughing at the ways in which time and absence has a way of fading memories, almost like death, and somehow in our memories we had killed each other off . . . but in that moment we realized that our memories of each other were very much alive, just suppressed—maybe like my immune system just waiting to be reminded or ignited . . . I guess we were also just laughing because instead of just fucking, we used to laugh a lot . . . and I still like to laugh . . . I haven't lost that.

I like these narrative moments and enjoyed interviewing these men. Jason and Thomas embraced life, even as they were very cognizant of the realities of their diagnosed condition. Each offered a counternarrative of optimism to the "death sentence" narrative of HIV/AIDS, and the particular reification and reminder of death that the AIDS Memorial Quilt represents—both as reminder for political argument and memorial for those lost. Each invoked the longevity of their lives after diagnosis and a particular zeal for life. Each make a distinction between having sex and being in love as correlate acknowledgments often associated with and not associated with gay life—in that way in which gay men are depicted as promiscuous without the sustainability of meaningful monogamous relationships. Jason is still searching for love and Thomas gives a sense of interpersonal knowing as a foundation for meaningful relational engagement.

In a practical and biblical sense, my father would always remind his seven children that we are mortal creatures and we are born to die, that the meaningfulness of who we are will be measured in the deeds accomplished in a fixed expanse of living. One of my father's best friends when I was growing up was a man named Mr. Walter. Mr. Walter worked for the church and maintained the cemetery. Often he would give me a couple of dollars to help him clean graves. Around Easter and All Saints Day people would pay him to scrape their loved ones' graves and apply a fresh coat of white paint as a sign of their continued care and dedication. Some of my friends thought it morbid, but I enjoyed the work. I enjoyed reading the stories told on each grave. The state of the grave reflected the presence or absence of living relatives. It told a story of care, concern, and diligence. The death markers, birth date, and death date symbolized the longevity of life, and the pictures of the deceased offered a faded glimpse of a life once lived. Some headstones, like obituaries, also listed surviving family: "She is survived by . . ." and then the names of a spouse or children or siblings. These are narratives fixed in stone that the passage of time cannot augment. I often wondered, *Is her husband still alive? Are her children still alive? Is she now a grandmother or great-grandmother?* The AIDS Memorial Quilt narrates such stories and timelines, but the commemoration of the death is also a commemoration of the disease; on the Quilt, rows of names in fixed plots, like veterans of war taken under the same conditions, establish a linear logic from diagnosis to death. The stories of Jason and Thomas give way to new possibilities in narrating the story of those *living with* HIV/AIDS. They are storylines that are not as fixed as those told on headstones or on the Quilt. They offer stories that narrate new adventures, stories that resist quick foreclosure because of the disease, stories that tell of people engaging the challenges of living.

EXIGENCIES AND POLITICAL NECESSITIES, OR "(NOT) FUCKING WITH WILD ABANDON"

When I use the word "exigencies," I am referencing situations that demand attention, that we ignore only at our own regret or peril. Exigencies straddle the borders between problems and opportunities. In the following short stories, these men comment and critique on exigencies of knowing and doing, offering critical reflections on being and becoming, and of knowing and acting. Their HIV-positive status is reframed as an exigency *to act,* not merely react. And the notion of *fucking (or not fucking) with wild abandon* becomes metaphor for a particular level of engagement in light of moral responsibility and reasoned acknowledgment of the potential consequences. While casual in nature, these short stories drawn from ethnographic interviews offer critical expressions within an interpretive community. Lives are laid bare, and responses to the exigencies are both personal and political. In the interview protocol, the question framing this response was "As someone living with HIV/AIDS, do you see yourself having a social role?"

> ALAN: I have heard older gay men tell stories of the heyday of gay life . . . variably marked somewhere in the 60s, 70s, and even the 80s for some. They tell stories of being able to "fuck with wild abandon" in parks, public bathrooms, and bath houses with little fear of painful consequences . . . short of, for them, contracting an "easily treated" venereal disease. I have always been curious as to why these stories are told . . . They are like the opposite of those . . . "we had to walk through sleet and snow, ten miles to get to school kinda-stories" . . . but, in this case, "fucking with wild abandon" is meant to be a story of advantage and not hardship. I used to think that if that was the case, then they were asking for it . . . not knowing what "it" was, and not wanting to say that they deserved to get sick—but shit . . . "fucking with wild abandon" and many of these old shits were now healthier than me . . .
>
> I came out at age twenty. I had my first sexual encounter with a man at age twenty-one, and I was diagnosed as HIV-positive at age twenty-two. I am now twenty-five. I didn't have a heyday of "fucking

with wild abandon." Before contracting the disease I was only with two guys. Being diagnosed made me feel like an object lesson, like someone was being taught a lesson, and I was the visual aid. I thought to myself that I did all the right things . . . I don't remember being careless in any other aspect of my life and not even in that moment . . . that moment when I contracted the virus, I didn't feel that I was being careless . . . I was making love with someone that I cared about, who wasn't honest with me about his own history . . . I now kinda wish that I had been "fucking with wild abandon," at least I would have good stories to tell . . . [*laughs*] . . . not really, that's not me . . .

So now I spend time volunteering . . . talking to young black gay boys who think that it can't happen to them, boys who "come on to me" while I am trying to talk to them about safe sex, . . . boys who don't think it can happen to them . . . I feel good about what I am doing, and while I am still healthy (and I plan to be for a long time) I want to dedicate my life to educating young people about the disease so that they don't become an object lesson.

TERRENCE: My mother used to laugh and say that I came out of her womb gay. "He was just born that way." That became a family joke that was librating in some ways—when compared to so many of my friends who lived their lives in the closet and heard their parents talking about hating fags . . . But it was not so funny when people didn't always take me seriously . . . like being gay was being mentally retarded or . . . being gay meant being "not all there," or not a "real man" . . . or assuming that I did when I didn't know the first thing . . .

But I have always been out, and for that I am proud that I have never pretended to be something that I am not. I am happy to have people who have always loved me for me—even if they didn't always take me seriously. Now I want to be taken seriously . . . because if they don't take me serious—then they don't take this disease serious and more boys like me die because no one is taking anything serious . . . and they assume that I know and I don't . . . and kids are told "not to fuck," so they fuck, instead of being told "if you're going to fuck, then use a condom" . . . That's what people say when they take it serious and they want to protect you.

Of course we all have a social role. A role within the larger matrix of culture and society, family and friends, place and space. But roles shift as the conditions of living change, and as the exigencies for action become immediate and contingent. Each of the men in the interviews paused on the wording of the question. Some asked for clarification, "*Do you mean, now that I am living with HIV/AIDS, has my sense of my social role changed?*" Each played with what might have been a loaded question that expected a shift in their social consciousness once they became aware of their diagnosis. This was an intentional lead on my part, one that had an anticipated rejection or capitulation as a test of attitudinal shift. The responses varied, but Alan and Terrence offered the expanse of these responses.

Alan's response reminds me of stories told by elders of any cultural community who reflect on past exploits with a sense of nostalgia that both celebrates and mourns the past. In Alan's case, the nostalgic turn was invoked by his queer elders in relation to random unprotected sex, even in light of known potential consequences of such actions, both pre- and post-AIDS. Alan playfully mourns an unlived past as he also narrates an alternative construction of gay life that does not invoke promiscuity and play—which are often associated with being gay and contracting HIV/AIDS through sexual transmission. He narrates a story of many gay men whose personal integrity and unfortunate circumstances are overshadowed by the specificity of their illness and the social construction or reduction of that meaning. By informing young black gay boys of the disease, Alan continues to claim and enact a social role of service and information sharing. His narrative helps to dissipate the miasma of the epidemic and the cultural ignorance that leads to young black boys living cloistered gay lives without caution.

The narrative that Terrence offers pivots on the notion of "taking it serious"—taking gay lives seriously, as well as taking the time to seriously talk about HIV/AIDS. Terrence invokes aspects of my own experience as a young black gay boy. In the midst of family friends and neighborhood kids, I remember being taken seriously as a good student and maybe taken seriously as a creative person or a relatively articulate person, but I was not taken seriously as a young man—not in the same ways that the more hyper-heterosexual boys, and even my three straight brothers, were.

That reality in my black cultural community, and maybe in Terrence's, reinforced a pernicious homophobia. It reinforced a hatred for what is reductively perceived as the feminine in the man, as well as a reductive perception of women altogether, establishing a sense of social value very early in our lives of what it means to be a man (to be straight) and the social positioning of that designation.

While Terrence speaks of a particular joy of having always been out and known, his not being taken seriously as a gay man living with HIV/AIDS presents a huge risk—the risk of the disease also not being taken seriously because of the population it seemingly most affects.[16] Terrance's call is a social position as well as a political position, one that sits at the intersections of assumed knowledge and necessary action, a place where "fucking with wild abandon" and not taking it seriously has consequences for self and society.

Self-Constructed Eulogies for the AIDS Quilt

As Vivian M. Patraka noted in "Spectacles of Suffering," "no historical referent is either stable, transparent in its meaning, agreed upon in its usage, or even engaged with in the same way by a large group of people."[17] The AIDS Memorial Quilt means different things to different people. The following short stories are responses to the question "What would you want your panel on the AIDS quilt to represent about you?" The responses are varied, from abject refusal of a panel to playful self-constructions, messages about self and other, self as other, and secret messages to private readers. I press these stories together without interceding analysis. Like the actual panels on the Quilt, they are designed to be read in relation to each other, in opposition to and in tension with each other, as collective and mediated memory of the diverse lives that have been taken by HIV/AIDS. These lives speak in their own voices, and the messages are not about an easy solidarity, but a tensive negotiation of being and the remembrance of being.

> DAVID: I don't want a fucking panel on the Quilt . . . I don't know what that would mean . . . So people could look at my name and my story as a fucking object lesson of what not to do? So my panel could end up

folded in some storage room collecting dust, the lost relevance of both my life and a political movement gone bust? Did you see that article in the *LA Times* a couple of months ago? That story about how the AIDS Quilt is stacked in a warehouse in Atlanta?[18] There is nothing worse than losing relevance, of becoming commonplace, or even complacent. AIDS for me is a reality—one that is only relevant to the people who are dying from it . . . and that's sad . . . it [AIDS] has become a part of our national consciousness, something that we have come to live with and die with as if commonplace. There needs to be another great symbol of the disease . . . like a Rock Hudson or Arthur Ashe or Magic Johnson. I am not wishing it on someone, but there needs to be a figure that brings AIDS back into the political consciousness as necessity of concern . . . the quilt was an emotional catharsis whose tears have dried . . . Maybe there should be a public burning of some of the panels . . . not as an act of blasphemy, but as an act of public outrage to mark this anniversary . . . like burning flags—burning banners of hope as a means of igniting a renewed attention.

JOHN: My panel would just say, "Be Careful, Protect Yourself, Protect Your Lover! John." Then the date of my death . . . I've thought about more political statements, like, "It's time for a cure" or "Pressure the Government for More Research," but in the meantime, people who are having sex just need to be safe . . . no exchange of fluids . . . suck, fuck, lick whatever with a condom or a dental dam . . . don't swallow . . . don't let anything in your body . . . I don't know what to say to those fucks who are sharing needles . . . that level of addiction ignores all logics of safety. If I had a panel I would just say, "Be Careful, Protect Yourself, Protect Your Lover!"

DANE: You know that sounds funny . . . [*singing*] "if I had a panel, I'd panel in the morning . . . I'd panel in the evening" . . . [*laughing*]. Do ya get it?[19] [*laughter*]. Okay, I'll get serious. I don't know . . . a couple of years ago my brother was killed by a drunk driver, and I helped my mother pick out a plot and a headstone . . . she bought one for me too. My mother knows that I am HIV-positive—and she's not in good health—so maybe she was mourning in advance for me too. The graveyard is probably one of the saddest places that I have ever visited, but trying to find words for his headstone was painful . . . born—died. What do you write in the middle? . . . Instead of his birth date and death date, we simply wrote—"He lived and he died." My mother thought that he would get a kick out that, and we laughed . . .

I feel good, and I am not planning on dying anytime soon, so I really don't want to plan a panel or a headstone . . . I have seen pictures of the quilt . . . Are they still accepting panels? I think that if I would want anything, maybe it would say, "if I had a panel, I'd panel in the morning . . . I'd panel in the evening" . . . [*laughing*] just kidding. I want to go laughing. I want to go kicking and screaming. What's that poem? I want to rail against the darkness. AIDS is an ugly disease that in my experience effects beautiful people, people looking for love and comfort, the dick or the needle . . . There needs to be more research . . . people need to care more about finding a cure, maybe my panel says something like, "Care more about finding a cure." Maybe it has a picture of my brother's headstone that reads "He lived and he died." My brother would like that.

These three brutally honest yet wonderfully endearing narratives offer bracing constructions of the tellers' orientation to the Quilt, and of the epidemic of HIV/AIDS and their own mortality. David's response is an act of political resistance against the current utility of the AIDS Quilt, but he also clearly articulates a radical repurposing of the Quilt to reignite a social consciousness about the disease that gives manifest meaning, not to the artifact but to the issue that the quilt signifies. John's response is a call for personal caution and responsibility that speaks with the power of testimony from an affected/infected party, the type of message that both speaks to and embodies the consequences of its opposite. And Dane's message is a playful response that invokes the resiliency of the human spirit in the face of terrible odds, and the compassion of care that advocates change.

These short stories serve as counternarratives in the ways in which they give voice to those for whom panels have been constructed. Panels mostly constructed with the best intentions by lovers and loved ones, by family and friends who articulate their own desire, regret, and remembrance; panels that document the dead and their lives. The brief narratives offered here of men living with HIV/AIDS mostly resist the fixity of the linear construction from diagnosis to death. And while each of these men understand the complications of their situation in relation to current research and the still-stalled race to a cure, they are not resigned to just lay down their lives. John and Dane, who have begun to figuratively construct their own panels for the Quilt, each offered memoirs of their personality and calls for a cure. In contrast, Joseph chose to address the question of his own panel in this way:

> JOSEPH: I know that a well-constructed quilt displays the skill of the person or persons crafting it. And I know that the aesthetics of a quilt often suggests or presents a recognizable pattern, a unified whole . . . but I wouldn't want to have a panel on a quilt like that or even the AIDS Quilt . . . I don't think I would fit . . . I know that AIDS attacks our bodies in similar ways, but all my life I have been described as a "black gay man" . . . Yeah, of course I am a black man, and I am a gay man, but the distinction of me being a black gay man has always been made—either by my family, who never accepted me as gay, or the general gay community, mostly white, . . . that has used race as a demarcater of difference within community . . . So I cringe when I don't see the distinction of black gay lives who have died from AIDS on the Quilt, and maybe they are on the Quilt and nothing is ever made of that . . . maybe if I had a panel it would just be a piece of kente cloth that symbolized all the lost black lives . . . maybe that would create a pattern with a pattern.

On Eulogies, Narratives, and Rhetorical Hybrids

I think of the AIDS Memorial Quilt as a *rhetorical hybrid,* a communicative act with complex and competing intentionalities in the performative moment of its presentation. Or as Kathleen Hall Jamieson and Karlyn Kohrs Campbell state, "'rhetorical hybrids' is a metaphor intended to emphasize the productive but transitory character of these combinations."[20] Jamieson and Campbell are addressing the concept of genre as dynamic fusions in the particular cases of political and presidential rhetoric in the context of the eulogy. I want to apply their heuristic metaphor to the AIDS Memorial Quilt, and the rhetorical messaging of its intent and presence as eulogy, as memorial. In particular, what makes the Quilt a rhetorical hybrid is the intertextual quality in which it engages the intensions of eulogies, mixed with the dynamic stillness of an artifact as visual rhetoric to invoke a narrative—both of a disease and the lives lost to that disease, engaging what Jamieson and Campbell refer to as the deliberative quality, an appeal to action.[21] In other words, in its complexity the AIDS Memorial Quilt serves as both memorial (eulogies for the dead and a rhetoric of remembrance), as well as an act of intervention. So while I want to address the contributing qualities of this hybridity, I will not tease these elements out as separate, but always and already as collaborative qualities of the rhetorical and narrative gestalt of the Quilt, "linking individual human actions and events into interrelated aspects of an understandable composite."[22]

In *Acts of Intervention: Performance, Gay Culture, and AIDS,* David Román writes: "Before the Names Project's unfolding of the AIDS Memorial Quilt at the 1987 March on Washington for Lesbian and Gay Rights, the most public AIDS memorializations were candlelight vigils." Hence the AIDS Memorial Quilt served as a particular *act of intervention* and a *performance of protest* in the crisis of AIDS to further publicize the disease, to quantify the magnitude of its effects, to take a public stance on needed research/money/legislation in finding a cure for the disease, and to memorialize if not eulogize the lives of the dead and HIV/AIDS infected gay men.[23]

The eulogy as performance fits under the more expansive umbrella of performance as commemoration—which is true of the AIDS Memorial Quilt. In this medium, performance is engaged as a means of documenting the life and character of an absent other, an absent experience, or an absent construct of the self. Specifically, commemoration is an act of remembrance and recovery. Eugene Vance defines commemoration as "any gesture, ritualized or not, whose end is to recover, in the name of collectivity, some being or even either anterior in time or outside of time in order to fecundate, animate, or make meaningful a moment in the present."[24] Performance as commemoration can include eulogy, testimony, personal narrative, ethnography, biography, autobiography, autoethnography, and

other performances of reflection, remembrance, remorse, and mourning
that the AIDS Memorial Quilt both engages and signifies.

Within the expressive ethnographies included in this chapter, we
see the ways in which personal experience and the relation to disease,
death, and despair are played out as a means of noting absence and simultaneously invoking the absence as presence. In particular, the narratives of men living with HIV/AIDS offer performative constructions that
animate the dead and make dynamic their own continued existence as a
contested sight of struggle and possibility. Linda Park-Fuller states, "All
performances, and indeed all arts give testimony to absences—even as
they manifest presence."[25]

The eulogy is always in relation to an absent other, thus it is a referen-
tial (auto)biographical performance that recounts the life of another in relation to the self, the person/circumstance/context of marking the death.
In the case of the AIDS Memorial Quilt, the individual stories—eulogies
and memorials of those who died—are sutured and stitched together to
amplify a shared experience or circumstance of death. In literal ways,
while the eulogy is often the process of unreading a life text in order to
recontextualize the life lived, the stitching of such stories into a collective
fabric of social consciousness frames the magnitude of common experience for political purposes. But Della Pollock asks a series of questions
that can appropriately be applied to the eulogy as I am now contextual-
izing it in relation to the AIDS Quilt:

> What happens when a story begins in absence? When it takes its
> momentum from a gap, a break, a border space, or element of differ-
> ence that violates laws of repetition and re-presentation even in the
> act of repeating, retelling, [and] representing [a life]? What happens
> when "the boundary becomes the place from *which something begins
> its presencing*"?[26]

In the case of the AIDS Memorial Quilt, the teller of the story, the one
who constructed the panel for a loved one or the one left behind, becomes a *stand between person,* helping others (and the self) to cross over,
mediating and bridging the chasm between life and death, presence and
absence, or the social reconstructions of memory and desire.[27] In fact,

the eulogizer for the individual person/panel is engulfed in the collective eulogy of the Quilt. And like the very nature of Pollock's query, the AIDS Memorial Quilt, as the moment and mode of eulogizing the dead, becomes the place in which the larger issues of the disease are illuminated.

The Quilt becomes that argument that seeks to halt the momentum; it becomes the public statement that articulates the violation of human laws in the slow responses to the disease. The Quilt serves as suture in the gap, bridging breaks and border spaces that might suggest elements of difference to halt the act of repeating, retelling, and representing the same patterns of disease, death, and loss. But like the experience told by some of the black gay men in this project, racialized difference in the epidemic of HIV/AIDS is not always present in the actual Quilt, though the sentiment of the collective struggle might suggest so. And unlike the oral performance of testimony or traditional eulogies, the silence of this visual rhetoric speaks volumes to the silence in HIV/AIDS research; it speaks volumes to the absent voices unable to speak. Yet their stories are made present in the graphic representation of mourning, an absence made present, a feeling made palpable.

The AIDS Memorial Quilt functions as eulogy, a commemoration of a life. It "responds to those human needs created when a community is sundered by the death of one of its members. In Western culture, at least, a eulogy will acknowledge the death, transform the relationship between the living and the dead from present to past tense, ease the mourners' terror at confronting their own mortality; console them by arguing that the deceased lives on, and reknit the community."[28] But in the political efficacy of the AIDS Memorial Quilt, a community of the dead is constructed and extended to encompass an entirety of humanity, and the consolation becomes not only that of containing emotions but also of igniting passions and urging action.

The eulogistic requirements can be teased out to show how the AIDS Memorial Quilt disrupts these traditional functions for broader political purposes:

- A eulogy responds to those human needs created when a community is sundered by the death of one of its members.
- A eulogy will acknowledge the death.

- A eulogy will attempt to transform the relationship between the living and the dead from present to past tense.
- A eulogy establishes the relationship between the speaker and the deceased and those on whose behalf the speaker speaks.
- A eulogy may attempt to reconcile the interpersonal relationship between the speaker and the deceased.
- A eulogy may attempt to ease the mourners' terror at confronting their own mortality.
- A eulogy will console the mourners by arguing that the deceased lives on.
- A eulogy will signal shared cultural beliefs about death.
- A eulogy will attempt to reknit the community.

The complex of these requirements of the traditional eulogy is to be accomplished in a manner fit for the solemnity of the occasion. Yet I suggest that the AIDS Memorial Quilt takes these particular acts for more public intentions. Yes, the Quilt *responds to those human needs created when a community is sundered by the death of one of its members,* but the Quilt takes the private deaths and coalesces them into a collective public mourning that transforms the actuality of death into a political call for action—linking deaths not exclusively to practices but also to lack of governmental action in finding a cure for AIDS. The AIDS Memorial Quilt does not *seek to move the reality of death from the present to past tense* as much as it magnifies in the present to make arguments for the future. The AIDS Memorial Quilt *establishes the relationship between the gay community* (those living and deceased) with a larger public and political agenda of human rights and protections.

The Quilt as eulogy *reconciles interpersonal relationships between the speaker and the deceased;* however, it also uses the occasion of death as a means of unsettling notions of governmental inaction toward the disease, especially as perceivably linked exclusively to the gay community. Hence, the actuality of death and the deceased are engaged in a public awareness campaign for the disease and needed action toward a cure. In essence, unlike traditional eulogies, the AIDS Memorial Quilt as eulogy does not make *attempts to ease the mourners' terror at confronting their own mortality.* In fact, the Quilt and the occasion of its display and presence attempt to ignite renewed awareness of the disease and how it is contracted, as well as force a particular confrontation between mourners and their own potentially unsafe practices (and that of hospitals, in the cases of HIV transmissions through tainted blood supplies).

The AIDS Memorial Quilt in its original construction and subsequent growth served to continually dramatize the disease and its potential to further devastate the gay community and beyond. The collective efforts of organizers and contributors to the NAMES Project invoked collective concerns and cultural beliefs about death, care, and humanity—coalescing a public memory for those who have died of AIDS. Thus the project works toward *reknitting community* through a call for action on the local level of safer sex practices and on the government level of increased funds for researching a cure.

Shifting from the AIDS Memorial Quilt to the NAMES Project redirects the focus of this analysis from the particular artifact (the Quilt) to the larger political project that the artifact signifies. Jamieson and Campbell argue that a "functional hybrid will occur when deliberative appeals are subordinate to the eulogy, when they can be viewed as a memorial to the life of the deceased, when they are compatible with positions advocated by the eulogist."[29] In this construction the reference is to an individual rhetor, one person responding to the particularity of an individual death, linking the death and the occasion of the eulogy to a larger political intent. Yet the NAMES Project is a collective political action offering response to a large-scale epidemic and a multitude of deaths.

The eulogizing and memorializing intent of the NAMES Project uses the Quilt as a vehicle for delivering the message. Hence, the deliberative appeal (in the campaign, in the Quilt) is not subordinate to the eulogy or the act of memorializing the dead. The politicized message and the medium are a coordinated effort. And in effect "deliberative elements fuse to form organic wholes when they are consistent with and contribute to the goals of the eulogy," or in the case of the NAMES Project, the larger campaign that the Quilt signifies. Jamieson and Campbell go on to state that "hybrids are called forth by complex situations and purposes and, as such, are transitory and situation bound."[30]

The epidemic of HIV/AIDS is a complex social crisis that has necessitated complex and concerted information campaigns and calls to action.

HIV/AIDS is still a bound circumstance, and the eulogizing aspects of the Quilt are still fixed—both as historical archive and performative repertoire. It is a host of rhetorical strategies that remember the dead, call for action, and narrate storied lives. The men interviewed in this project present their stories as affective rhetors, men narrating aspects of their own lived and living experience in relation to HIV/AIDS and the AIDS Memorial Quilt, as artifact to the disease and their predicament of living. Their narratives are eulogies for the dead and for the living; the narratives are deliberate and deliberative—intentional and careful, appealing and advocating—both for those who have died and for their own situated being. And, in this sense, their participation in this ethnographic project, like the NAMES Project that gave way to the AIDS Memorial Quilt, is a functional and effective rhetorical hybrid working toward common goals with an emphasis on the future.

The AIDS Quilt as a Continued Performance of Possibilities: A Conclusion

Since the inception of the NAMES Project, and in particular the political campaign that is the AIDS Memorial Quilt, no cure for HIV/AIDS has been found. While the political potency of the project stands as a historical testament to collective political action, both as demand for increased research funding and as an information campaign on the spread of the disease, the Quilt has become *archival memory*, static and fixed. In *The Archive and the Repertoire: Performing Cultural Memory in the Americas*, Diana Taylor writes: "What changes over time is the values, relevance, or meaning of the archive, how items it contains get interpreted, even embodied . . . Bones might remain the same, even though their story may change, depending on the paleontologist or forensic anthropologist who examines them."[31] To what degree is the AIDS Memorial Quilt still relevant? How might we, like paleontologists or forensic anthropologists, reexamine *the body of* and *the bodies in* the Quilt to find renewed understanding and a renewed conviction to the motivating impulse of the project as a whole, giving continued credence to the roll call of names that the project narrates?

The voices in this ethnoperformative text serve as testimony to desire and the continued efficacy of political activism on issues related to HIV/AIDS research that at once commemorates the historical significance of the NAMES Project while resisting the historicizing of lives still living in hope. Each story and the brief analyses that stitch them together throughout this project serve as hypothetical entries in a renewed NAMES Project; they serve as rhetorics of possibility: strategically constructed communications drawn from ethnographic interviews that articulate the dense particularity of the respondent living in the present, speaking of both the past and the future with the intent to motivate action, assuage the grief of loss, and perform a particular resistance to the social stigma of living with HIV/AIDS.

To what degree might an expanded ethnographic project collecting the stories of those living with HIV/AIDS serve as a foundation to invigorate a new NAMES Project, one that does not memorialize the dead but narrates and expands the repertoire of enacted possibility while meaningfully reinterpreting the archive (the Quilt)? How might such a project celebrate possibility, reanimating the abject bodies of those who have died in relation to their living counterparts, all while reinforcing the continued need for research, not just to extend lives but also to save lives? How might such a project also illuminate the diversity of experiences within HIV/AIDS—including the stories of raced others, accidental transmissions, children born with the disease, rape survivors, women who have contracted the disease from their husbands, men who are intravenous drugs users and/or are living on the down low, and "bug chasers," those who seek the disease as an act of fatal commitment or activism. As with the men in this study, the articulation of stories that implicate race, culture, and community in the social construction of gendered identities sometimes results in alienation—both before and after diagnosis.

In "Performance, Personal Narratives, and the Politics of Possibility," D. Soyini Madison identifies a list of prescriptions for a "performance of possibilities."[32] Madison's work is grounded in building an ethic for embodied performance as a tool for social change in the realm of performance and critical ethnography. In many ways, the NAMES Project and the AIDS Memorial Quilt engage in performance as critical ethnography. Broadly constructed performance ethnography is literally the staged reenactment of ethnographically derived notes. This approach to studying and staging culture works toward lessening the gap between a perceived and actualized sense of self and the other. This is accomplished through the union and practice of two distinct yet interrelated disciplinary formations—*performance studies* and *ethnography*. Practitioners of performance ethnography acknowledge the fact that culture travels in the stories, practices, and desires of those who engage it.[33] In this sense, the AIDS Memorial Quilt is just that—an aggregate of stories, practices, and desires that provided a particular vision of a cultural landscape. Through the efforts of friends, families, and lovers, the stories of the deceased are told to make real the loss associated with AIDS and to politicize the disease in human terms.

Madison's construct of a *performance of possibilities* speaks to the intentions of the AIDS Memorial Quilt in palpable ways. As a *performance of possibilities,* the NAMES Project functions as a politically engaged pedagogy that never has to convince a predefined subject—whether empty or full, whether essential or fragmented—to adopt a new position. Rather, the task is to win over an already positioned, already invested individual or group to a different set of places, a different organization of *the space of possibilities*. A renewed NAMES Project that focuses on the voices of those living with HIV/AIDS would reignite political activism that focuses on future possibility and not exclusively on loss.

A renewed NAMES Project as a *performance of possibilities* would take the stand that performance matters because it does something in the world. And what it does for the audience, the subjects, and those engaged in it must be driven by a thoughtful critique of assumptions and purpose. It must be grounded in politics for social change, both on the level of governmental intervention and personal practice. The voices of those living with HIV/AIDS should serve as the new representative members of the campaign, not a list of names of those lost, narrated for effect by family, celebrities, and politicians—but actual narratives voiced from the embodied place of experience.

A renewed NAMES Project as a *performance of possibilities* and as an interrogative field would aim to create or contribute to a discursive space where unjust systems and processes are identified and interrogated. What has been expressed through the illumination of voice and the encounter with subjectivity motivates individuals to some level of informed and strategic action. The voices of those living with HIV/AIDS are the voices most significant to a renewed activism; through embodied, emotional, and affective testimony, the actualization of those living in the liminality caused by a lack of cure and the social constructions of gender and disease can be more effectively illustrated.

A renewed NAMES Project as a *performance of possibilities* would motivate performers and spectators to appropriate the rhetorical currency they need, from the inner space of the performance to the outer domain of the social world in order to make a material difference. In this sense, as David suggested in his resistance to formulating a panel, whether in a literal or figurative sense, the rhetorical currency of the Quilt as archive can be appropriated as critical reflection on progress in an invigorated repertoire of performative activism.

A renewed NAMES Project as a *performance of possibilities* is moral responsibility and artistic excellence that culminates in the active intervention of unfair closures, *remaking* the possibility for new openings that bring the margins to a shared center. Such an endeavor would bring a wider range of cultural others affected by the disease into a more unified presence, thereby truly illuminating the magnitude of the disease.

Invoking the work on U.S. Holocaust museums, "within the physical and conceptual envelope of its democratic discourse,"[34] the AIDS Memorial Quilt offered viewers a display of lives as documentation of the disease; documentation as a death toll, documentation as carefully constructed messages from loved ones that bore the weight of their loss; documentation as formal pieces of writing on cloth that provided information, context, and history of a happening; documentation as evidence of action or inaction; documentation as a database or spreadsheet chronicling the particularity of an experience of loss. The AIDS Memorial Quilt, like the Holocaust Memorial Museum, has become an archive—a museum that reinforces "the ethical ideal of American political culture by presenting the negation of those ideals," as well as our historical response to them, on public display for inspection, reflection, contemplation, and mourning.[35]

Like the "dilemma of resisting the total erasure of represented absence" that chronicles the brutality of rapes and butchery in Jewish concentration camps, the short stories in this chapter offer counternarratives to the unspoken stories the Memorial Quilt could not capture.[36] These stories are told in the present voice by *mourning subjects* who have not fully laid down their burden. They understand the efficacy of struggle and the necessity of survival. In this project, I have offered only a minimal representation of their narratives (coupled with my own story of loss)—narratives that are not trapped in what could be constructed as the "blindly optimistic goal of reconciliation" that is often a response to the public display of trauma. These stories, gathered through ethnographic methods, are everyday constructions of living with HIV/AIDS that do not ignore the infrastructure of culture in the narrating of experience.[37] The stories and, more important, the men who tell them, are active agents in the ongoing narrative of HIV/AIDS. Their voices are like new panels for an invigorated NAMES Project that would promote rhetorics of living.

NOTES

Throughout this chapter I use narrative entries drawn from ethnographic interviews with black gay men living with HIV/AIDS. My initial encounter was through a member of a HIV/AIDS men's support group who invited me to address the collective about this project. Subsequently, ten members volunteered to meet with me privately for a discussion. Pseudonyms are used to protect their privacy. For a more extended oral history on the experiences of black gay men, see E. Patrick Johnson, *Sweet Tea: Black Gay Men of the South* (Chapel Hill: University of North Carolina Press, 2008).

The section titled "Standing at the Cross Roads" was originally published as "Standing at the Crossroads" in *Callaloo: A Journal of African American and African Arts and Letters* 22 (Spring 1999): 343–345. It was republished in Edwidge Danticat, ed., *Beacon Best 2000: Best Writing of Men and Women of All Colors* (Boston: Beacon Press, 2000), 72–75.

1. Maude Southwell Wahlman and John Scully, "Aesthetic Principles of Afro-American Quilts," in *Afro-American Folk Art and Crafts*, ed. William Ferris (Boston: G. K. Hall, 1989), 79–97.
2. Elsa Barkley Brown, "African-American Women's Quilting: A Framework for Conceptualizing and Teaching African-American Women's History," in *Black Women in American Social Science Perspectives*, ed. Micheline R. Malson, Elisabeth

Mudimbe-Boyi, Jean F. O'Barr and Mary Wyer (Chicago: University of Chicago Press, 1990), 14.

3. Brown, "African-American Women's Quilting," 10.

4. Vivian M. Patraka, "Spectacles of Suffering: Performing, Presence, Absence, and Historical Memory at U.S. Holocaust Museums," in *Performance and Cultural Politics,* ed. Elin Diamond (New York: Routledge, 1996), 89.

5. See Cindy Ruskin, *The Quilt: Stories from the NAMES Project* (New York: Pocket Books, 1988).

6. D. Soyini Madison, *Critical Ethnography* (Thousand Oaks, CA: Sage, 2005), 13.

7. Ruskin, *The Quilt.*

8. Patraka, "Spectacles of Suffering," 99.

9. See Henry Giroux, Colin Lankshear, Peter McLaren, and Michael Peters, eds., *Counternarratives: Cultural Studies and Critical Pedagogies in Postmodern Spaces* (New York: Routledge, 1996). Giroux uses the construct of "short stories" as a reference to counternarratives. See also Norman Denzin, "Emancipatory Discourses and the Ethics and Politics of Representation," in *Handbook of Qualitative Research,* 3rd ed., ed. Norman K. Denzin and Yvonna S. Lincoln (Thousand Oaks, CA: Sage, 2005), 933–958.

10. Patraka, "Spectacles of Suffering," 106

11. See Cindy J. Kistenberg, *AIDS, Social Change, and Theater: Performance as Protest* (New York: Garland Publishing, 1995); Michael Hunter, ed., *Sojourner: Black Gay Voices in the Age of AIDS, Other Countries,* vol. 2 (New York: Other Countries Press, 1993); Jose Esteban Muñoz, *Disidentifications: Queers of Color and the Performance of Politics* (Minneapolis: University of Minnesota Press, 1999).

12. Charles I. Nero, "Black Queer Identity, Imaginative Rationality, and the Language of Home," in *Our Voices: Essays in Culture, Ethnicity, and Communication,* ed. Alberto Gonzalez, Marsha Houston, and Victoria Chen (Los Angeles: Roxbury Publishing Co., 1997), 66–67.

13. Conceptualizing through the work of Barry Brummett, *A Rhetoric of Style* (Carbondale: Southern Illinois University Press, 2008), visual rhetorics can be described as powerful messages that embody a system of *signification grounded largely in image,* what is seen as a representation of thought and style and its political signaling. Olson suggests that visual rhetorics may have common qualities—a pictorial representation, a motto in the vernacular of the time or situation, and a resulting moral lesson. Lester C. Olson, *Benjamin Franklin's Vision of American Community: A Study in Rhetorical Iconology* (Columbia: University of South Carolina Press,

2004), 3.

14. Richard Schechner, *Performance Theory* (New York: Routledge, 1988), 123.

15. Judith Butler, *Gender Trouble: Feminism and the Subversion of Identity* (New York: Routledge, 1999), 179.

16. Homosexuality becomes the origin of the disease, not a location of its affect, in a homophobic environment, even though gay men are statistically shy of intravenous drug users, babies born with AIDS, and those who contract the disease through blood transfusions.

17. Patraka, "Spectacles of Suffering," 90.

18. David is referencing "Politics Sewn to Art, Panel by Quilt-like Panel," *Los Angeles Times,* June 9, 2007, E12. The article focuses on LA-based artist Andrea Bowers's video installation, *The Weight of Relevance,* a piece that focuses on the artist's "interest in the relationship between art and activism and archival process."

19. Dane is referencing the old Trini Lopez song "If I Had a Hammer."

20. Kathleen Hall Jamieson and Karlyn Kohrs Campbell, "Rhetorical Hybrids: Fusions of Generic Elements," *Quarterly Journal of Speech* 68 (1982): 147. Also see "Form and Genre in Rhetorical Criticism: An Introduction," in *Form and Genre: Shaping Rhetorical Action,* ed. Karlyn Kohrs Campbell and Kathleen Hall Jamieson (Falls Church, VA: Speech Communication Association, 1978), 18–25. The authors also draw heavily on Kathleen M. Jamieson, ed., *Critical Anthology of Public Speeches* (Chicago: Science Research Associates, 1978); James O. Payne, "The American Eulogy: A Study in Generic Criticism" (master's thesis, University of Kansas, 1975).

21. See Jamieson and Campbell, "Rhetorical Hybrids,"147–148.

22. Donald E. Polkinghorne, *Narrative Knowing and the Human Sciences* (Albany, NY: State University of New York Press, 1988), 13.

23. David Román, *Acts of Interventions: Performance, Gay Culture, and AIDS* (Bloomington: Indiana University Press, 1998), 27. See Kistenberg, *AIDS, Social Change, and Theatre.*

24. Eugene Vance, "Roland and the Poetics of Memory," in *Textual Strategies: Perspective in Post-Structuralist Criticism,* ed. Josué V. Harari (Ithaca: Cornell University Press, 1979), 374–375.

25. Linda Park-Fuller, "Performing Absence: The Staged Personal Narrative as Testimony," *Text and Performance Quarterly* 20 (2000): 20.

26. Della Pollock, *Telling Bodies/Performing Birth* (New York: New York University Press, 1999), 27.

27. In developing his notion of a useful queer mythology, Scott Dillard cites Andrew

Ramer's construct of the "Stand Between Person." Suggesting the social positionality of gay people, Ramer states, "We stand between genders. We stand between the living and the dead. We stand between night and day. We stand between matter and spirit. Our job is to scout that terrain for the main body of the tribe, and to bring back all that information for the main body of the tribe." Scott Dillard, "Breathing Darrell: Solo Performance as a Contribution to a Useful Queer Mythology," *Text and Performance Quarterly* 20 (2000): 74–83; Andrew Ramer, "Keynote Address," First Annual Celebrating Gay Spirit Visions Conference, 1998, www.mindspring. com/~gayspirit/key_1990.htmramer.

28. Jamieson and Campbell, "Rhetorical Hybrids," 147.

29. Ibid., 149.

30. Ibid., 150.

31. Diana Taylor, *The Archive and the Repertoire: Performing Culture Memory in the Americas* (Durham, NC: Duke University Press, 2003), 19.

32. D. Soyini Madison, "Performance, Personal Narratives, and the Politics of Possibility," in *The Future of Performance Studies: Visions and Revisions*, ed. Sharon. J. Dailey (Annandale, VA: NCA, 1998), 276–286.

33. Bryant K. Alexander, "Performance Ethnography: The Reenacting and Inciting of Culture," in *The Sage of Handbook of Qualitative Research*, 3rd ed., ed. Norman K. Denzin and Yvonne S. Lincoln (Thousand Oaks, CA: Sage, 2005): 411–441.

34. Patraka, "Spectacles of Suffering," 93.

35. Here Patraka is citing work from Philip Gourevitch, "Behold Now Behemoth: The Holocaust Memorial Museum: One More American Theme Park," *Harpers,* July 1993, 55–62.

36. Sonja Arsham Kuftinec, "Bridging Haunted Places: Performance and the Production of Mostar," in *Opening Acts: Performance in/as Communication and Cultural Studies*, ed. Judith Hamera (Thousand Oaks, CA: Sage, 2006), 84.

37. Kuftinec, "Bridging Haunted Places," 84; Hamera, *Opening Acts*, 12.

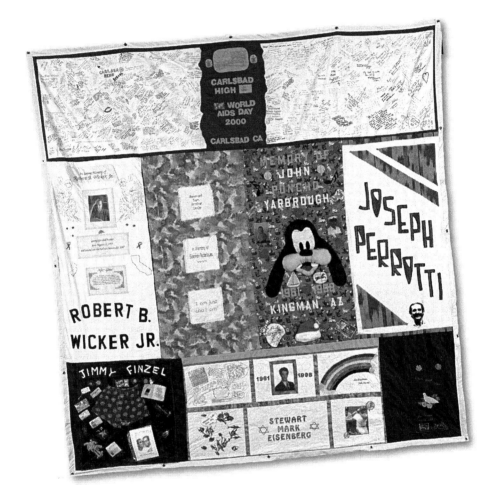

Repeated Remembrance: Commemorating the AIDS Quilt and Resuscitating the Mourned Subject

Erin J. Rand

The NAMES Project AIDS Memorial Quilt celebrated its twentieth anniversary in 2007. Marking this occasion is undoubtedly bittersweet, perhaps inspirational or humbling, but also rather troubling. Commemorating the Quilt recognizes the many thousands of people who have been lost to AIDS and testifies to the power of individual efforts to come together as a community in times of staggering loss and sadness. The trouble of the anniversary of the Quilt, however, emerges from the fact that the Quilt itself is already a project of remembering and memorializing. What does it mean, then, to commemorate a memorial? If those included in the Quilt have already been named and remembered, what incites us now to name and remember the means of their memorial? This doubled commemoration—the remembering of a project designed to remember—leads me to two questions. First, it prompts an investigation of the apparent compulsion to commemorate: what effects—in terms of the nation's relationship to AIDS and homosexuality, as well as the subject positions afforded to gay men—are produced by this repeated remembrance? Second, by situating the Quilt within the realm of memorials, to what extent are the potential political interventions of the Quilt disarticulated from discourses of activism and opposition?

The first of these questions suggests that the repeated ritual of memorializing those who have died of AIDS (and the Quilt that marks these deaths) serves to maintain a particular "mourned subject" position. Arising from the nation's ambivalent reaction to gay men in the late 1980s—shock and grief mounting apace with homophobia—the mourned subject is the subject position through which gay men were incorporated into the national imaginary during the early years of the AIDS crisis. Considering both the social and psychic mechanisms through which this subject position was created, this position enables social recognition and at least a tenuous sort of tolerance; ultimately, however, it radically circumscribes the agency of the subject constituted as such. With respect to the second question, and as an alternative to the limitations of the mourned subject position, the Quilt must also be situated in relation to activist discourses. That is, as both a memorial and an activist project—or more accurately, activism in the form of a memorial—the Quilt participates in a larger conversation regarding the roles of mourning and grief versus militancy and anger in AIDS activism. Thus, when the Quilt's activism is taken seriously and its rhetorical force considered in terms of the activist agency it enables, the mourned subject position it produces is revealed not only as being conservative in the sense that it maintains a particular kind of oppressive subjection, but also as actually preventing legitimate mourning of the dead.

Importantly, the mourned subject position is not self-fashioned by those who occupy it, but becomes intelligible and inhabitable through national discourses about AIDS and homosexuality. The Quilt, therefore, also must be considered as a public memorial or site of ritualized mourning, since it participates in shaping national sentiment and public memory, and in working out the nation's relationship to the AIDS crisis. As studies of public memory tend to emphasize, the presumption of shared values and identity of the "nation" is rhetorically built, in part, through the construction and consumption of public memorials. Blair, Jeppeson, and Pucci, for example, argue that in addition to their more

obvious epideictic function, public memorials also work politically or de-
liberatively, acting as "registers of present and future political concern,"
and instructing visitors in national values.[1] Similarly, Barbara Biesecker
suggests that reconstructions of the past play an important role in (re)
crafting a sense of national identity or belonging: "what we remember and
how we remember it can tell us something significant about who we are
as a people now, about the contemporary social and political issues that
divide us, and about who we may become." For Biesecker, the popular
texts through which public memory functions do not simply reflect national values, but also work persuasively as "civics lessons" that instruct
citizens in particular understandings of and relationships to the nation.[2]
When public memory is thus understood to be rhetorical, the contested
nature of any memorial object or event is highlighted. As Stephen Browne
points out, not only do public memories often result from processes of
struggle and contention, but they also serve as resolutions to perceived
national problems. That is, commemorations can alleviate the national
anxieties that emerge from demographic and historical change.[3] Marita
Sturken argues that it is through cultural memory texts such as the Quilt
that "definitions of the nation and 'Americanness' are simultaneously
established, questioned, and refigured." The Quilt's form, she contends,
"evokes a sense of Americana, yet it also represents those who have been
symbolically excluded from America—drug users, blacks, Latinos, gay
men." Sturken goes on to explain that the tensions woven through the
Quilt intersect with "contemporary battles over identity politics and political correctness," and that they raise questions about difference, inclu-
sion/exclusion, and who is able to speak about particular memories.[4] As a
public memorial that negotiates national identities and national struggles,
the Quilt most certainly is situated within a matrix of discourses that, as
Sturken observes, have consistently troubled the American public. One
of the Quilt's most significant rhetorical effects for the nation, then, is
the stitching together of the national identity and values whose integrity
have been threatened by these conflicting discourses of homosexuality,
disease, drug use, race, and poverty.

However, as a memorial to those who have died of AIDS, the Quilt
is significantly different than memorials that commemorate, for example,
the veterans of World War II or Vietnam, or the victims of the 9/11 attacks.

Specifically, by remembering those who have died, the Quilt also reminds us that many more continue to die; unlike veterans' or 9/11 memorials, the Quilt is still expanding, and those living today may yet have their names added to the list of AIDS-related deaths. Therefore, the Quilt is always an incomplete memorial, marking not the end of the epidemic, but its perpetual presence. Remembering those who have died of AIDS certainly involves a construction of the past, but it also necessarily entails particular understandings of the present and of those who remain alive. In other words, while the Quilt clearly does important work for the nation—by providing a site for ritualized mourning and absolution—it also directly affects (indeed *effects*) the living by producing a subject position through which certain people are able to be socially recognized and to act.[5]

In what follows, the Quilt, as a public memorial, is understood to participate significantly in discourses of national identity; however, focusing primarily on the construction of the mourned subject position—especially as it relates to AIDS activism—highlights the process of subjectivation, by which subjects are constituted rhetorically through the discourses surrounding the Quilt. That is, the mourned subject position is both produced by and is necessary to the national identity formed in relation to AIDS. The commemoration of the Quilt's anniversary resuscitates the mourned subject and reinforces the nation's earlier relationship to AIDS and homosexuality.

As a significant cultural text, the Quilt is a highly recognizable site at which to explore the fraught relationship between mourning and activism during the AIDS crisis. The potential for forging activism from mourning is engaged both theoretically and practically in three key critical interventions. First, in his 1989 essay, "Mourning and Militancy," Douglas Crimp cautions that activist groups like ACT UP, with their penchant for militancy, lead to a denial of the melancholic incorporation of sexual shame. However, because he is hesitant to embrace activists' anger and aggression, his use of the Freudian concepts of mourning and melancholia offers only an incomplete account of ego formation during the AIDS crisis. Second, Judith Butler's examination of the process of subjectivation highlights both the psychic and the social mechanisms of subject formation, suggesting that it is only by radically risking the dissolution of the subject that the terms of subjugation can be resisted or resignified.

Finally, Andrew Sullivan's 1996 "When Plagues End," written seven years after Crimp's essay and at a very different point in the AIDS crisis, attempts to imagine a gay male subject free of his attachment to mourning. Sullivan argues that an embrace of "responsibility" and "life" is the means for changing both gay male subjectivity and a homophobic and AIDS-phobic society; however, the aggressive impulses that Sullivan and Crimp both eschew are crucial to the possibility of resubjectivation. That is, the militant AIDS activism that emerged in the late 1980s may have been a means of both responding to oppressive social conditions and shifting the terms of subjectivity available to gay men.

The possibilities for transformation available through risking the subject may be glimpsed in the political funerals of ACT UP and a 1989 protest in Montreal. Unlike the mourned subject position afforded by the Quilt, militant activist practices like these may actually serve to disrupt the terms of subjection and create the condition of possibility for both mourning and resubjectivation.

Activism through Mourning:
The Beginnings of the Quilt

When President Ronald Reagan addressed the opening ceremonies of the Third International Conference on AIDS on May 31, 1987, he publicly uttered the word "AIDS" for the first time. Having blatantly ignored the AIDS epidemic for six years after the HIV virus had been identified, Reagan finally acknowledged it only to suggest the implementation of repressive and discriminatory testing procedures. By the time Reagan delivered this speech, over 40,000 Americans had already died from AIDS, a vastly disproportionate number of whom were gay men.[6] Of course, Reagan's lack of attention is only one instance of the overwhelmingly callous and homophobic attitude that characterized the nation's response to the AIDS epidemic. Though the pervasive homophobia and systemic neglect of the federal government, drug companies, and medical institutions is by now well documented, its significance to the activist practices of the gay men who continued to live through the AIDS crisis cannot be underestimated.[7] As Douglas Crimp suggests, "there is an all but inevitable connection between the memories and hopes associated with our lost friends and the daily assaults on our consciousness. Seldom has a society so savaged people during their hour of loss."[8]

It is not surprising, then, that some of the earliest AIDS activism focused on providing a dignified and public forum for mourning the deaths of the men whose disease was often understood to be synonymous with— or worse, justified by—their sexuality and therefore viewed with revulsion and hatred. The NAMES Project Memorial Quilt was formally organized by Cleve Jones in June 1987 in order to counter the anonymity and secrecy that surrounded AIDS deaths by specifically naming—and by naming, providing a means for mourning—the dead. Only two months later, the Quilt already contained almost two thousand panels and was displayed on the National Mall in Washington, D.C. By 1992 it included over 21,000 panels, and today it has expanded to over 47,000 panels. Not only did the Quilt serve as a memorial to the dead and a site for ritual mourning, but it also provided an opportunity for protesting the nation's mismanagement of the AIDS epidemic and rallying for more research and support. In fact, as Jones maintains, the Quilt specifically was intended to confront the nation's apathy: "The Quilt was and is an activist symbol—comforting, yes, but mortally troubling. If it raised a single question, it was, What are we going to do about it? That was the challenge we laid at the national doorstep." However, the kind of activism that was made possible through the Quilt—an activism based on mourning—existed simultaneously, and sometimes in tension with, another activist reaction to the rapidly increasing number of dying gay men: to be enraged rather than saddened, to fight instead of grieve. For instance, the group of activists who founded the AIDS Coalition to Unleash Power (ACT UP) in March of 1987 in New York City sought to put their anger and frustration to use through confrontational protests and "zaps." Calling themselves "a diverse, non-partisan group united in anger and committed to direct action to end the AIDS crisis," ACT UP enacted loud, visible demonstrations primarily at the local level and often utilized bold, eye-catching graphics (such as the "Silence = Death" emblem) to attract attention.[9]

Both of these activist responses to the AIDS crisis rely upon a certain communal relationship to mourning, either by providing an outlet for sadness or by converting the pain of loss into militancy. The process of mourning for gay men in the late 1980s and early 1990s was not simply a reaction to the loss of the lives of their friends and their lovers—and to the potential loss of their own; it actually functioned in the formation of particular activist subject positions.[10] Furthermore, as the nation mourned—even if diffidently—for a population toward which it was decisively ambivalent, gay men found themselves being accorded, at the moment of their deaths, a dubious acceptance and social recognition.[11]

Mourning or Militancy?

As AIDS claimed more and more lives, rituals of mourning—candlelight vigils, the Quilt, funerals, and private ceremonies of remembrance—became common fixtures of gay communities. The tension between the need to mourn for lost friends and lovers and the need to organize forceful protests against the political and medical institutions that did not prevent their deaths thus became increasingly significant throughout the 1980s. Some activists, such as the vituperative Larry Kramer, were alarmed by the quiescence these events seemed to condone. In his characteristic polemic style, he goads his fellow gay men: "You are going to die and you are going to die very soon. Unless you get off your fucking tushies and fight back. Unless you do, you will forgive me, you deserve to die."[12] While candlelight vigils often provided a means for gay men to unite as a community in their mourning, AIDS activist leaders such as Roger McFarland worried that they did not move their attendees to participate in more politically oriented actions. Speaking at a vigil, McFarland explains his own turn from sadness to anger:

> I never want to forget my pain, or what my friends endured. I embraced that pain, I took it to heart, and I use it to feed the bilious rage that has taken root in my soul. I know I would lose my mind, if not my life, if all these people we love so much ended up dying for nothing but the ineptitude of a racist, sexist, classist, homophobic political regime and an apathetic public. That's why I fight instead of cry.[13]

Shifting the focus from mourning to anger, and engaging in actions aimed at social transformation rather than demonstrations of grief, activist organizations such as ACT UP hoped to replace feelings of devastation and fatalism with rage and courage.[14]

Reacting to the tendency for gay activism to be dominated and defined by these calls to anger, Crimp suggests that gay men must also find a way to incorporate mourning into their activism. In his now seminal essay "Mourning and Militancy," Crimp describes the rising suspicion with which mourning is met in the gay community. The violence wreaked by the AIDS virus, Crimp explains, demands a vindication of the dead: it is not only through death that people are brutalized, but also through the widespread homophobia that prevents their friends and lovers from properly remembering and grieving for them. In the face of this violence, mourning therefore becomes militancy.[15] However, drawing on Freud's distinction between mourning and melancholia, Crimp suggests that this militancy may operate as a form of denial and come at great psychic cost to gay men.

According to Freud, mourning is a normal process of reacting to the loss of a loved person or ideal. Melancholia, on the other hand, is a pathological state of dejection, inability to love, self-reproach, and lowered self-esteem. Freud notes that most of the features of melancholia are also present in extreme grief; mourning and melancholia therefore appear to be analogous, and the process of normal mourning can be used to understand the mechanisms of melancholia. The work of mourning involves the withdrawal of the libido from the lost object. This process is always a struggle that can only be carried out gradually over time, but once the libido has been detached from each memory of the lost object, "the ego becomes free and uninhibited again." While the similarities between mourning and melancholia would suggest that melancholia also involves the loss of a loved object, Freud explains that the melancholiac's loss is "one in himself." The loved object is internalized, or transferred onto the individual's ego; unlike the process of mourning, in which the libido is withdrawn from the object and eventually shifted to a new object, in the case of melancholia, the libido is "withdrawn into the ego" and "establish[es] an *identification* of the ego with the abandoned object." This internalization has the additional effect of constituting the ego, or the conscience, in its self-reflexive capacity: "in this condition one part of the ego sets itself over against the other, judges it critically, and, as it were, looks upon it as an object." Whereas the mourner is conscious of her or his loss, the melancholiac is not, or cannot be, conscious of the loss with which she or he identifies and through which her or his ego is constituted.[16]

Furthermore, when the loved object is turned inward onto an individual's ego, the criticisms and reproaches directed toward the object then become self-criticisms and self-reproaches of her- or himself. It is through this internalization of ambivalence that Freud explains the tendency in melancholiacs toward low self-esteem and self-reviling. He elaborates, "If the object-love, which cannot be given up, takes refuge in narcissistic identification, while the object itself is abandoned, then hate is expanded upon this new substitute-object, railing at it, depreciating it, making it suffer and deriving sadistic gratification from its suffering."[17] In other words, the self-punishment of melancholia is a means of expressing the ambivalent feelings originally intended for the loved object.

It is through this notion of ambivalence that Crimp makes his argument for the importance of mourning to AIDS activism. He insightfully suggests that the lost object of the gay male community is not only the thousands of actual lives, but also "the ideal of perverse sexual pleasure," or "a culture of sexual possibility: back rooms, tea rooms, bookstores, movie houses, and baths; the trucks, the pier, the ramble, the dunes."[18] The uninhibited sexuality that is missed, however, is fraught with ambivalence: it was never generally tolerated and is often repudiated by gay men themselves. In other words, the reactions of gay men to the devastation of AIDS are similar to what Freud describes as melancholia. Not only are gay men prevented from consciously mourning the loss of their sexual culture—because of both internal and external prohibitions against that culture—but their feelings of ambivalence toward their own promiscuity are turned inward onto themselves. Crimp argues that this self-imposed misery must be acknowledged along with the obvious misery inflicted by contemporary social conditions: "By making all violence external, pushing it to the outside and objectifying it in "enemy" institutions and individuals, we deny its psychic articulation, deny that we are effected, as well as affected, by it." The tendency for activists to embrace rage and militancy, then, may operate as a mechanism of disavowal; rather than facing their own ambivalence toward safe sex and HIV testing, Crimp suggests, their self-criticisms are simply directed outward. Crimp does not deny the importance or validity of the anger of militant activist groups; instead, he calls for an activism that includes mourning: "Militancy, of course, then, but mourning too: mourning *and* militancy."[19]

The Melancholic Ego and the Mourned Subject

Crimp's essay focuses primarily on the melancholic effects of an un-acknowledged, ungrievable loss and the internalization of ambivalence toward the loved object. Though he begins to gesture toward the way in which this ambivalence constitutes the self (recall his comment that "we are *effected,* as well as affected, by it"), he does not explore fully the rhetorical process by which gay men come to be recognized as subjects.[20] His argument that activist militancy represents a form of denial or disavowal rests upon an incomplete account of the subjectivation of gay men during the AIDS crisis. In order to understand the psychic rationale for the turn toward militancy, we must first investigate more fully the constitution of the subject—and its enabling and constraining elements—that might make this turn.

While Crimp rightly identifies the importance of the self-inflicted violence resulting from the inability to grieve a lost gay male sexual culture, he implies that this violence is directed against the ego but does not elaborate the process through which it also *constitutes* the ego. As Judith Butler explains, the turning inward of the lost object onto the ego presumes the preexistence of the ego, but is also said to produce the ego: "it is unclear that this ego can exist prior to its melancholia. The 'turn' that marks the melancholic response to loss appears to initiate the redoubling of the ego as an object; only by turning back on itself does the ego acquire the status of a perceptual object." According to this account, the ego never has been, nor ever can be, free of melancholia, since melancholic loss is the very condition for the emergence of a self-reflexive subject. Furthermore, since the loss of the loved object is an unconscious loss, it "*institutes* the ego as a necessary response to or 'defense' against loss," and must remain unconscious in order to fulfill this function.[21] Thus, when Crimp suggests that gay men need to acknowledge the psychic violence they inflict upon themselves, he does not account for the fact that the ego is premised upon—and therefore remains unconscious of and actually preserves—this violence.

Of course, understanding the subjectivity of gay men during the AIDS crisis cannot be limited to a consideration of the intrapsychic processes of melancholia and ego formation; one must also address the social conditions and particular form of the Quilt that rhetorically constituted a certain subject position. While the gay male community was continually blamed for the transmission of AIDS, and the effects of the disease were assumed at the time to be confined largely to this demographic, the AIDS epidemic nevertheless became an occasion for mourning on a national scale. This is due in no small part not only to the existence of the Quilt as a public memorial, but also to its particular resonance with traditional Americana: by utilizing a symbol of American folk art and mythology— the patchwork quilt—the Quilt was able to encourage nationwide mourning, even if those being mourned continued to be reviled. According to Hawkins, "It was also a brilliant strategy for bringing AIDS not only to public attention but into the mainstream of American myth, for turning what was perceived to be a 'gay disease' into a shared national tragedy." Furthermore, Hawkins suggests that by grouping thousands of individual memorials into a single enormous fabric, especially when it is displayed near other national monuments in Washington, D.C., the Quilt reformulates and contextualizes individual losses as national devastation.[22]

Though the Quilt does position the deaths due to AIDS as a national loss, it does not necessarily redefine the "deaths of gay men" as "deaths of Americans." That is, while AIDS might be viewed as a tragedy that should be mourned by the nation as a whole, those who have died are still regarded as part of a specific—and marginalized—gay male community.[23] In fact, during the Quilt's early years, many panels used only partial names, nicknames, or were left blank in order to protect the anonymity of the deceased; being represented on the Quilt was tantamount to being "outed" as a gay man. Noting the divisiveness marked and reinforced through the Quilt, Crimp suggests that it functions, in part, as "the spectacle of mourning, the vast public-relations effort to humanize and dignify our

losses for those who have not shared them." Rather than encouraging a
sense of national responsibility for *all* citizens, Crimp wonders, "Does it
provide a form of catharsis, an easing of conscience, for those who have
cared and done so little about this great tragedy?"[24] In fact, Americans
may be uniquely predisposed to engage in precisely this form of mourning
of gay men. Butler suggests that a "culturally prevalent form of melancholia" might be expected to exist when societal regulations strictly prohibit
the grieving of a loved object. In this case, the unrecognized and therefore
ungrievable loss to which she refers is the "homosexual cathexis," or the
possibility of homosexual attachment and love.[25] The spectacle of mourning provided by the Quilt and similar rituals, then, may be a means of
performing grief for that unconscious and ungrievable loss that homosexuality represents in America, and therefore of negotiating the tensions
that it produces in the imagined national identity.

While Butler's explanation clarifies the way in which such performances of mourning serve the nation (when it is understood to exclude the
group for which it mourns), it does not address the effect of this mourning in the constitution of a subject position that gay men themselves are
able to occupy. The scholarship on public memory is again useful here,
since the Quilt as a memorial helps define the nation's relationship to
those who are being remembered and as such also produces them as a
particular kind of citizen. As Browne explains, instances of public commemoration not only create an "official" version of history, but also have
bearing on "who counts as an American and who does not."[26] Thus, the
process by which one becomes intelligible as a citizen is explicitly rhetorical: the ways in which gay men are positioned in discourses surrounding
the Quilt is not merely a question of representation, then, but a question
of the kinds of agency afforded to particular kinds of subjects. If the
gay male community is situated as the cathected object that the nation
mourns, it is granted a certain kind of social recognition, and gay men are
able to occupy a subject position that is not otherwise available. To put it
differently, gay men—codified as a group that is dying of AIDS—become
socially recognized subjects by being mourned. This does not mean that
they are "subjects who are mourned," which would imply that this subject position existed prior to the mourning process, but that they become
"subjects through mourning," or more precisely, "mourned subjects." The

mourned subject can only exist, then, on the condition of a mourning that has the ability to grant validity and subjectivity to those mourned. Clearly, gay men as a group occupied (and continued to occupy) particular subject positions before being positioned as mourned subjects; however, the nation's (limited) empathy and compassion for gay men during the AIDS crisis led to the production of a gay male subject position that was not defined primarily by perversion and secrecy.

Being constituted as mourned subjects, then, is enabling insofar as it confers visibility, identification, and recognition. When Andrew Sullivan writes about the shift from "fearful stigmatization" to "awkward acceptance" of homosexuality in America, it is the enabling capacities of "mourned subjectivity" that he is identifying. He explains,

> AIDS and its onslaught imposed a form of social integration that may never have taken place otherwise. Forced to choose between complete abandonment of the gay subculture and an awkward first encounter, America, for the most part, chose the latter . . . What had once been a strong fear of homosexual difference, disguising a mostly silent awareness of homosexual humanity, became the opposite. The humanity slowly trumped the difference. Death, it turned out, was a powerfully universalizing experience.[27]

For some gay men during the AIDS crisis, the kind of recognition and even acceptance that being mourned by the nation provided was, at the least, a relief from constant invisibility and hostility. As Crimp concedes, the Quilt "is one of the few efforts of our community that has been generally granted exemption from opprobrium."[28] In fact, as Hawkins demonstrates by juxtaposing the Quilt with the Vietnam Veterans Memorial, the untimely, tragic deaths of gay men can even be construed—like the deaths of soldiers—as heroic and especially suited for memorializing.

On the other hand, when they are constituted as mourned subjects, the agency of gay men is significantly constrained, and their potential for activism is severely limited. After all, the range of activities accorded to one who is mourned is essentially restricted to suffering and death. As Steve Abbott contends, the message of the Quilt, which he reads as a "memorial to a dying subculture," is "We didn't like you fags and junkies when you were wild, kinky and having fun. We didn't like you when you were angry, marching and demanding rights. But now that you're dying and have joined 'nicely' like 'a family sewing circle,' we'll accept you."[29] Again, it is significant that the Quilt as a memorial is always necessarily incomplete. As Abbott's comment illustrates, the Quilt attests to a "dying" subculture rather than to a subculture that is already "dead." Even those still living, in other words, are being identified by the Quilt as those whom it will name in the future, and their fates, it seems, are inescapable. The subjectivity provided to gay men through mourning, therefore, depends not only on being always already ill or dead, but also on a tenuous acceptance that is maintained only through appropriate behavior. Returning to Butler's contention that the mourning of AIDS is a performance of the loss denied by a cultural melancholia, it is clear that the nation's sentiments toward this loss—because it is melancholic—will always be deeply ambivalent. Hence, love will be mixed with hatred, and acceptance tinged with violence. Crimp suggests that along with assuaging the nation's guilt, then, the Quilt may also provide a means of expressing secret abhorrence: "It would, of course, be unseemly for society to celebrate our deaths openly, but I wonder if the quilt helps make this desire decorous."[30]

The shackles of the mourned subject position cannot merely be thrown off at will, since the subject cannot act prior to its own constitution, and since it necessarily maintains a psychic attachment to its own subjection. According to Butler, subjection is a paradoxical form of power since it "signifies the process of becoming subordinated by power as well as the process of becoming a subject." She uses the term "subjectivation" for the French *assujetissement* to denote "both the becoming of the subject and the process of subjection—one inhabits the figure of autonomy only by becoming subjected to a power, a subjection which implies a radical dependency." The process of subjectivation, therefore, is marked by the same peculiarity as Freud's description of the melancholic formation of the ego: the subject that is subordinated to power is also constituted by that power and cannot preexist it. Any agency or possibility of resistance that may be available to the subject, then, must always originate in the power that it is said to resist. The subject always maintains, according to

Butler, a "passionate attachment" to the terms of its subjection, precisely because it relies upon this subjection in order to exist, but must deny its attachment to preserve its apparent autonomy. This does not mean, however, that the subject is doomed to simply replicate the conditions of its own subjection; instead, the power assumed as the agency of the subject may be discontinuous with the power that led to the subject's formation. As Butler explains, "Where conditions of subordination make possible the assumption of power, the power assumed remains tied to those conditions, but in an ambivalent way; in fact, the power assumed may at once retain and resist that subordination."[31]

The conservative nature of power in subjectivation arises from the subject's desire for its own continued existence: the attachment to subjection protects the subject from dissolution. It is for this reason, then, that gay men cannot simply refuse to be mourned subjects; any alteration of subjectivity must have recourse to what Butler calls the "unconscious of power itself." In other words, the unconscious attachment to subjugation is the condition of possibility for resisting and resignifying the terms of subjection. Attempting to resist necessarily entails the risk of the annihilation of the subject, but it is in this risk that Butler locates the opportunity for the reorganization of subjectivation. She queries, "What would it mean for the subject to desire something other than its continued 'social existence'? If such an existence cannot be undone without falling into some kind of death, can existence nevertheless be risked, death courted or pursued, in order to expose and open to transformation the hold of social power on the conditions of life's persistence?"[32] Butler is essentially calling for the necessity of risking desubjectivation in order to create real change in practices of systemic oppression. For gay men engaged in activism during the AIDS crisis, this means placing in jeopardy their subjectivation through mourning in both the psychic and social realms: the formulation of the ego through the melancholic incorporation of their ambivalence toward a lost sexual culture, as well as the social recognition conferred by a nation ready to mourn—for ambivalent reasons of its own—the tragedy of AIDS in the gay male community. That is, theorizing the possibility for desubjectivation requires attention to both the psychic and the social mechanisms through which subjectivity is formed.

Sullivan's Solution

For the first fifteen years of the AIDS epidemic, the annual number of AIDS deaths relentlessly increased with each year. It was not until 1996, due in large part to the introduction of protease inhibitor drugs, that the death toll was actually lower than the previous year.[33] For the first time, it was possible to imagine AIDS as an illness with which one could live relatively normally, rather than as an inevitable death sentence. In response to this hopeful attitude, Andrew Sullivan wrote his now in-famous *New York Times Magazine* article, "When Plagues End," which proclaimed the foreseeable end of the epidemic. Sullivan was widely criticized by AIDS activists for discounting the astronomical numbers of people who were still dying of AIDS (after all, there were approximately 47,000 more deaths in the United States in the next three years alone), for ignoring the expense of the new drugs that prohibited many people with AIDS from having access to them, and for imposing moral stan-dards on gay men that denied and sought to undermine the uniqueness of their sexual culture.[34]

Sullivan's article, in spite of its reprehensible claims, is interesting here because it seems to push toward precisely the kind of desubjectivation of gay men that Butler might suggest, and which might be an alternative to the mourned subject position produced by the Quilt. Sullivan argues that the devastation of AIDS has led to an unprecedented solidarity within the gay community; while this solidarity was necessary during the crisis, he sees gay men clinging to the tragedy of AIDS because they are frightened of the prospect of living without it. He writes, "the solidarity of the plague years is becoming harder and harder to sustain. For the first time, serious resentment is brewing among HIV-positive men about the way in which AIDS has slowly retreated from the forefront of gay politics." Faced with returning to the "normalcy" of life that does not revolve around AIDS, Sullivan suggests that many gay men feel threatened. Some, "sensing an abatement of the pressure, have returned, almost manically, to unsafe sexual behavior, as if terrified by the thought that they might actually survive, that the plague might end and with it the solidarity that made it endurable."[35] In short, according to Sullivan, the gay male community is fixated on death and dying; it stubbornly refuses to let go of the disease that has nearly decimated it, because it can no longer imagine life without terror and grief. This position clearly resonates with Freud's description of melancholia: rather than mourning the losses incurred by AIDS, gay men have internalized the loved object. Not only is their ambivalence toward the virus therefore turned upon themselves, but it is also the foundation of their subjectivity; hence, gay men maintain a passionate attachment to the very terms of their deaths and misery.

Sullivan's answer to this impasse offers an implicit critique of a form of activism, like that of the Quilt, that occurs through the process of grieving for the dead. He suggests instead an embrace of responsibility and the possibilities of life. He contends that the AIDS crisis required gay men to become more responsible for themselves and for one another: "Men who had long since got used to throwing their own lives away were confronted with the possibility that they actually did care about themselves and wanted to survive . . . A culture that had been based in some measure on desire became a culture rooted in strength." He advocates putting this responsibility to use in shifting the terms of gay male subjectivity, for "gird[ing] yourself . . . for the possibility of life" rather than for the possibility of death.[36] In other words, Sullivan exhorts gay men to risk the terms of their subjugation and subjectivity—the all-consuming fight against AIDS, their irresponsible and self-loathing sexual practices, the solidarity that arises among an oppressed and suffering minority group—in order to take up new subject positions that are rooted in self-respect and responsibility, freedom from stigmatization, and survival. Unlike the Quilt, then, which constitutes for gay men a subject position premised on death and mourning, Sullivan envisions a form of subjectivity that intentionally eschews this morbid attachment.

Ultimately, Sullivan is perhaps correct in identifying the unconscious attachment to death and mourning as a basis for gay male subjectivity during the AIDS crisis. However, his solution, though it appears to offer an opportunity for resubjectivation, in fact merely reinforces the terms of gay male subjection in both the psychic and social domains. First, by characterizing pre-AIDS sexual practices as irresponsible and promiscuous, Sullivan contributes to the ambivalence that many gay men feel toward the loss of this sexual culture. As Crimp points out, it is the inability to grieve for these pleasures—because they are prohibited—that leads to resistance to safe sex: "safe sex may seem less like defiance than resignation, less like accomplished mourning than melancholia."[37] In other words, Sullivan's suggestion that gay men renounce their sexual pasts does nothing to move them toward more "responsible" sexual behavior, but actually deepens the ambivalence through which the ego is constituted, thereby effectively *strengthening* the unconscious attachment to the lost sexual culture.[38] Second, Sullivan's position is based on the assumption that the AIDS crisis has effected a transformation in the nation's stigmatization of homosexuality; he claims that this tragedy has led to a newfound empathy for gay men.[39] What he does not acknowledge is that this acceptance is extended only to those willing to occupy the position of the mourned subject: it precludes activities supposedly not suited to the ill or dying, such as expressing anger, fighting homophobia, engaging in activism, and, of course, having gay sex. Far from attempting to modify this subject position, Sullivan encourages gay men to occupy it and implies that a refusal to embrace tolerance in this way amounts to immaturity and irresponsibility.

Thus, I offer this extended reading of Sullivan's position because he recognizes that what he calls the "possibilit[ies] of life" are simply not available to those whose subjectivity is constituted through mourning. However, Sullivan's solution, in which gay men are encouraged to embrace life, depends upon the very mourned subject position produced by the Quilt and to which he claims to object. To put this differently, the rhetorical form of activism enacted by the Quilt serves to stitch together the conflicting national sentiments that are wrought by AIDS. That is, the Quilt makes possible a suturing of the wounds that the AIDS crisis inflicts on the identity of the American nation: it allows the mourning and grief for those named by the Quilt panels to cover over the underlying homophobia and neglect that sustained the severity of the epidemic in the early years. And as a consequence of the Quilt's affirmation of the nation's apparent tolerance and compassion, the mourned subject position becomes available as a means for gay men to access a previously impossible acceptance. Though Sullivan criticizes the culture of death and mourning that supposedly sustains the gay community during the AIDS crisis, then, his suggestion that gay men embrace the tolerance that the nation extends to them necessarily requires occupying the mourned subject position through which this tolerance is offered.

Risking the Subject: Resubjectivation

In the midst of a trenchant critique of Sullivan's position in "When Plagues End," Crimp laments, "I sometimes get the claustrophobic feeling that Andrew Sullivan and I inhabit the very same world."[40] The world to which Crimp refers is a relatively privileged one, where he and Sullivan are both able to spend time thinking, writing, and speaking about AIDS, and yet where—in spite of being well-informed and habitual practitioners of safe sex—both have become infected. His cognizance of his privilege, Crimp admits, only adds to the shame attending his sero-conversion. Crimp and Sullivan are caught in a similar bind: though they each strive to transform their world (admittedly with quite different ends in mind), their attempts are continually frustrated by the conservative nature of subjectivity—that is, by the passionate and unconscious attachments that secure one to the terms of one's subjection because it is only by maintaining these bonds that one has access to a recognizable position as a subject. The fact that Crimp and Sullivan continually find themselves subject to a return to this claustrophobic space suggests that neither has successfully theorized the ego's severing of its attachment to the terms of its melancholic formulation. Their shared hesitancy to attend to anger and militancy—for Crimp they are a denial of mourning; for Sullivan, a sign of immaturity—indicates, I contend, that it is precisely in these factors that the greatest risk of desubjectivation and the most fertile ground for activism is located.

Similarly, the Quilt, as a project of remembrance, simply cannot enact the anger and aggression that might break this melancholic attachment. This is not to say that particular panels of the Quilt do not speak loudly and vehemently of the rage that the AIDS virus and its mismanagement can elicit. As Cleve Jones argues in response to activists who claim that the Quilt is not angry enough, "Anger is released at the Quilt, it is expressed in the Quilt. Anger can be a great motivator if it's communicated in a creative way such as in the Quilt; it helps move us on with life and brings us together."[41] For instance, a panel dedicated to Billy

Donald reads, "My anger is, that the government failed to educate us," while Roger Lyon's panel states, "I came here today to ask that this nation with all its resources and compassion not let my epitaph read he died of red tape."[42] And the infamous panel created for the closeted and homophobic Roy Cohn both outs him in death and indicts him in life: "Bully. Coward. Victim."[43] As eloquently as these panels—and many others like them—may speak of individuals' feelings of anger and frustration, they do little to change the overall rhetorical force of the Quilt, which, in the form of a memorial on a national scale, deals in discourses of mourning and national identity. In other words, it is through the rhetorical form of the Quilt as a whole, not through the contents of individual panels, that the particular melancholic effects of the Quilt are produced.

The only way for the ego's attachment to the lost object to be broken, and for conscious mourning to take place, according to Butler, is to marshal the aggression that was internalized when the object was withdrawn into the ego. As she explains, "the aggression instrumentalized by conscience against the ego is precisely what must be reappropriated in the service of the desire to live." If, as Freud asserts, the ego absorbs the ambivalent feelings—both love and aggression—toward the lost object so as to protect it from hostility, then the aggression that serves as a founding condition for the ego was originally directed outward and was meant for an other. Butler argues that it is only by turning this aggression back onto the loved object and ceasing to shield it that the "melancholic bind" can be fractured: "Survival, not precisely the opposite of melancholia, but what melancholia puts in suspension—requires redirecting rage against the lost other, defiling the sanctity of the dead for the purposes of life, raging against the dead in order not to join them." Clearly, the prescription for change described here is, if not antithetical to the mission of the Quilt, at least representative of a distinct interruption in the assumption that mourning will move the nation toward compassion and transformation. Furthermore, it is not only the "sanctity of the dead" that is risked by this re-externalization of aggression. Turning outward the aggression that served to consolidate the ego essentially forfeits the melancholic construction of conscience, or, as Butler says, "'uncontains' the ego." In other words, the re-externalization of aggression is the possibility for resubjectivation, or for the subject, as described earlier, to "desire something other than its continued 'social existence.'" Hence, ironically, when Crimp argues that the militancy of AIDS activists is a means of denying internalized violence and protecting themselves from self-inflicted misery, he fails to note the potential for the converse effect.[44] Rather than protecting the subject, the expression of aggression and rage—when the ego is constituted through their incorporation—radically risks the subject.

In fact, some of the militant activist tactics of groups like ACT UP, which focus on channeling internalized aggression and anger onto their proper external objects, might usefully be viewed as a response to the need for transformation of both social conditions and gay male subjectivity. These practices open the possibility for shifting the terms of subjectivation, not only refusing the mourned subject position but also potentially unraveling the psychic bond to melancholia. Furthermore, if the melancholic attachment to the lost gay male sexual culture is broken, it therefore becomes available for mourning. Mourning, as Gregg Horowitz points out, does not entail forgetting or ceasing to care about the object; instead, it separates the self from the object, thereby making the object accessible to memory: "The mourner decathects the psychic traces of the lost object not to forget them, but to detach them from the lost object and thus render them memorable for the very first time. In this way, grieving preserves the intimacy with the lost object . . . despite its being lost to us."[45] Therefore, not only is the gay male community's ambivalence toward its lost sexual culture ejected from the ego and redirected onto its proper object, but the sexual culture itself can be mourned and remembered, rather than unconsciously preserved through the troublesome attitudes toward safe sex that Sullivan and Crimp discuss. This is not to suggest a particular moral stance regarding the practice of safe sex during the AIDS epidemic but merely to recognize that its equivocal adoption is both performed and described by Sullivan and Crimp as a cause for concern (though, again, for quite different reasons). As Freud tells us, self-imposed violence arises only when violent impulses against an other are redirected against the self;[46] therefore, the self-abasement of the melancholic, in the form of the sexual shame of gay men during the AIDS crisis, is certainly intended for a different target. However, if the aggression that motivates that shame can be re-externalized through angry, militant activism, it need not continue to be a founding condition of the ego.

The connection between severing melancholic attachments and activism is not coincidental. As Greg Forter argues, the process of extracting the lost object from the self (and therefore remembering it) has a "political corollary": "it is only once we can consciously articulate, as fully as possible (though never of course completely), what racism or homophobia or sexism has destroyed that we can build a collective memory of it and seek to do battle in its name."[47] In other words, the apparent "mourning" that is provided by the Quilt may be more accurately described as melancholic attachment and may, in fact, preclude the possibility for legitimate grief at the loss of thousands of lives and a unique sexual culture. Not only is aggression necessary to free the lost object, then, but its separation allows for an attack against the very systems that prohibited it from being mourned in the first place.

Unstitching the Quilt

The possibilities for mourning the dead need not exclude anger and aggression; indeed, the process of mourning may actually serve as an opportunity for the externalization of aggression that serves to constitute the subject in a new way. To illustrate this process of re-externalizing aggression and fighting political battles, I turn now to two examples of activism—ACT UP's political funerals and a demonstration at the Fifth International AIDS Conference—that suggest a different relationship between mourning, militancy, and subjectivity.

Part somber processional and part angry demonstration, ACT UP's political funerals not only provide a space in which grief and rage can coexist, but also alter the terms of subjectivity, effectively refusing the limited recognition provided by the mourned subject position. Political funerals take the ceremonies associated with death—the display of the coffin and possibly the deceased, the funeral procession, the scattering of ashes, the delivery of eulogies—and invest them with the anger and spirit of activism. One of the most jarring elements of political funerals is their publicness: rituals that are usually performed privately are conducted in places that are not only public but also sites of immense national power. For instance, Steve Michael, founder of the Washington, D.C., chapter of ACT UP, was remembered in 1998 with a political funeral that consisted of a half-mile walk down Pennsylvania Avenue with ACT UP members acting as pallbearers and carrying the group's trademark signs calling for an end to the government's neglect of the AIDS crisis. The procession concluded in front of the White House, where Michael's casket was opened and speakers eulogized Michael and criticized President Clinton for failing to follow through with promises to increase spending to expedite AIDS research.[48] Mark Lowe Fisher, another AIDS activist, in his request that his death be marked with a political funeral, articulates some of the important work that might be done by emphasizing the shame and anger that accompanies grief:

> I suspect—I know—my funeral will shock people when it happens. We Americans are terrified of death. Death takes place behind closed doors and is removed from reality, from the living. I want to show the reality of my death, to display my body in public; I want the public to bear witness. We are not just spiraling statistics; we are people who have lives, who have purpose, who have lovers, friends and families. And we are dying of a disease maintained by a degree of criminal neglect so enormous that it amounts to genocide.
>
> I want my death to be as strong a statement as my life continues to be. I want my own funeral to be fierce and defiant, to make the public statement that my death from AIDS is a form of political assassination.[49]

Even as he anticipates his own death, then, Fisher identifies the violence of AIDS as originating in a homophobic culture, and he sacrifices the modicum of respect and recognition that he may receive in his passing. In its place he imagines his political funeral as an opportunity for a new kind of existence, in which death and mourning need not preclude activism, opposition, and social transformation.

While less directly concerned with rituals of mourning, the 1989 demonstration at the Fifth International AIDS Conference in Montreal, which drew several AIDS activist groups (including ACT UP) from Canada and the United States, elegantly exhibits the possibilities for resubjectivation

made possible by risking the subject.[50] Beginning outside the conference
center with chants and placards, the demonstration quickly moved inside the building and seized control of the opening plenary itself. Later,
when New York City's health commissioner, Stephen Joseph, proposed
nonanonymous HIV testing and aggressive sexual contact tracing—policies that ACT UP firmly opposed—he was drowned out by protesters
yelling that he had provided only two hundred clean needles for the city's
500,000 intravenous drug users. These cries eventually coalesced into a
single roar, as protesters literally pointed fingers and shouted repeatedly,
"Shame! Shame! Shame!"[51]

It is difficult to judge the effects of this protest on the AIDS policy
makers and researchers that it targeted. Once the demonstration ended,
the conference presumably proceeded as planned, though hopefully with
a heightened awareness of some of the most pressing issues affecting
people with AIDS. What is significant about this protest for my purposes,
however, is the relationship between the mode of activism and the kind
of subjectivity it seems to constitute. The protesters, displaying obvious
rage, directly identify and indict Commissioner Joseph as a representative
of a homophobic institution. The shaming of Joseph re-externalizes the
aggression that had been turned inward in the form of social sanctions
against a specifically gay male sexual culture. The protesters mine their
own sexual shame for the power through which it constitutes the ego,
but redirect it—with pointing fingers to guide the way—onto its rightful
object: the social systems that prohibit the expression of (and mourning
for) homosexual desire.

The demonstration in Montreal and ACT UP's political funerals
therefore provide a vivid, albeit brief, glimpse of the resubjectivation that
might be achieved through aggression. This is, of course, not to say that
any individual protest leads to a complete reconstitution of subjectivity;
rather, it is to point to a set of practices that offer a possibility—though
as yet unfulfilled—of radical transformation of the psychic and social
mechanisms through which subjects come to be recognized. Not only
does the angry, confrontational activism of these protests create the possibility to mourn the loss of gay male sexual culture, but it also makes available—by radically risking the terms of subjectivation—different forms
of gay male subjectivity. That is, by projecting outward aggression and

ambivalence (the internalization of which was the founding condition of the ego), the ego is "uncontained" and therefore available to new terms of psychic and social subjectivation. It is this resubjectivation through militancy, I contend, that the Quilt's form, with its emphasis on mourning and memorializing, cannot offer. After all, the Quilt as a public memorial performs a suturing of national identity—it stitches together the tatters of tolerance and equality that have been rent by the traumas of AIDS and homophobia—and as such it constitutes rhetorically a subject position for gay men that does not threaten this imagined compassionate nation. It is only by figuratively unstitching the Quilt, by risking desubjectivation and loss of social acceptance, that the possibilities emerge for reimagining the nation's relationship to AIDS and homosexuality and for facilitating the legitimate mourning of the dead.

When we commemorate the Quilt's anniversary, then, we memorialize not only the Quilt's ability to name and remember the dead while comforting and providing a space for grieving for the living, but also its production of a mourned subject position. Since new names continue to be added to the Quilt, though, it does not merely mark a historical moment; rather, that history—of the Quilt, of AIDS, and of the nation's relationship to homosexuality—is repeatedly reinscribed in the present. As we memorialize the dead, so we constitute the living, and as we remember the memorial, so we reconstitute the subject position that it effects. It is this resuscitation of the mourned subject position—a position that confers social recognition and acceptance, perhaps, but has not in the past and will not in the future lead to progressive shifts in national discourses about AIDS or sexuality—that is one of the troubling effects of the celebration of the Quilt's anniversary.

By participating in this doubled commemoration, as this essay inevitably and paradoxically does, I hope for the possibility that its contribution might not be merely replicative, but also transformative. After all, if the Quilt provides a particular "framework of recognition," then it need not be the case that the militant tactic of an activist, the sewing of a quilt panel, or even the writing of an essay are invariably determined by this framework; instead, it is in relation to this framework that these actions come to make sense, and it is here that the resources for risking the subject, for resubjectivation, and for acting differently might be found.[52]

Thus, if the mourned subject can make sense in relation to the Quilt, then it is equally possible that another subject position—one that also incorporates militancy and sex and that enables activism—may become recognizable and inhabitable through the discourses of AIDS, homosexuality, and nation, from which the Quilt initially emerged and within which it continues to work.

NOTES

The author would like to thank Daniel Brouwer, Rafael Cervantes, Charles E. Morris III, and Barbara Biesecker for their helpful comments on earlier versions of this manuscript.

1. Carole Blair, Marsha S. Jeppeson, and Enrico Pucci Jr., "Public Memorializing in Postmodernity: The Vietnam Veterans Memorial as Prototype," *Quarterly Journal of Speech* 77 (1991): 263–288.

2. Barbara Biesecker, "Remembering World War II: The Rhetoric and Politics of National Commemoration at the Turn of the 21st Century," *Quarterly Journal of Speech* 88 (2002): 393–409.

3. Stephen H. Browne, "Remembering Crispus Attucks: Race, Rhetoric, and the Politics of Commemoration," *Quarterly Journal of Speech* 85 (1999): 169–187.

4. Marita Sturken, *Tangled Memories: The Vietnam War, the AIDS Epidemic, and the Politics of Remembering* (Berkeley: University of California Press, 1997), 3, 13. Sturken uses the term "cultural memory" to designate shared memories that are not inscribed through official historical discourse. Also, cultural memory is a particular kind of collective memory that is produced and reinforced through the mediums and artifacts of popular culture.

5. Dickinson, Ott, and Aoki note that particular subject positions are produced by museums, memorials, and other public historical sites through their construction and reconstruction of national identities and histories. However, the subject position with which these authors are concerned is that of the *viewer,* rather than that of the individuals named by the memorial; that is, the viewer is invited to view a display from a particular perspective, thereby shaping their understanding of the world. Greg Dickinson, Brian L. Ott, and Eric Aoki, "Spaces of Remembering and Forgetting: The Reverent Eye/I at the Plains Indian Museum," *Communication and Critical/Cultural Studies* 3 (2006): 27–47.

6. "Positive," VHS, directed by Rosa von Praunheim (New York: First Run Features,

1990); "HIV/AIDS Timeline," http://www.co.monterey.ca.us/health/Communi-tyHealth/pdfs/123101HIVTimeline.pdf (accessed April 24, 2004). Of the cumulative cases of AIDS reported to the CDC between 1981 and 2000, male-to-male sex was by far the most common mode of exposure (46 percent), compared to injection drug use (25 percent) and heterosexual sexual contact (11 percent). "HIV and AIDS—United States, 1981–2000," *MMWR Weekly* (2001): 430–434.

7. See, for example, Douglas Crimp, "Melancholia and Moralism: An Introduction," *Melancholia and Moralism: Essays on AIDS and Queer Politics* (Cambridge: MIT Press, 2002), 1–26; Douglas Crimp and Adam Rolston, *AIDS Demo Graphics* (Seattle: Bay Press, 1990); Michael A. Hallett, *Activism and Marginalization in the AIDS Crisis* (New York: Haworth Press, 1997); Cindy Patton, *Inventing AIDS* (New York: Routledge, 1990); "Positive"; Brett C. Stockdill, *Activism against AIDS: At the Intersections of Sexuality, Race, Gender, and Class* (Boulder, CO: Lynne Rienner Publishers, 2003).

8. Douglas Crimp, "Mourning and Militancy," in *Melancholia and Moralism: Essays on AIDS and Queer Politics* (Cambridge: MIT Press, 2002), 136–137.

9. Peter S. Hawkins, "Naming Names: The Art of Memory and the Names Project AIDS Quilt," *Critical Inquiry* 19 (1993): 752–779; "The AIDS Memorial Quilt," http://www.aidsquilt.org/index.htm (accessed April 1, 2009); Cleve Jones, *Stitching a Revolution: The Making of an Activist* (San Francisco: Harper Collins, 2000),138; Crimp and Rolston, *AIDS Demo Graphics,* 13. ACT UP still exists today and is still involved in activist demonstrations designed to draw attention to the political nature of the AIDS epidemic, and to encourage awareness and increase funding and support for AIDS prevention and treatment. This essay is not intended to provide a comprehensive history of ACT UP, nor to address the ways in which its activism has developed and changed since its early years. It is the kind of militant activist tactics with which ACT UP is often associated that I am interested in discussing here; that is, ACT UP uses various modes of activism to accomplish its goals, and I do not claim that militant tactics are the most characteristic of the group or the most instrumentally effective. For extensive information about ACT UP's history, as well as its current activities, see http://www.actupny.org.

10. Though this chapter deals exclusively with gay male subjectivity during the AIDS crisis, this is not to imply that women did not die of AIDS; did not mourn the deaths of friends, lovers, and family members; or were not involved in AIDS activism. In fact, women played a critical role in supporting the sick and dying gay men in their communities, as well as in agitating for better standards of care, better

access to drugs, etc. For more information on women and AIDS, see, for example, Katie Hogan, *Women Take Care: Gender, Race, and the Culture of AIDS* (Ithaca: Cornell University Press, 2001); Sarah Schulman, *My American History: Lesbian and Gay Life during the Reagan/Bush Years* (New York: Routledge, 1994); ACT UP / NY Women and AIDS Book Group, *Women, AIDS, and Activism* (Boston: South End Press, 1990).

11. I use the terms "gay men" and "the gay male community" throughout this chapter cautiously and provisionally in order to preserve the language used by Crimp, Sullivan, and other authors of the texts I examine. I want to point out, however, the problems of homogenization and essentialism that accompany such references to a diverse group of individuals. It should be understood that the gay men who were involved in ACT UP—and who are being described in this chapter—were primarily white, middle-class, and urban. The gay male subjectivities constituted within nondominant positions of race, class, religion, etc. cannot be presumed to be equivalent. However, I also preserve this potentially problematic language to point intentionally to the homogenizing force of the limited acceptance granted to gay men at this time; that is, one's access to the mourned subject position depended on one's ability to conform to the nonspecific descriptor "gay man." For an analysis of race and class in AIDS and AIDS activism, see Phillip Brian Harper, "Eloquence and Epitaph: Black Nationalism and the Homophobic Impulse in Responses to the Death of Max Robinson," in *Fear of a Queer Planet: Queer Politics and Social Theory,* ed. Michael Warner (Minneapolis: University of Minnesota Press, 1993), 239–263; Brett C. Stockdill, *Activism against AIDS: At the Intersections of Sexuality, Race, Gender, and Class* (Boulder, CO: Lynne Rienner Publishers, 2003).

12. "Positive."

13. Ibid.

14. This is not to suggest that activist groups such as ACT UP saw no place for mourning or did not support the Quilt as an important activist move. On the contrary, ACT UP has called the Quilt "the largest, most creative, most personal, and most explicit memorial for people with AIDS ever," and even in the group's criticisms of the Quilt (for instance, ACT UP protested the inclusion of pharmaceutical company booths in a "wellness pavilion" at the Quilt's 1996 display in Washington, D.C.) ACT UP continues to affirm and support its purpose. See ACT UP / New York, "Names Project Foundation Letter," http://www.actupny.org/campaign96/NAMESltr.html (accessed January 10, 2007); ACT UP / New York, "We Know When We're Well, and When We're Not," http://www.actupny.org/campaign96/

PWAChand.html (accessed January 10, 2007). In addition, by considering the Quilt in relation to ACT UP, I do not mean to suggest that these two activist projects are antithetical in their objectives or in their effects. Rather, I want to highlight the differing rhetorical modes through which their tactics typically are carried out.

15. Crimp, "Mourning and Militancy," 137.
16. Sigmund Freud, "Mourning and Melancholia," in *A General Selection from the Works of Sigmund Freud,* ed. John Rickman (New York: Liveright Publishing Corp., 1957), 124–140. For a different account of mourning, in which mourning is cast not as a desirable goal, but as an unfortunate closing off of future possibilities, see Joshua Gunn, "Review Essay: Mourning Humanism, or, the Idiom of Haunting," *Quarterly Journal of Speech* 92 (2006): 77–102; Jacques Derrida, *Specters of Marx: The State of Debt, the Work of Mourning, and the New International,* trans. Peggy Kamuf (New York: Routledge, 1994).
17. Freud, "Mourning and Melancholia," 130, 132.
18. Crimp, "Mourning and Melancholia," 140–141. The notion that the practices and sites of gay male sexuality may be viewed as a cultural development is also explored by Patrick Moore, who characterizes gay male sexual culture of the 1970s as a "social experiment" and as "art." Patrick Moore, *Beyond Shame: Reclaiming the Abandoned History of Radical Gay Sexuality* (Boston: Beacon Press, 2004).
19. Crimp, "Mourning and Melancholia," 140–41, 147, 149.
20. Ibid., 147 (emphasis added).
21. Judith Butler, *The Psychic Life of Power: Theories in Subjection* (Stanford: Stanford University Press, 1997), 169.
22. Hawkins, "Naming Names," 757, 776.
23. As AIDS relentlessly expands today to affect other American demographics (e.g., youth and African American women) and becomes a worldwide pandemic, the original presumed connection of AIDS to gay men is demonstrated to be false. However, in the late 1980s and early 1990s, the association between AIDS and homosexuality was still powerful; arguably, regardless of epidemiological trends, AIDS will always be understood in America as a "gay disease."
24. Douglas Crimp, "The Spectacle of Mourning," *Melancholia and Moralism: Essays on AIDS and Queer Politics* (Cambridge: MIT Press, 2002), 195–202.
25. Butler, *The Psychic Life of Power,* 138–139.
26. Browne, "Remembering Crispus Attucks," 172.
27. Andrew Sullivan, "When Plagues End: Notes on the Twilight of an Epidemic," *New York Times Magazine,* November 10, 1996, 52+.

28. Crimp, "Spectacle of Mourning," 197. Even this exemption, however, is conditional. Crimp makes this comment in order to point out the unexpectedness of a cartoon that callously ridicules the Quilt and viciously attacks a grieving community.

29. Quoted in Hawkins, "Naming Names," 772.

30. Crimp, "Spectacle of Mourning," 201.

31. Butler, *The Psychic Life of Power*, 2, 9, 13, 83.

32. Ibid., 28, 104.

33. Lawrence K. Altman, "Hope vs. Hype: A Special Report," *New York Times,* January 19, 1997, 1+. The declaration of protease inhibitor regimens as a miracle cure fostered unrealistic expectations and obscured serious problems involved in the administration and effectiveness of the drugs.

34. "HIV and AIDS—United States, 1981–2000." For criticisms of Sullivan's article, see, for example, Douglas Crimp, *Melancholia and Moralism: Essays on AIDS and Queer Politics* (Cambridge: MIT Press, 2002), 5–16; Phillip Brian Harper, *Private Affairs: Critical Ventures in the Culture of Social Relations* (New York: New York University Press, 1999), 89–104.

35. Sullivan, "When Plagues End," 58.

36. Sullivan, "When Plagues End," 62, 76. Sullivan does not take a stance on the Quilt in "When Plagues End"; in fact, it is only mentioned once in passing in the entire article. By discussing Sullivan here in relation to the politics of the Quilt and ACT UP, I do not mean to align him with (or position him in opposition to) either activist endeavor; rather, I offer his "solution" as a way to illuminate the ways in which the mourned subject position may both enable and constrain the agency of the subject who occupies it.

37. Crimp, "Mourning and Militancy," 141.

38. Indeed, Sullivan's own well-publicized brush with sexual hypocrisy (he was revealed to have solicited unprotected anal sex through an anonymous online ad) is a poignant example of the extent to which the renunciation of "shameful" behavior merely strengthens the unconscious attachment to the loss that cannot be grieved. Richard Kim, "Andrew Sullivan, Overexposed," *Nation,* June 18, 2001, http://www.thenation.com/doc/20010618/kim20010605 (accessed March 1, 2007).

39. Sullivan, "When Plagues End," 56.

40. Crimp, *Melancholia and Moralism*, 11.

41. Jones, *Stitching a Revolution,* 168.

42. Cindy Ruskin, *The Quilt: Stories from the NAMES Project* (New York: Pocket Books, 1988), 98, 34.

43. The NAMES Project Foundation, "The AIDS Memorial Quilt," http://www.aids-quilt.org (accessed March 1, 2007).

44. Butler, *The Psychic Life of Power*, 28, 192, 193; Freud, "Mourning and Melancholia," 133; Crimp, "Mourning and Militancy," 149.

45. Gregg M. Horowitz, *Sustaining Loss: Art and Mournful Life* (Stanford: Stanford University Press, 2001).

46. Freud, "Mourning and Melancholia," 133.

47. Greg Forter, "Against Melancholia: Contemporary Mourning Theory, Fitzgerald's *The Great Gatsby*, and the Politics of Unfinished Grief," *differences: A Journal of Feminist Cultural Studies* 14 (2003): 134–170.

48. "Steve Michael Political Funeral," http://www.actupny.org/reports/SteveMichael.html (accessed March 1, 2007).

49. Mark Lowe Fischer, "Bury Me Furiously," http://www.actupny.org/diva/polfunsyn.html (accessed March 1, 2007).

50. One of the keynote speakers at the conference in Montreal was Cleve Jones, and his display of international Quilt panels was intended as "a symbol of international cooperation"—a cooperation that was, as he notes, "fractured from the first" by divisiveness amongst various factions of the audience and American policies that prevented HIV-positive travelers from entering the country. Jones, *Stitching a Revolution*, 177–178.

51. "Positive."

52. Judith Butler, *Giving an Account of Oneself* (New York: Fordham University Press, 2005), 22.

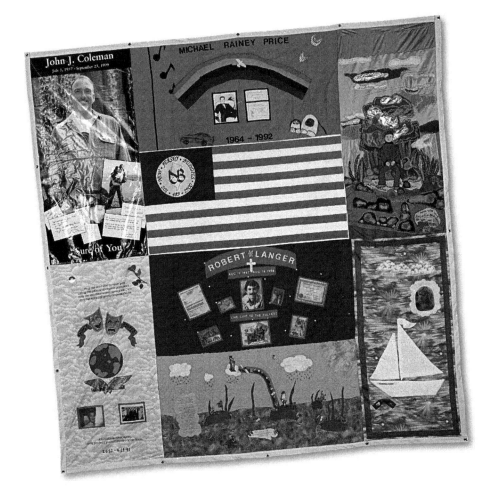

How to Have History in an Epidemic

Kyra Pearson

In 2006 the California senate approved a bill that would require all
public schools to adopt social studies textbooks that portray the sexual
diversity of society and avoid material that "reflects adversely" upon a
group based on sexual orientation. By proposing this legislation, the bill's
author, state Senator Sheila Kuehl (D-Santa Monica), the first out lesbian
member of the legislature, sought to enhance the quality of education
for all students and the safety of lesbian, gay, bisexual, and transgender (LGBT) students in particular.[1] Recognizing the "contributions" of
LGBT individuals and communities in U.S. history, as the bill espoused,
would extend existing state law requiring the "accurate inclusion of 'men,
women, black Americans, American Indians, Mexicans, Pacific Island
people and other ethnic groups.'" Though quite compatible with a sanitized, "age appropriate" civil rights model of history, the bill predictably
ruffled the feathers of conservative Christian groups and some California
newspapers that accused the bill of "political meddling" and a "twisting of

history." After the state assembly had passed a water-downed version, one that omitted the "positive role model" feature, Governor Arnold Schwarzenegger vetoed the bill, claiming that the phrase "reflects adversely" was too vague.[2]

Upon hearing the news, I wondered, if the bill had passed, how would public schools have reconciled a state legislated commitment to sexual diversity with an existing mandate (in some schools) to teach abstinence-only sex education? Within such a climate, how might the narration of AIDS activism, including the creation of a safe-sex culture, to which gays, lesbians, bisexuals, and queers have "contributed" immensely, unfold? How might the narration of AIDS, a mode of signification historically hostile (not simply "adverse") to LGBTQ people, proceed? These questions do not simply go away with Schwarzenegger's veto of the bill. Indeed, they demonstrate some key rhetorical and corporeal dilemmas that face us, as scholars, students, teachers, and activists, making our way through the third decade of the AIDS epidemic.

In *Tangled Memories: The Vietnam War, the AIDS Epidemic, and the Politics of Remembering,* Marita Sturken argues that "American political culture is often portrayed as one of amnesia, and the media seem complicit in the public's apparent ease in forgetting important political facts and events. However, this definition of American culture is highly superficial, relying on evidence of memory in traditional forms and narratives." Sturken continues by stating her central premise—that "American culture is not amnesiac but rather replete with memory, that cultural memory is a central aspect of how American culture functions and the nation is defined."[3] While cultural memory indeed has proven instrumental to nation building, Sturken's premise might be difficult to accept for queer historians and activists whose intellectual and political labor continues to demonstrate the manifold ways that sexual dissidents are exiled from the National Symbolic—that archive of icons and images that populate the nation's storehouse of cultural memory. California's attempt to expunge from the history books gay and lesbian contributions to political life reflects only a recent attempt to police the boundaries of this "official" repository. Such *mnemonicide*—Charles E. Morris's provocative term for the "assassination of memory"—contracts the discursive space available for resurrecting a queer past in the service of cultivating contemporary queer lives and futures. Moreover, nearly three decades of AIDS have "contributed profoundly to the material and political depletion of public memory." Absent "institutions for common memory," queer pasts are vulnerable to a counternostalgia that has rewritten the 1970s values of sexual liberation as immature and deadly.[4]

From a rhetorical perspective, the available means of persuasion are severely compromised if the past cannot serve as a resource for present and future activism. This is especially the case if we define cultural or collective memory, with David Zarefsky, as a "storehouse of common knowledge and belief about history that forms the premises for arguments and appeals." One need only imagine how differently Martin Luther King's canonical oration "I Have a Dream" would sound without the ethos of Abraham Lincoln and the nation's constitutional documents that King summoned on the steps of the Lincoln Memorial during the 1963 March on Washington for black civil rights. By calling upon material from the National Symbolic, King's speech illustrates, as Bruce Gronbeck observes, the strategic appropriation of the "past for guidance of present-day concerns or problems." How do activists appropriate a past that is not commonly shared? With few, if any, similarly canonical speeches or manifestoes, and with few, if any, "iconic photographs" that circulate with the same regularity and force as, say, the photo of U.S. soldiers erecting the American flag at Iwo Jima, it is no wonder that ephemerality has been named a hallmark of queer discourse. And it is no wonder that queer scholarship has made a self-conscious "archival turn," documenting and interpreting material from the past, producing an "archive of the ephemeral," to be used as resources for future activists and historians "who may want to interpret the lives we have lived from the few records we have left behind."[5]

If there *is* anything like an institution for *queer* memory, one that is not only publicly accessible but that circulates publicly, it is perhaps the NAMES Project AIDS Memorial Quilt, founded by gay activist Cleve Jones in the mid-1980s for two purposes: to commemorate the lives lost to AIDS, the overwhelming majority of whom were gay men, and to challenge the negligent indifference that characterized the federal government's response to AIDS. President Ronald Reagan's infamous silence on AIDS until 1987—six years into the epidemic and nearly 50,000 American AIDS diagnoses and 28,000 deaths (and counting) later—made the need for such a memorial in an AIDS-phobic and homophobic culture palpable. Since its first display on the National Mall in 1987, the AIDS Memorial Quilt seems to have achieved institutional status. After all, it is repeatedly heralded within the mainstream media as the "most powerful icon in the history of AIDS," the "world's most vivid symbol of the enormity of the AIDS pandemic," and the "most effective and enduring symbol of the fight against the epidemic," its size "dwarfed only by the magnitude of the epidemic itself." Arguably the most publicized form of the Quilt—aerial photographs of tens of thousands of panels laid out on the National Mall in Washington, D.C.—accentuate the Quilt's "spectacular" function: disarming viewers with the sheer enormity of the epidemic. Simultaneously, the individual panels dedicated to loved ones who have died from AIDS have been praised for "humanizing the statistics" and putting a "face on this epidemic." As Capozzola has put it, "The people memorialized in the quilt are commemorated as unforgettable individuals embedded in social relationships rather than statistical representation of forgotten risk groups." For its commemorative role, the Quilt is often recognized as offering a blanket of intimacy in the face of cold statistics. For its activist role, the Quilt has been credited with no less than "shaking the government and priming the funding pipeline that has poured billions of dollars into AIDS research."[6] With these credentials, the Quilt would likely make a seamless entry into a California textbook narrating AIDS activism and LGBTQ history.

And yet, splashed among the debate over California's history curriculum were headlines about "AIDS at 25" years old, a temporal benchmark that brought under scrutiny the Quilt's relevance within a changing epidemic.[7] Calling it an "aging snapshot of the first decade of AIDS, when gay white men were dying in the tens of thousands," the *Los Angeles Times* in 2006 pronounced the Quilt's obsolescence. Out of nearly 6,000 blocks of panels (totaling 40,000 individual panels), the Quilt's 616 blocks dedicated to women no longer mirrored the demographics of the epidemic in the United States, where women account for 27 percent of new infections, highest among African American women. The 260 blocks memorializing African Americans as of 2006 meant they comprised 4 percent of the Quilt's blocks, even though African Americans accounted for nearly 50 percent of all new infections.[8]

Predictions that the AIDS Quilt would fade into obscurity consequently signaled a possible shift in the symbolic value of the Quilt. For Cleve Jones, such predictions are unacceptable in light of staggering rates of new infections. The Quilt, he believes, can counter the perception that AIDS is a treatable, chronic condition, a view he sees prevalent among young people today. Jones's rallying cry against this complacency represents a growing concern, and shift in rhetorical exigencies, among AIDS educators and activists. Kevin Fenton, chief of HIV/AIDS at the Centers for Disease Control and Prevention (CDC), announced in 2009, "There is a serious health threat to our nation—and that threat is complacency." Ephen Glenn Colter, one of the contributors to *Policing Public Sex: Queer Politics and the Future of AIDS Activism,* put the problem this way: "change is epidemic, complacency is the real disease, because it dulls thinking about what kinds of safer sex knowledge are livable in an ongoing epidemic and ever-changing world." Indicative of the "ongoing epidemic and ever-changing world," the CDC in 2008 revised its statistics for the rate of new infections in the United States; previously estimated at 40,000 per year, it is now hovering at 56,300 per year.[9]

Consequently, the juxtaposition of California's education bill in 2006 with media attention to the AIDS Memorial Quilt that same year produces for me a context in which to ask an additional set of questions about the place of historical claims within the rhetoric of this public health crisis: What might it mean to have a *history* in an epidemic? *How* might we historicize an epidemic that is now within Western nations considered a "manageable," chronic condition (at least for those who can afford treatment)? And *why* might a sense of the past be important now?

My focus on history within and about the AIDS epidemic is not without precedent. In fact, historians of public health Elizabeth Fee and Daniel M. Fox have argued that AIDS has "stimulated more interest in history than any other disease of modern times."[10] As their book, *AIDS: The Burdens of History,* illustrates, this "interest in history," demonstrated by journalists, scientists, public officials, and professional historians, has been motivated by a desire to know both the social and epidemiological history of AIDS (when and where it emerged). In contrast to Fee and Fox, I am interested in examining the function of history within the rhetoric of AIDS activism—rhetorical appeals to the past and in the rhetoric of historiography about social movements more broadly. I argue that although the AIDS Quilt would likely make a seamless entry into a California textbook narrating AIDS activism and LGBTQ history, it also poses challenges to the temporality of progress that often underwrites such histories. This is because the Quilt is an artifact of progression, not one of progress. I submit that this is one of its most valuable rhetorical features, but it is also the feature that makes it vulnerable to charges of obsolescence. While the significance of the Quilt can be discerned by analyzing the rhetorical features of the Quilt and its ceremonial displays, the rhetorical and political import of the Quilt can also be fruitfully gleaned from analysis of the media coverage of it. Rather than offer an interpretation of the Quilt panels themselves, then, I examine the discourse of history that circulates alongside the Quilt as the "most powerful icon in the history of AIDS" enters—and recedes from—the mass-mediated public sphere.[11]

The first section of the essay situates the AIDS Quilt within the context of two competing understandings of history, one that narrates the past as exerting inescapable influence on the present, and the other that narrates the past as elusive. This context helps me demonstrate in the second section of the essay that the Quilt is not only a rhetorical response to the AIDS epidemic, but also a rhetorical response to the *historicizing* of the AIDS epidemic. Here I analyze U.S. media coverage of the AIDS Memorial Quilt to demonstrate the Quilt's status as an artifact of progression within an AIDS public sphere, a status that places a drag on narratives of progress. The third section examines accounts of the Quilt's "diminishing future," including the controversy over its seeming obsolescence, a topic debated on the pages of the *New York Times,* the *Los Angeles Times,* the *Advocate,* and *Poz* magazine, inspiring even the creation of independent art. The essay concludes by exploring the implications the Quilt's status as an artifact of progression has on the study of the history and rhetoric of social movements. I suggest that grappling with the Quilt as a rhetorical figure of progression within public discussions of AIDS activism may require developing a model of history that breaks from historiographies of rupture.

History in an Epidemic

For readers familiar with cultural criticism on representations of AIDS, my speculation about the practice of history in the AIDS epidemic should recall Paula Treichler's book-length chronicle analyzing the discourse surrounding AIDS, *How to Have Theory in an Epidemic,* as well as Douglas Crimp's essay "How to Have Promiscuity in an Epidemic," initially published in a special issue of *October* on AIDS activism. Just as Crimp warns against the moralizing dismissals of desire and sexual pleasure in AIDS education,[12] Treichler highlights the danger of abdicating theory in discussions of the prevention and treatment of HIV/AIDS. In her view, theory leads to practical action. Focusing on debates over the AIDS drug AZT, Treichler argues that out of "available resources [AIDS treatment activism] assembled a complex conception of the body and a multi-layered strategy for rescuing it from disease and death."[13] Theory is necessarily "provisional," facts contingent upon context. Community research experiments could, over time, contribute to processes of knowledge production. In this case, the strength of such activism lay "not in a resistance to orthodox science but in strategic conceptions of 'scientific truth' that leave room for action in the face of contradiction."[14]

Treichler and Crimp's calls remain as urgent as ever, especially given the accelerated rate of new infections and the virus' spread around the world. Of course, debates over knowledge production are not restricted to the domain of biomedicine or health; they can also impact historical work, as the recent challenge posed to California's history curriculum helps illustrate. Despite its failure, California's bill affirms the importance of the project Scott Bravmann calls for in *Queer Fictions of the Past*: a queer cultural studies of history. Extending queer theory's commitment to challenging "regimes of the normal," Bravmann proposes that scholarship occurring under the sign of LGBTQ history challenge not only heteronormativity but the academic practices of *historiography*.[15] I would add that such work could be explored by turning to invocations of the past within public discourse about AIDS.

Within public and scholarly discourse about AIDS (particularly AIDS in the context of sexual transmission), invocations of the past animate two competing trajectories. In one trajectory, history is said to exert a gravitational pull on the present, impacting contemporary understandings of AIDS and those afflicted with it. In the other, history is considered an elusive narrative slipping away as time marches on. Each of these trajectories offers a way of thinking about history in an epidemic.

The first trajectory can be found in interdisciplinary studies of AIDS discourse that have well documented the striking resemblance that establishment responses to AIDS in the 1980s bear to prior responses to social epidemics such as cholera and syphilis. In this work, the past functions as a context for understanding the contemporary AIDS crisis. So entrenched in prior sense-making devices, such as iconographies and narratives of disease, some industrialized nations responding to AIDS have become, in the words of historian Peter Baldwin, "slaves to the past." Baldwin argues that, in the arena of public policy, industrialized nations in Europe and North America adopted different approaches to prevention methods that "corresponded to the preventive tactic they adopted during the nineteenth century" when dealing with cholera, smallpox, and syphilis. Because these divergent responses are due to precedence, he claims, they indicate the existence of a "deep historical public health memory." Similarly, Fee and Fox argue that AIDS was first historicized as discontinuous from modern history, enabling a plague model of disease to dominate.[16]

The circulation of this public health memory within biomedicine and popular media has had devastating consequences for women, gay men, people of color, and "foreigners," as Treichler and Sander Gilman demonstrate. Less indebted to a legal concept of precedence than to a cultural studies concept of "articulation" theory, Treichler shows how the "semantic baggage" within gendered representations of AIDS tend to bear "complex historical burdens."[17] Long-standing images of women as vectors of disease within Western medicine were momentarily resurrected in AIDS discourses and displaced onto female sex workers in the early 1980s, while constructions of AIDS as a "gay disease" or "male disease" rendered information about women's susceptibility virtually and dangerously invisible. Female-to-female sexual transmission was hardly on the biomedicine radar screen and thus further precluded the gathering of accurate information. Making a similar move in his 1987 essay, "AIDS and Syphilis: The Iconography of Disease," Gilman shows that the vocabulary of syphilis provided a lens through which AIDS was understood and the perceived "boundaries of pollution" delimited. By comparing early 1980s media representations of AIDS to artistic renderings of syphilis that appeared in Europe some 500 years earlier, he illustrates the way the stigmatization of STDs and the construction of the diseased body as sexually excessive and "foreign" occurred. So great was the force of history in these narratives that "despite appearances of the syndrome among hemophiliacs and IV drug users, sexual orientation persisted as the defining characteristic of the person with AIDS." For Gilman, recognizing this continuity between past and present "may not eliminate it," but it can lead to understanding the "regularity with which it recurs historically." From this perspective, there is a lesson to be learned about the "burdens of history," the "inescapable significance of events of the past." If inventional resources that could intervene within a punitive public health memory are not readily accessible as counternarratives, we remain "burdened," haunted by the ghosts of history.[18]

If the first trajectory finds the past inescapable, the second trajectory, by contrast, views the past as elusive. This perspective can be seen in work that crosses both AIDS activism and queer scholarship. Testimony offered by Cleve Jones himself in 1987 is illustrative. He describes how his idea for the Quilt emerged: Overwhelmed by grief upon watching so many fellow gay men in San Francisco, including his best friend, succumb to AIDS, he explains, "I went through a period of real despair. My past has been wiped out. I've lost all my friends from my youth."[19] The vanishing past to which he refers is not, significantly, restricted to his own personal history. It is instead very much rooted in the collective loss of a gay culture, a point he develops in his memoir, *Stitching a Revolution.* Jones, a longtime resident of San Francisco's Castro area, recalls reading newspaper headlines in 1985 that the death toll from AIDS in San Francisco had surpassed 1,000. Since the predominantly gay area of the Castro was disproportionately decimated, there was, he writes, a "deep yearning not only to find a way to grieve individually and together but also to find a voice that could be heard beyond our community, beyond our town."[20]

Whereas Jones is impacted by the disappearance of "the familiar faces of the neighborhood—the bus drivers, clerks, and mailmen,"[21] AIDS activist and cultural critic Douglas Crimp laments the loss of a more sexually explicit public sex culture: "Alongside the dismal toll of death, what many of us have lost is a culture of sexual possibility: back rooms, tea rooms, bookstores, movie houses, and baths; the trucks, the pier, the ramble, the dunes."[22] The contracted physical space of erotic possibilities would be further contained with rezoning laws in major urban cities such as New York in the 1990s. The reasons that these losses are lamentable are not trumpeted very easily these days for a variety of reasons: the institutionalization of abstinence-only sex education policies for young people, the lexicon of celibacy and monogamy upon which those policies are based, and a gay media conservatism possessing the power to revise history.

The need to be "heard beyond" the enclave of San Francisco's Castro is a testament to the towering obstacles impeding the circulation of knowledge about queer lives in the United States. Without "institutions for common memory," writes Michael Warner, queers lack the resources to circulate the ethics, politics, and pleasures of queer culture. "No institutions—neither households, nor schools, nor churches, nor political groups—ensure that this will happen."[23] What is lost in the process is not only the lively sex culture and accompanying promiscuity to which Crimp refers, but the recognition that it is precisely this promiscuity, not its abandonment, that led to the invention and circulation of safe sex by gay people.[24]

What these two trajectories can tell about having history in an epidemic has provided a profound nexus for understanding the AIDS Memorial Quilt and its role in AIDS activism. In the first trajectory, the past influences present understandings, such that "having a history" means carrying the weight of the past into the present. As it has played out in the context of AIDS, this has not been an especially liberating form. The second trajectory, however, makes clear that evacuating the present of the past entails some important bodily and affective risks as well.

Bodies, Memories, and the Quilt

The AIDS Memorial Quilt, in many respects, can be seen as a response not only to the AIDS epidemic but to the historicizing of AIDS—where past epidemics function as a burdensome weight and where the past is an elusive, vanishing presence. As a response to the inadequate public health policies underwriting the government's negligent inattention to AIDS, the Quilt addressed the burdensome weight of the past. In addition to homophobia enabling the federal government's inattention to AIDS, the historicizing of AIDS as analogous to earlier models of disease also explains this inattention. Reagan reportedly considered AIDS as analogous to "measles and it would go away," a view his biographer aptly characterized as "halting and ineffective."[25] While reflecting on his original idea for the Quilt, Jones has written, "When I thought of the quilt, I was thinking in terms of evidence." He recalls telling a friend, "If this were a meadow and there were one thousand corpses lying out here and people could see it, they would have to respond on some level."[26] The Quilt's central commemorative function responds to the sense of the past as elusive—to preserve the memories of the lives lost to AIDS, a purpose captured in the slogan "Remember the Names." The Quilt reconstituted those killed by AIDS and government neglect as "bodies that matter."[27] The AIDS Quilt, Jones hoped, would challenge the "nation to speak a new political tongue."[28]

In 1987, the unmasking function Jones hoped the Quilt would perform went largely unheeded by the federal government, despite the kairotic dimensions of its national debut. The Quilt's first full display on the National Mall in Washington, D.C., took place during the weekend of the October 1987 National March on Washington for Gay and Lesbian Rights, which was timed to capitalize on the presidential election campaign season. Indeed, for some who visited the Quilt that day, it would seem that the federal government was more concerned about preserving the grass on the Mall than protecting the lives of the country's citizens. As one visitor remembers, "The National Park Service was on hand to enforce that the quilt was shaken every so many hours so that the grass could breathe. I remember thinking, 'How typical of our government, to care more about the grass on the Mall than the lives that were lost.'"[29] Within days of the March, Congress passed the Helms Amendment, which prohibited the spending of federal tax dollars on AIDS education programs that "promote or encourage, directly or indirectly, homosexual activities."[30]

To suggest a causal relationship between the Quilt display and the Helms Amendment, or to call the Quilt a rhetorical failure would be too facile, for the obstacles to generating a sustained federal response to AIDS had long been in place. Testimony from CDC official Don Francis, which he gave before a congressional committee March 16, 1987, is illustrative:

> Much of the HIV/AIDS epidemic was and continues to be preventable. But because of active obstruction of logical policy, active resistance to essential funding, and active interference with scientifically designed programs, the executive branch of this country has caused untold hardship, misery, and expense to the American public. Its efforts with AIDS will stand as a huge scar in American history, a shame to our nation and an international disgrace.[31]

National print and television media arguably exacerbated the neglect. In their analysis of nightly television news about AIDS, Timothy Cook and David Colby suggested that television's relative silence on AIDS until 1983—two years into the epidemic—and its subsequent ebb and flow of stories "enabled the government to overlook the gravity of the epidemic." Between 1987 and 1989, the number of nightly news AIDS stories decreased by half. "So scarce were the stories about AIDS in the late 1980s and early 1990s that the September 24, 1991, headline in the weekly health supplement of the *Washington Post* asked, "Whatever Happened to AIDS?"[32]

As a strategic response to the historicizing of AIDS as analogous to epidemics of the past, the Quilt functioned to document the progression of the epidemic. As an artifact of progression, the Quilt functioned to place a drag on the temporality of progress that often characterized public discussions of AIDS. Cook and Colby argue that beginning in 1983, television networks, like news magazines, started to "express cautious hope, reassuring the audience that scientists were inexorably progressing toward a treatment, cure, or vaccine."[33] The progression of the epidemic, as illustrated by the Quilt's growth, runs counter to the cultural practice of telling progress narratives.

Commonly found in media accounts of the national displays in Washington is the exponential increase in its size from its initial full display.

What was once described as a "giant quilt" of 1,920 panels, spanning the length of "two football fields" in 1987, became 40,000 panels in 1996, an "exhibit the size of twenty-four football fields." Calling attention to the growth of the Quilt had already begun by its second national display in 1988, when it was "five times bigger" than the one in 1987, the size of "nearly eight football fields." Having "grown with dizzying speed," the Quilt was, in 1992, "more than 10 times the size it was during its first display in Washington five years ago." Writing for the *New Republic,* Andrew Sullivan observed that it had grown so large that it could no longer be contained within the Ellipse in front of the White House. "At 26,000 panels, it filled most of the vast space between the Washington Monument and the Reflecting Pool." Such growth would no doubt earn the Quilt its reputation as a "potent symbol of the continuing epidemic."[34]

The Quilt has also circulated as a symbol of continued government inattention to AIDS. Capturing both the continued expansion of the Quilt's size and the continued neglect, the *San Francisco Chronicle*'s coverage of the 1996 display reported: "The Reagan White House ignored the 2,000 [panel] quilt display brought to Washington in 1987, as well as when it grew to 8,000 panels in 1988. The Bush White House paid it little attention as it expanded to 11,000 panels in 1989 and 20,000 in 1992." The persistence of the Quilt—the way it continued to return to Washington for displays in 1987, 1988, 1989, and 1992—is a feature the *Los Angeles Times* described in its coverage of the 1992 display as a model of American citizens' "refusal to be silent in the face of government inadequacy." The Quilt becomes as much a measure of resilience as it is a measure of the government's negligence. Descriptions of some of the panels also draw attention to discrimination, cultural indifference, and government inaction. The *San Francisco Chronicle,* for example, explains that a panel made for Joe Del Ponte features a picture of him "holding up a sign that read[s], 'Homophobia Kills, Cure Hate, Stop AIDS,'" with the White House standing behind him. The *New York Times* describes a different panel depicting a "syringe dripping with blood and bearing the words, 'Another Victim of 3rd World Genocide.'"[35]

In short, media accounts of Quilt displays occasion assessments of failed progress. This is true even in accounts of the 1996 display, which is commonly regarded as a turning point in the history of the Quilt and AIDS activism, as it was the first time the Quilt was visited by a president of the United States. Bill and Hillary Clinton both walked among the panels, finding panels dedicated to friends they knew. In his memoir, *Stitching a Revolution,* Cleve Jones remarks that the 1996 display was the first time he felt hope, a feeling occasioned in part by the president's visit to the Quilt. About that year's display, the *New York Times* similarly announced: "for the first time" the grief that blanketed the Mall was "tempered by the growing hope that AIDS might be transformed into a manageable disease through antiviral drug therapies and genetic research." This hope radiated from David Varala, an HIV-positive man visiting the Quilt in 1996 for World AIDS Day. He told the *San Francisco Chronicle* that "we're seeing an incredible change." "No more chemo. No more IV infusions. I'm moving to pills." After seven months of protease inhibitors, he had become virtually asymptomatic. The *Washington Post*'s coverage of the 1996 national display of the Quilt also celebrated the new AIDS drugs for their "dramatically slow[ing] the course of the disease and even seemingly revers[ing] its effects." And yet a crucial difference between the *New York Times* and the *Washington Post* articles is that the latter counters a narrative of hope with a narrative of the fatality of AIDS. After explaining that "many people live seven, eight, 10 years or longer with AIDS" because of the new drugs, the *Post* points out, "but it still kills: sooner, in the case of some; later for others. There is no cure." The fatality of AIDS is imagined as inevitable, just a matter of time. This feature of AIDS was a chief reason one high school teacher used to explain why she organized a field trip for her students to visit the 1996 Quilt display on Youth Day. She stated, "We want them to realize that right now AIDS is 100 percent fatal, but it's also 100 percent preventable." Obvious though it may be, the Quilt facilitates the perception of AIDS as a death sentence, a view that by 1996 was beginning to compete with the emerging historical model of AIDS as a chronic, manageable disease. Thus, despite the optimism circulating in 1996 due to the president's visit and the availability of protease inhibitors, the Quilt's contribution to the AIDS public sphere that year served in part to interrupt these political and scientific advancements.[36]

The *San Francisco Chronicle* perhaps goes even further than the *Washington Post* by tempering a narrative of hope with a sobering narrative of the global epidemic AIDS has become. Its byline, "Despite progress, epidemic spreading," captured the ambivalence that springs from a mixture of optimism and despair. While new treatment options gave Western nations reason to hope in 1996, the *San Francisco Chronicle* reminded its readers that, according to the World Health Organization, AIDS was "spreading at an explosive rate in developing countries, especially those in Asia and Africa, home of 63% of the world's estimated 23 million HIV-infected people." In recognition of World AIDS Day, it continued, Uganda newspapers reported a decline in the number of new cases since a nationwide effort had encouraged men to use condoms, whereas in Paris, AIDS activists displayed signs reading, "Zero equals the number of AIDS survivors." Also cited was Robin Avant, an African American woman who worked for the San Francisco AIDS Foundation. She pointed out that "black and Latino women are the fastest-growing group of new AIDS cases in [the United States]." Testimony from the executive director of the NAMES Project, Anthony Turney, concluded the *Chronicle*'s coverage of World AIDS Day with a sobering account made possible by the AIDS Quilt. He recalled that in 1987 the Quilt comprised 40 panels displayed in San Francisco's Civic Center. In 1996 it had 39,000 panels and weighed forty-six tons, a stark reminder that "in his office he sees evidence that the struggle against the pandemic is far from over." This textual globetrotting through Uganda, France, Thailand, and the United States reveals uneven results of AIDS activism. In the process, a drag is placed on attempts to mark progress on the commemorative World AIDS Day.[37]

In this way, the discourse is burdened not by representations of past epidemics, as in other AIDS discourses described earlier, but a cautionary reminder that this continues to be a worldwide struggle. In their analysis of network television nightly news, Cook and Colby argue that the media's coverage of AIDS between 1983 and 1989 generally followed an "alarm-and-reassurance" pattern, whereby stories would lead off with dramatic fear tactics and conclude with reassuring stories that quelled fears of the epidemic, usually by reporting on advancements in treatments or research on a cure or vaccine.[38] Accounts of the Quilt displays tend to alter this trend, shrinking the discursive space for reassurance by interrupting the forward march of progress. As the "most powerful icon in the history of AIDS" enters—and recedes from—the mass mediated public sphere, the reputation of the Quilt as a symbol of a continuing epidemic would become more difficult to sustain.

From Large to Largely Forgotten

Even before the accounts of "AIDS at 25" had questioned the Quilt's relevance in AIDS activism, the Quilt's ability to circulate had already become an issue. The twin forces of expansion and ephemerality are said to threaten the circulation of the Quilt, and thus its continued function as both a memorial and educational tool. Despite serving as one of its greatest rhetorical resources, the Quilt's increasing size has been cited as reason to halt its future display. As early as 1989, two years after its first full display in Washington, D.C., activists and journalists predicted that soon the Quilt would be too large to display in its entirety. The 1989 headline of the *Washington Post* read, "Ever-Growing AIDS Quilt Set for Finale." Michael Bento, board member of the National Capital chapter of the NAMES Project, was quoted as saying, "as with the epidemic, [the Quilt] outpaced our ability to keep up." Another affiliate concurred, stating, "now it's just growing too large to show the whole thing." In 1996 the *Washington Post* predicted that that year's display might be the "last time any one site will be able to accommodate the ever-growing memorial." By 2006 it weighed in as a "54-ton albatross," burdened by the weight of its own history.[39]

Activists and journalists alike have worried not only about expansion but its ephemerality—the Quilt's durability as panels decay from age or from exposure to rain or sun. Unlike its granite or marble counterparts, the Quilt, when displayed, is more vulnerable to the elements. From this vantage point, it is, as Flavia Rando puts it, "transient, perishable, conditional." This aspect of the Quilt has led, in part, to the personification of the memorial. For example, one reporter at the 1989 display who found himself overwhelmed by the fourteen acres of Quilt observed, "So delicate and vulnerable to nature's elements, each fiber became the very embodiment of the AIDS victim that it represented." Evelyn Martinez, one of the Quilt repair crew members at the time, similarly reflected on its frailty. Though she worked full time on the panels, she "always feel[s] like they are not going to hold up. It's as if they were human beings. As they get older, they begin to fall apart." Restoring them, therefore, becomes more than an act of memorializing; it is an act of caregiving.[40]

Nearly twenty years later, the need to mend panels was a focal point in a front-page story of the Quilt in the *Los Angeles Times*. For the *Times*, the literal withering away of the Quilt is analogous not only to the bodies of those who have succumbed to AIDS, but to the Quilt's place in history. The byline reads, "Once a mighty symbol of love and loss, the tribute to victims with AIDS had gone from large to largely forgotten." In a story mostly centered around the Quilt's dedicated seamstress of nineteen years, Gert McMullin, the *Los Angeles Times* leads off with a description of McMullin hunched over a panel, repairing a section of the Quilt's "fraying edges." "There are some spots that are really faded, that you can barely see anymore," she explains. Like Evelyn Martinez, McMullin personifies the Quilt panels, calling them her "boys." These panels are reportedly where "all [her] friends are." Late at night, when tired or depressed, she sometimes, we are told, "climbs into the shelves, covers herself with a section of quilt and falls asleep." To be touched, cloaked, and comforted by her "friends" is to be blanketed in affective and corporeal intimacy. In this scenario, the direction of caregiving reverses itself. It isn't the panel deriving care from the Quilt repair worker, but rather the Quilt repairer deriving comfort from "her friends" who literally blanket her. The logic of this narrative implies that to forget the Quilt is to forget those who died from AIDS. Moreover, if the panels symbolize friends from her past, as they do for Cleve Jones, the past in this scenario reaches into the present moment. The role it is said to perform, however, is primarily a therapeutic one inside the warehouse where the Quilt is stored, invisible from the public eye. Such a role allows the *Los Angeles Times* to narrate the Quilt as forgotten and increasingly out of step with the changing face of AIDS.[41]

Despite its preoccupation with restoration narratives, the *Los Angeles Times* nonetheless invokes the Quilt's alleged growing obscurity: "The Quilt has gone the way of AIDS itself in the United States—swept into the background as new drugs have driven down the death rate here and shifted the epicenter of anguish abroad, where the disease kills 2.8 million people a year." Mending a wounded panel is depicted as both important and less important as advancements in science seemingly call the Quilt's value into question. Like the bodies whose lives it honors, the Quilt purportedly faces a "diminishing future."[42]

The Quilt resists usage in AIDS activism, not merely because it is too large, too fragile, or too expensive to display, but because it cannot be folded easily into a chronic model of disease. If AIDS is historicized as a chronic ailment, we recognize that "we are dealing not with a brief, time-limited epidemic but with a long, slow process more analogous to cancer than with cholera," and that treatment options would more likely extend life than offer a cure. Fee and Fox date the widespread acceptance of this historical framing among medical professionals to June 1989, at an international AIDS meeting in Montreal. In their 1992 book, *AIDS: The Making of a Chronic Disease,"* Fee and Fox argue, "As contemporary perceptions of AIDS change, so too does its history; historical accounts that at one time seemed most relevant to understanding the epidemic need to be replaced by new interpretations." The adoption of this newer historical model has not been without rhetorical consequence, for it has fueled the debate over the Quilt's seeming obsolescence.[43]

Forgetting the Quilt

In his September 2000 article in *Poz*, David Groff summarized what were still popularly held beliefs about the Quilt: "Whether you think of it as America's largest work of folk art or biggest piece of AIDS kitsch, moveable cathedral, international cult or do-rag of death, there's no arguing that Cleve Jones' brainchild, the AIDS Memorial Quilt, is not only the epidemic's most recognizable symbol but probably its most enduring."[44] Despite continued references to the Quilt as the "most enduring" symbol of the AIDS epidemic, its relevance within AIDS activism has fallen under scrutiny. Commentators and activists alike have made the case for the Quilt's obsolescence by depicting the Quilt as temporally backward, a relic of the past. Characterizations of the Quilt as a relic highlight both the Quilt's connection to gay men and history and consequently its seeming irrelevance. As such, it is depicted as incapable of adequately addressing the needs of today's activism.

One primary strategy used to question the Quilt's utility as a rhetorical tool is to characterize it as a memorial that no longer mirrors the changing face of the epidemic. In 2006, NAMES Project Executive Director Julie Rhoad cited the Quilt's representational makeup as a "political problem" associated with displaying the Quilt. The fact that it does not "represent the current face of the epidemic," she explains, is reason not to pursue full displays of the Quilt.[45] Because the current face of the epidemic now disproportionately includes African Americans and heterosexual women, the Quilt, she implies, is too gay, white, and male. Although she also cites financial limitations affecting the organization's ability to display the Quilt in full, the "political problems" she sees would arguably still exist absent the financial constraints. The more recent concern with the Quilt's representational makeup manifested in 2004, when the NAMES Project decided not to go forward with plans to display the full Quilt in Washington, D.C., prior to the 2004 presidential election. Former NAMES Project manager Mike Smith defended the decision, stating, "I don't think it is appropriate to do big Quilt displays these days. . . . It needs to go to the communities where the epidemic is spreading."[46] Since Washington, D.C., is one such community where the epidemic is spreading, particularly among African Americans, Smith's opposition to full displays appears to rest on the assumption that more can be accomplished if the Quilt is segmented into smaller displays targeted to the communities currently affected by AIDS. Accordingly, in 2004, for National HIV Testing Day in June, the NAMES Project elected to display the 1,000 panels made since 1996, when it was last displayed in full.[47] Thus, Smith's logic suggests that the pre-1996 Quilt's representational makeup conflicts with, if not hinders, contemporary AIDS activism. This is a striking conclusion given that the CDC reports that male-male sexual contact is still the leading cause of transmission for all adults and adolescents (53 percent) as of 2006, the last year for which figures are available; and that of all *male* adults and adolescents, 72 percent of men diagnosed with HIV or AIDS contracted the virus through male-male sexual contact.[48]

A one-hour 2006 ABC television news report titled "Out of Control: AIDS in Black America" likewise questioned the Quilt's role in AIDS activism due to its representational makeup.[49] Although the majority of the report examines reasons for the lack of public attention to AIDS among African Americans, the news report ends with a segment on the Quilt. "Remember the Quilt?" asks the narrator, while aerial photographs of the Quilt from the 1996 display on the National Mall appear on screen. Shots of visitors walking slowly among the panels, and close-ups of panels themselves, function to corroborate the narrator's claim: "But the Quilt, even then, represented only a fraction of the number of Americans that died of AIDS and most of the faces were white." The segment then cuts to close-ups of the inside of the building, where the Quilt now resides, "tucked away in a non-descript warehouse in Atlanta." By showing only the aerial photos of the last full display and then shots of the Quilt "tucked away," the segment lends credence to activists' critique that the NAMES Project has let the Quilt languish in Atlanta. Indeed, the narrator points out that the Quilt's invisibility is a "reflection of the attitudes of most Americans toward AIDS—that it's no longer an issue in this country, not something we have to worry about. But this year, nearly 20,000 Americans will die of AIDS and most of them will be Black." At the same time, however, it casts doubt on the Quilt's ability to reach "communities where the epidemic is spreading," because it is too white.

As these critiques of the Quilt's representational features begin to suggest, what also contributes to the perception of the Quilt's obsolescence is its attachment to white gay male lives and history. This connection is advanced most explicitly by the *Los Angeles Times,* which describes the Quilt as an "aging snapshot of the first decade of AIDS, when gay white men were dying in the tens of thousands." Moreover, it points out that in 2005, the NAMES Project received 609 panels, the "majority of them for gay men who died in the 1990s." Because we are told that the panels, which "once arrived by the thousands each year, now trickle in at a few dozen a month," 609 panels for an entire year seem substantially small. Why has the flow of panels ebbed? The reason the *Times* offers is the advent of antiretroviral drugs in 1996 that significantly extend the lives of people with AIDS: "More than any factor, the drugs have transformed the quilt." With the "annual deaths [of Americans] peak[ing] in 1995 at 51,000, [t]he desperation that had driven the growth of the quilt seemed to fade away. New panels stopped arriving in large numbers," and "so did the donations of $200 or more that often accompanied them." Gay men and their families and friends are described as the major source of fund-raising for the Quilt. Absent their support, the Quilt has seemingly remained frozen in time, an "aging snapshot." The Quilt, which once grew feverishly as the epidemic grew, now is portrayed as a relic. The ABC report on "AIDS in Black America" furthered this image of the Quilt by using footage from the 1996 display in Washington, D.C., to illustrate the Quilt's association with gay white men, despite the availability of the more recent display in 2004, in which the 1,000 panels made since 1996 were shown on the Ellipse for National HIV Testing Day.[50]

Not only is the Quilt portrayed as a relic, those who advocate for displaying the Quilt in full are discredited as chasing the past. This can be seen in debates over the NAMES Project's small-scale displays of the Quilt. To refute charges that the Quilt simply languishes in a warehouse in Atlanta, Julie Rhoad points out that the NAMES Project "tripled the display activity of [the] Quilt" since moving to Atlanta. This has been achieved by loaning sections of the Quilt to hundreds of schools, places of worship, charities, and companies each year. Nevertheless, this smaller scale circulation has garnered criticism. As the *Los Angeles Times* put it, "those who want to rekindle the fire of the past say parceling out the quilt for tiny displays is like letting a sword rust in its scabbard." Here, the *Times* refers largely to Cleve Jones's efforts to display the entire Quilt in 2004 before the presidential elections. About the NAMES Project's decision not to display the Quilt at that time, Jones argues, "The people with the Quilt have a weapon that they have decommissioned."[51] Casting the desire for a full display of the Quilt as a "rekindling [of] the past" implies a less serious rhetorical and political act, as if such a display is merely "for old time's sake." Here, the past is understood as an impediment to progress rather than a viable rhetorical resource for social change.

Accordingly, some activists render the Quilt obsolete by locating its rhetorical value in the past, thereby questioning its relevance in today's AIDS activism. For example, San Francisco AIDS activist Michael Petrelis argues, "The quilt was very effective in the late 80s and early 90s for AIDS awareness." Similarly, Robert McMullin, executive director of the Stop AIDS Project, said the Quilt, like the red ribbon campaign, "might have 'lost its punch' over time." Neither McMullin nor Petrelis name the Quilt's perceived representational shortcomings—that it does not represent the changing face of the epidemic—as reason to question its utility in AIDS activism today. Instead, they use the Quilt's status as a memorial to do so. For Petrelis, the Quilt's memorializing function competes with other, more pressing priorities: "There's hundreds and thousands of people that need a housing subsidy, just trying to keep a roof over their head. Should we be putting our time and money into another vigil? I don't know." Similarly, for McMullin, whose organization focuses on HIV prevention among gay, bisexual, and transgender men, "The quilt is about loss." "And while people are still dying," he continues, "for most of us, the most important part of our message may not be about people dying." Even if the Quilt were to mirror the current face of the epidemic, such a representational change most likely would not satisfy those who believe the Quilt's message is about dying.[52]

To rescue the Quilt from charges of obsolescence, advocates point to the Quilt's role in an AIDS public sphere and less to its status as a memorial. Cleve Jones, for example, counters these charges by contending, "It's not intended as a passive memorial." Indeed, the Quilt's ability to both participate in and generate contexts of safe-sex education is elided in the reasoning used by Petrelis and McMullin. Significantly, as Jones makes the case for the Quilt's continued relevance, he shifts the terms of the debate from the language of "vigil" to the language of "vigilance," advocating, "We have got to constantly be vigilant against the idea that AIDS is over—that's what the quilt can do, particularly for young people who think this is just a treatable chronic condition."[53] For Jones, maintaining vigilance means using the Quilt for two purposes: preventing new HIV infections and pressuring political and medical institutions to develop new drugs to treat those who are already infected. If "vigil" privileges the Quilt's memorializing function, "vigilance" privileges the Quilt's activist function, serving once again as a stark reminder that the epidemic is far from over. Placed in these terms, Jones shares more in common with Stop AIDS than on first glance, as both are committed to HIV prevention measures, in particular combating the perception among gay men that AIDS is treatable.

In addition to using the Quilt to prevent new infections, Jones seeks to recommission the Quilt to battle bureaucracy within the institutions that oversee the creation and distribution of new drug treatments. As a veteran of earlier AIDS activism, Jones anticipates that there "won't be more effective drugs to treat HIV if we don't keep the pressure on the system that creates them."[54] On one hand, his argument reflects knowledge of the gains borne of AIDS activism from earlier decades, when getting "drugs into bodies" was a key goal, but it does not answer the critique that the Quilt may have limited ability in achieving these goals. Nonetheless, the need to pressure the system is a view corroborated by more recent testimonials from doctors who specialize in HIV/AIDS medicine. For example, Dr. Michael Gottlieb, the author of the CDC's now famous 1981 *Morbidity and Mortality* article documenting the "first" cases of AIDS, was quoted in the *Los Angeles Times* series on "AIDS at 25" as saying, "I've always looked at AIDS therapy as a series of leaky lifeboats. . . . You stay in the first one until you're sinking, then you jump to another one. But you don't give up looking for others."[55] Whether the "you" he refers to are patients or doctors (or both), the metaphor of "leaky lifeboats" emphasizes the scarcity of resources—including time—for extending the lives of people with AIDS.

For some advocates, limiting the Quilt's circulation to small-scale displays signifies a re-silencing of the disease. This is a view found in the pages of *Poz,* a magazine for HIV-positive readers, in response to the NAMES Project's decision not to show the Quilt in full in 2004. Concerned with the transmission of HIV among crystal meth–using men who practice unsafe sex, one reader responded to the news of the decision by arguing the following:

> I am disgusted that the NAMES Project is refusing to tour the AIDS Quilt—locking it up and showing only a few sections here and there, as if that will impact anything. . . . [D]on't the Quilt handlers think the loud statement and free press from a full display would be a wake-up call? They have decided to silence more than a million voices when these voices need to be heard. Someday, my name may end up as a patch on that Quilt, and I'll be damned if it will be kept silent.[56]

For Andrea Bowers, a Los Angeles–based feminist visual artist, the lack of publicity paid to AIDS now that women, especially brown and black women, constitute a significant percentage of HIV/AIDS diagnoses also signifies a re-silencing of the disease.[57] Her video installation, *The Weight of Relevance,* includes a three-part video segment of the inside of the NAMES Project warehouse, where stacks and stacks of folded panels sit. Departing from the mainstream news media coverage, Bowers's video does not reproduce the spectacular aerial photographs of the Quilt that we have become accustomed to seeing. Nor does her video include any footage of an unfolded Quilt. Instead, she juxtaposes documentary interviews with NAMES Project staff members with still photographs of folded Quilt panels in storage. Her strategy to depict the Quilt as "still life" while staff members discuss the shifting demographics allows her to call attention to the simultaneous spread of the epidemic among women and a furled Quilt. Denying viewers images of the Quilt unfurled echoes Jones's concern that the NAMES Project has "decommissioned the most powerful weapon against AIDS." Unlike Jones, however, Bowers indicts a culture that has once again allowed AIDS to disappear from public eye at the precise moment when ethnic minority women are among the fastest growing demographic affected. Of course, her use of slow-moving still-photography images of the Quilt in storage obscures the fact that the NAMES Project sends out sections to hundreds of organizations each year. Like Jones and others, she implies that these smaller sectional displays are insufficient in the continued fight against AIDS.

The critique of the NAMES Project's smaller displays negates the importance of those displays to its HIV prevention education programs. In 1995 the NAMES Project rebranded itself by announcing, in the words of then Executive Director Anthony Turney, "Two or three years ago, the quilt was a memorial, a means for grieving. Today, we have a much more active role to play in ending the epidemic." About the NAMES Project's plans to rebrand the identity and purpose of the Quilt, a 1995 article in the *San Francisco Chronicle,* "The AIDS Quilt Comes of Age," stated that the Quilt had been "transformed from an icon of mourning and emotional reaffirmation into a powerful, pragmatic instrument for prevention and education programs about AIDS."[58] Since 1994 the NAMES Project has conducted its outreach programs to high school and college campuses, reporting success with stimulating young people's knowledge of transmission and prevention. Its revamped National Youth Education Program reaches young people in both schools and community centers. And in 1999, with Coretta Scott King as keynote speaker, the NAMES Project launched its nationwide Historically Black Colleges and Universities Tour, which included Quilt displays as well as HIV prevention education, on-site testing, and counseling, a program that is now formalized among the NAMES Project's ongoing educational efforts.[59]

This educational role of the Quilt, pursued in displays smaller than those on the National Mall, is all but absent in the debates over its obsolescence. When once the smaller displays signaled the Quilt's "coming of age," they now register the Quilt's diminishing role in AIDS activism. The smaller displays do not produce the spectacular aerial photographs of the Quilt laid out on the National Mall, but they do allow the Quilt to enter more intimate spaces and temporalities of the everyday. This mode of circulation can create contexts for AIDS awareness and education that may not otherwise occur, a need that is palpable today in light of the prevalence of federally funded abstinence-only sex education programs.

The same "AIDS at 25" *Los Angeles Times* article that pronounced the obsolescence of the Quilt also announced that the NAMES Project had recently written a new strategic plan, suggesting that the Quilt has "outgrown its activist roots and should now serve as an inspiration to those living with AIDS."[60] Because the *Times* does not go on to explain how the NAMES Project intends to enact its strategic plan, the future of the Quilt is cast as bleak.

Consequently, those who believe the AIDS Memorial Quilt's message is primarily "about dying" may doubt the Quilt's ability to fulfill the NAMES Project's new strategic plan to be an "inspiration to those living with AIDS." They might instead find the Southern AIDS Living Quilt more suited to this goal.[61] Launched in October 2008 as a project of the Southern AIDS Coalition, the Southern AIDS Living Quilt is an online quilt featuring stories of women living with HIV and AIDS in the South, the region of the United States with the highest number of adults and teenagers with HIV and AIDS, and where AIDS is the leading cause of death for African American women between ages twenty-five and thirty-four. In contrast to the AIDS Memorial Quilt, the Southern AIDS Living Quilt features people who are living with HIV and AIDS. It also distinguishes itself from its NAMES Project counterpart in form; rather than a fabric quilt, it is an online video quilt, "stitched" together via the technologies of video editing and Web site design. In these video "panels," HIV-positive women, most of whom are African American or Latina, testify to what it means to them to be HIV-positive, making this both a visual and an oral history project.

As many testify to living with HIV since the 1980s and the importance of "knowing your [HIV] status," the women featured on the panels literally embody the organization's commitment to "empower, encourage, and educate." Currently featuring over 100 video "patches," the Living Quilt does not seek to reach its audience through its size and scale, as the AIDS Memorial Quilt does, but through its audio/video testimony. Rich in hope and optimism, the testimonies in many of the panels I viewed compare AIDS with diabetes or a similarly chronic condition, adopting a chronic model of disease. Rather than attest to continued fatalities, then, the memorial's growth will confirm the continued spread of infections among women in what is now the hardest-hit region of the United States. It remains to be seen whether or how the Southern AIDS Living Quilt might inform the future displays of the AIDS Memorial Quilt as the latter seeks to inspire those living with AIDS.

History Revisited

By discussing the AIDS Memorial Quilt as an artifact of progression, I have been gesturing to temporality as a key rhetorical feature in AIDS activism, AIDS discourse, and in social movements more broadly. Indeed, temporality shapes our understanding of AIDS. This is evident in its classification as an "epidemic," a term describing the *rapid* progression of a disease through a population. The rate at which HIV-infected bodies succumb to AIDS has also marked public narratives about AIDS. Progress is measured by the speed with which scientific developments occur and by the slowing down—if not complete arrest—of the epidemic. Like speed, duration is a central temporal logic. Expanding the life expectancy of an HIV-positive person is an indicator both of a drug's success and one's access to those drugs. The publication of "AIDS at 25" and other milestone stories bespeak the continued need to mark the duration of the epidemic.

At the heart of the debate over the Quilt's seeming obsolescence is a temporal conflict. Despite continued "advancements" in scientific knowledge—or perhaps *because* of these advancements—AIDS activism, including the AIDS Memorial Quilt, is placed in a curious rhetorical position. The availability of the chronic model of disease and the very drugs that have extended life have made it more difficult to engage in the crisis rhetoric that fueled much of the first fifteen years of activism. If, as James Darsey argues, AIDS catalyzed a shift in the rhetoric of the gay liberation movement, making appeals to health a significant priority, then the advent of antiretroviral drugs in 1996 signals a subsequent catalytic moment, altering the temporality of AIDS discourse and the temporality of AIDS activist rhetoric.[62]

Consequently, if we read the AIDS Quilt as a response to the historicizing of AIDS as a plague, we can begin to understand how the displacement of that historical model with a chronic model of disease produces its own set of rhetorical entanglements. As a "potent symbol of continuing epidemic," the Quilt's continued growth has been a recurrent feature of public discussion of the national displays. It once grew with "dizzying speed." If panels now only "trickle" in, the Quilt risks losing its reputation as a "symbol of a *continuing* epidemic." But if it does circulate as a symbol of a continuing (and fatal) epidemic, it makes itself vulnerable to charges of obsolescence, as it competes with the prevailing view that AIDS is a chronic, manageable condition.

To view the AIDS Quilt as representationally flawed because of the number of panels dedicated to gay white men is to miss the way it is marked as temporally "backward" within AIDS activism. Indeed, the perception that it has failed to keep up with the "current" face of AIDS only reinforces its status as "backward." Queer scholar Heather Love offers the term "backwardness" as both a queer historical structure of feeling and a model of historiography. She argues, "it is important to note the persistence of conditions that lead contemporary queers to experience their identity through the modalities of shame, secrecy, and self-hatred." By drawing our attention to the ways that pre-1970s liberation era feelings such as shame and stigma still manifest in a postliberation era, Love builds a persuasive case for a "model of history that sees a less defined break between past and present." She proposes this model of history as a challenge to an "affirmative historiography" and to a politics of affirmation that underwrites queer critics' attempts to turn shame into a creative, performative force. One way critics and historians produce an affirmative historiography is by "illuminat[ing] isolated moments of resistance in the larger story of homophobic oppression and violence." California's textbook legislation could be regarded as promoting an affirmative historiography, one that narrates acts of resistance by LGBTQ people, such as the 1969 Stonewall uprising. In such a narrative mode, the discourse of pride replaces a discourse of shame that all too often circumscribes experiences of queer people and people with HIV/AIDS.[63]

By contrast, to account for "bad feelings" would require a mode of narrating history that cannot be subsumed under a "progressivist view of history." By grappling with negative affects such as shame and loss, we can "find the clues to understanding the social, corporeal, and affective difficulties of queer existence."[64] While shame, loss, and mourning shape encounters with (and critical studies of) the AIDS Quilt, accounting for the persistence of these feelings may not be the only reason to question a progressivist model of history.

Accounting for the persistence of the AIDS epidemic in an era in which HIV is considered a "manageable" condition is also reason to question a progressivist model of history. If the development of drugs that prolong the health and lives of those with HIV is leading to complacency in some communities, as Cleve Jones and other AIDS activists suggest, is this progress? When lives in the United States and abroad hang in the balance of AIDS research and government funding of that research, we cannot afford to refuse the trope of "progress." But it is worth elaborating and questioning both the rhetorics with which we seek such advancements and the rhetorics that historicize such activism. I have sought to do so by discussing the Quilt as an artifact of progression. By accounting for the AIDS Quilt as an artifact of progression, one that is, like the preliberation literary texts Love analyzes, marked as temporally backward, I have highlighted the Quilt's ability to interrupt progress narratives endemic to both science and LGBTQ history and explained how the most "enduring" symbol of the epidemic could paradoxically recede from public view.

Casting the Quilt's changing roles in AIDS activism in metaphors of development has not produced long-term benefits. When the Quilt was said to "come of age" in 1995, it acquired a more activist status by designing the youth HIV education programs. This is a shift that mimics the trope of "maturity" within historical narratives about the gay and lesbian movement "maturing" from sexual liberation to activist issues such as same-sex marriage, a shift that has also been accompanied by AIDS declining in priority. Given this developmental logic, we could anticipate the rhetoric that suggested the Quilt had "outgrown its activist roots." If the Quilt came of age in 1995, then it seemed to have entered its golden years by 2006. In 2006 the *Los Angeles Times* linked the "activist roots" of the Quilt with immaturity by suggesting the organization had "outgrown" them. By implication, the Quilt's current role as a "curator of history" becomes associated with maturity. Given these rhetorics of development, it is no wonder the Quilt faces the possibility of retirement. As Cleve Jones reminds us, though, to retire the Quilt in a permanent home while the AIDS epidemic persists, as the NAMES Project once considered doing, would be like "building a Holocaust Museum in 1939."[65]

In 1995 Anthony Turney, then executive director of the NAMES Project, announced that the foundation's mission "is to put ourselves out of business."[66] The idea that the NAMES Project would aim to put itself out of business, while fittingly hyperbolic, nonetheless implies that the Quilt will lack purpose once there is a cure or vaccine. After all, there wouldn't be a need to use the Quilt as an activist tool, no need to remain "vigilant." What might become of the Quilt if a cure or vaccine does become available? Assuming something like the NAMES Foundation still exists to accept panels and add them to the archive, the Quilt could realistically continue to grow even after the "end of AIDS." In this way, the Quilt could still assert its status as an artifact of progression. Perhaps then it would symbolize even more than it does now the government neglect and cultural indifference that has marked the long history of this epidemic.

NOTES

I thank Martin Medhurst and the two anonymous reviewers for their critical engagement with this essay. Jeffrey Sens, Monica Bellflower, and Erin Sahlstein also provided invaluable feedback and conversations about the ideas herein. Finally, a special thanks goes to Charles E. Morris III for his editorial vision in developing this volume, his generous and critical insight, and especially his leadership in the area of queer rhetorical studies.

1. Kuehl authorized her claim by citing studies indicating that a "bias-free and LGBT-inclusive curriculum fosters tolerance, resulting in greater feelings of student safety and less bullying of students who are perceived to be lesbian, gay, bisexual, or transgender." See Denise Penn, "LGBT Legislators Making a Difference in Sacramento," *Lesbian News,* June 2006, 14.

2. Penn, "LGBT Legislators," 14; "Politically Correct History," *Los Angeles Times,* May 9, 2006, B12.

3. Marita Sturken, *Tangled Memories: The Vietnam War, the AIDS Epidemic, and the Politics of Remembering* (Berkeley: University of California Press, 1997), 2.

4. Lauren Berlant, *The Queen of America Goes to Washington City: Essays on Sex and Citizenship* (Durham: Duke University Press, 1997), 103; Charles E. Morris III, "My Old Kentucky Homo: Abraham Lincoln, Larry Kramer, and the Politics of Queer Memory," in *Queering Public Address: Sexualities in American Historical Discourse,* ed. Charles E. Morris III (Columbia: University of South Carolina Press, 2007), 95, 103; Michael Warner, *The Trouble with Normal: Sex, Politics, and the Ethics of Queer Life* (Cambridge: Harvard University Press, 1999), 51; Christopher Castiglia, "Sex Panics, Sex Publics, Sex Memories," *Boundary* 2 27 (Summer 2000): 149–175.

5. David Zarefsky, "Four Senses of Rhetorical History," in *Doing Rhetorical History: Concepts and Cases,* ed. Kathleen J. Turner (Tuscaloosa: University of Alabama Press, 1998), 28; Bruce E. Gronbeck, "The Rhetorics of the Past: History, Argument, and Collective Memory, *Doing Rhetorical History,* 54; Robert Hariman and John Louis Lucaites, *No Caption Needed: Iconic Photographs, Public Culture, and Liberal Democracy* (Chicago: University of Chicago Press, 2007); José Esteban Muñoz, "Ephemera as Evidence: Introductory Notes to Queer Acts," *Women and Performance: A Journal of Feminist Theory* 8 (1996): 5–16; Michael Warner and Lauren Berlant, "Sex in Public," *Critical Inquiry* 24 (1998): 547–566; Charles E. Morris III, "Archival Queer," *Rhetoric and Public Affairs* 9 (2006): 145–151; Morris, *Queering Public Address*; Ann Cvetkovich, *An Archive of Feeling: Trauma, Sexuality, and Lesbian Public Cultures* (Durham: Duke University Press, 2003); Judith Halberstam, *In a Queer Time and Place: Transgender Bodies, Subcultural Lives* (New York: New York University Press, 2005), 46.

6. Cleve Jones, *Stitching a Revolution: The Making of an Activist* (New York: HarperSanFrancisco, 2000), 260; Alan Zarembo, "AIDS at 25: The Quilt Fades into Obscurity; Once a Mighty Symbol of Love and Loss, the Tribute to Victims of AIDS Has Gone from Large to Largely Forgotten," *Los Angeles Times,* June 4, 2006, A1;

Jerry Roberts, "The AIDS Quilt Comes of Age," *San Francisco Chronicle,* December 3, 1995, A9; Jen Christensen, "A Rip in the Quilt," *Advocate,* February 28, 2006, 28; Marita Sturken argues that the Quilt is an "image of spectacle," not one of "intimacy or yielding space, but of impressive size and stature" (Sturken, *Tangled Memories,* 205); Todd Allan Yasui, "AIDS Quilt on the Ellipse," *Washington Post,* September 11, 1989, D7; Marc Sandalow, "AIDS Quilt Covers National Mall," *San Francisco Chronicle,* October 1, 1996, A1; Christopher Capozzola, "A Very American Epidemic: Memory Politics and Identity Politics in the AIDS Memorial Quilt, 1985–1993," in *The World the Sixties Made: Politics and Culture in Recent America,* ed. Van Gosse and Richard Moser (Philadelphia: Temple University, 2003), 225.

7. Throughout 2006 national and regional print news media ran stories recognizing AIDS at twenty-five-years-old. This periodizing reflects the media's proclivity to date the beginning of AIDS to 1981, the publication year of the Centers for Disease Control's *Morbidity and Mortality Weekly Report.* In June 2006, the twenty-fifth anniversary of the report's publication, the *Los Angeles Times* published a series of articles titled "AIDS at 25." The following is a snapshot of similar articles published that year: Zarembo, "AIDS at 25"; Jose Antonio Vargas, "D.C. Gay Group Battles 'AIDS Fatigue'; At 25, the Epidemic Presents a New Set of Complications," *Washington Post,* August 13, 2006, A1; Anita Gates, "The Epidemic as Avalanche: A Two-Part Series Documents 25 Years of AIDS," *New York Times,* May 30, 2006, E5; Paul H. B. Shin, "The Scourge that Shook the World: 25 Years of HIV Peril, Hope," *Daily News,* May 28, 2006, 6; Frankie Gamber, "NAACP Partners with Black AIDS Institute," *Crisis,* May/June 2006, 52–53; David Jefferson, "How AIDS Changed America," *Newsweek,* May 15, 2006, 36; Hannah Tucker, "AIDS: 25 Years Later," *Entertainment Weekly,* June 16, 2006, 161; "An Evening of Remembrance and Hope," *Jet,* June 19, 2006, 37.

8. Zarembo, "AIDS at 25," A1. As of 2010, the Centers for Disease Control and Prevention states that the 2006 figures on new infections among women and African Americans are the most recent available. See Centers for Disease Control and Prevention, "HIV in the United States," July 2010, http://www.cdc.gov/hiv/resources/factsheets/us.htm (accessed 3 December 2010).

9. Jen Christensen, "A Rip in the Quilt," *Advocate,* February 28, 2006, 28; Betsy McKay, "U.S. News: New Effort to Warn of HIV Risk in U.S.," *Wall Street Journal,* April 8, 2009, A3; Ephen Glenn Colter, "Discernibly Turgid: Safer Sex and Public Policy," in *Policing Public Sex: Queer Politics and the Future of AIDS Activism,* ed. Dangerous Bedfellows (Boston: South End Press, 1996), 161; McKay, "U.S. News,"

A3; Centers for Disease Control and Prevention, "HIV in the United States," July 2010, http://www.cdc.gov/hiv/resources/factsheets/us.htm (accessed 3 December 2010).

10. Elizabeth Fee and Daniel M. Fox, eds., *AIDS: The Burdens of History* (Berkeley: University of California, 1988), 1.

11. I examined about seventy-five news articles published in U.S. media about the AIDS Quilt. Given the hundreds of news articles published about local displays occurring any given month around the United States and recurring World AIDS Days, I narrowed my scope to national and major regional newspapers and magazines such as the *Washington Post, New York Times, San Francisco Chronicle, Los Angeles Times, Time, Newsweek,* and the *Advocate.* I also examined two prominent media outlets with HIV-positive readers: *Poz* and *The Body.com.* The time frame includes the displays of the Quilt in Washington, D.C., in 1987, 1988, 1989, 1992, and 1996; two partial displays on the National Mall in 1993 and 2004; the controversy over the Quilt's obsolescence; and, more selectively, the controversy about the NAMES Project decision not to display the full Quilt in 2004. The term "AIDS public sphere" comes from Gere's ethnographic analysis of the AIDS Memorial Quilt. David Gere, *How to Make Dances in an Epidemic: Tracking Choreography in the Age of AIDS* (Madison: University of Wisconsin Press, 2004), 177.

12. Douglas Crimp, "How to Have Promiscuity in an Epidemic," *Melancholia and Moralism: Essays on AIDS and Queer Politics* (Cambridge, MA: MIT Press, 2002).

13. Paula Treichler, *How to Have Theory in an Epidemic: Cultural Chronicles of AIDS* (Durham, NC: Duke University Press, 1999), 298.

14. Treichler, *How to Have Theory in an Epidemic,* 298. Treichler further explains the parallel she is drawing: "Like that for the right to experience pleasure, the struggle for the right to preserve health is founded on a political and theoretical analysis of the body—how it works, what it experiences, and how it exists and is valued in society" (311).

15. Scott Bravmann, *Queer Fictions of the Past: History, Culture, and Difference* (Cambridge: Cambridge University Press, 1997), 15, 25.

16. Peter Baldwin, *Disease and Democracy: The Industrialized World Faces AIDS* (Berkeley: University of California, 2005), 1; Elizabeth Fee and Daniel M. Fox elaborate that the widespread acceptance of a plague model indicated a belief in history as "pertinent to understanding the epidemic and that the events in the past that were most pertinent were those surrounding sudden, time-limited outbreaks of infection. . . . Because the history of visitations of plagues was the only history

that appeared relevant to the new epidemic, most people ignored the alternative historical models that were available," such as a chronic model of disease. I am suggesting that a chronic model is also problematic for it has enabled a complacency that impedes AIDS activism. Elizabeth Fee and Daniel M. Fox, eds., *AIDS: The Making of a Chronic Disease* (Berkeley: University of California Press, 1992), 3.

17. Treichler, *How to Have Theory in an Epidemic*, 6, 45.

18. Sander L. Gilman, "AIDS and Syphilis: Iconography of Disease," *October* 43 (1987): 90; Gilman, "AIDS and Syphilis," 88; Elizabeth Fee and Daniel M. Fox, eds., *AIDS: The Burdens of History* (Berkeley: University of California, 1988), 4.

19. Katherine Bishop, "Denying AIDS Its Sting: A Quilt of Life," *New York Times* October 5, 1987, C16.

20. Jones, *Stitching a Revolution*, 107.

21. Ibid., 105.

22. Douglas Crimp, "Mourning and Militancy," *Melancholia and Moralism: Essays on AIDS and Queer Politics* (Cambridge, MA: MIT Press, 2000), 140.

23. Warner, *The Trouble with Normal*, 51, 52. For the purposes of this essay, I am defining queer as an anti-assimilationist politics that challenges sexual mores and practices otherwise considered "normal" (as in heteronormativity).

24. See Cindy Patton, "Resistance and the Erotic: Reclaiming History, Setting Strategy as We Face AIDS," *Radical America* 20, no. 6 (1986): 68–78.

25. Craig A. Rimmerman, *From Identity to Politics: The Lesbian and Gay Movements in the United States* (Philadelphia: Temple University Press, 2002), 88.

26. Jones quoted in Sturken, *Tangled Memories*, 196.

27. This is David Gere's reading of the Quilt. Those memorialized on the Quilt, he suggests, are never rendered completely abject, for the Quilt turns them into citizens, constituents. Obviously, Gere is borrowing Judith Butler's phrase. Gere, *How to Make Dances*, 178–179.

28. I am borrowing this phrase from Lauren Berlant and Elizabeth Freeman, "Queer Nationality," in Lauren Berlant, *Queen of America*, 150.

29. Personal conversation with Monica Bellflower, December 9, 2007.

30. Quoted in Rimmerman, *From Identity to Politics*, 94.

31. Ibid., 89.

32. Timothy E. Cook and David C. Colby, "The Mass-Mediated Epidemic: The Politics of AIDS on the Nightly Network News," *AIDS: The Making of a Chronic Disease*, ed. Elizabeth Fee and Daniel M. Fox (Berkeley: University of California Press, 1992), 111; Cook and Colby, "The Mass-Mediated Epidemic," 122; Edward Alwood,

Straight News: Gays, Lesbians, and the News Media (New York: Columbia University Press, 1996), 238.

33. Cook and Colby, "The Mass-Mediated Epidemic," 103.

34. Sandra Boodman, "Giant Quilt Names 1,920 AIDS Victims; Memorial Will Be Unfurled on Mall," *Washington Post,* October 10, 1987, A1; Sandalow, "AIDS Quilt Covers National Mall," A1; Lynne Duke, "D.C. Crowds Recall AIDS Victims through a Common Thread," *Washington Post,* October 9, 1988, B1; "American Notes Washington," *Time,* October 10, 1988, http://www.time.com/time/magazine/article/0,9171,968617,00.html (accessed July 6 2009); Christopher Knight, "A Stitch in Time: The NAMES Project AIDS Memorial Quilt Returns to Washington, Its 21,000 Panels Casting a Shadow that Reaches the White House," *Los Angeles Times* October 4, 1992, Calendar, 8; Andrew Sullivan, "Washington Diarist: Quilt," *New Republic,* November 2, 1992, 43; John Gallagher, "Naming Names," *Advocate,* October 15, 1996, 53–55.

35. Sandalow, "AIDS Quilt Covers National Mall," A1; Knight, "A Stitch in Time," 8; Yumi Wilson, "Tragedy Transformed," *San Francisco Chronicle,* November 3, 1996, Z1; David W. Dunlap, "AIDS Quilt of Grief on Capitol Mall," *New York Times,* October 13, 1996, A22.

36. Jones, *Stitching a Revolution,* 236; Dunlap, "AIDS Quilt of Grief on Capital Mall," A1; Teresa Moore, "On AIDS Day, Gloom and a Ray of Hope: Despite Progress, Epidemic Spreading," *San Francisco Chronicle,* December 2, 1996, A1; Doug Struck, "Visitors Marvel, Grieve Over a Living Monument to the Tragedy of AIDS," *Washington Post,* October 13, 1996, A33; Victoria Benning, "AIDS Quilt's Moving Message; Mall Exhibit Awakens Students to Human Toll of Disease," *Washington Post,* October 12, 1996, B1.

37. Moore, "On AIDS Day," A1.

38. Cook and Colby, "The Mass-Mediated Epidemic," 99–100.

39. Elizabeth N. Aoki, "Ever Growing AIDS Quilt Set for Finale," *Washington Post,* August 19, 1989, D1. Struck, "Visitors Marvel," A33. The "54-ton albatross" characterization appears in the *Los Angeles Times* and is attributed to UCLA professor David Gere, author of *How to Make Dances in An Epidemic,* cited earlier. See Zarembo, "AIDS at 25," A1.

40. Flavia Rando, "The Person with AIDS: The Body, the Feminine, and the NAMES Project Memorial Quilt," in *Gendered Epidemic: Gendered Representations of Women in the Age of AIDS,* ed. Nancy L. Roth and Katie Hogan (New York: Routledge, 1998), 200; Courtland Milloy, "A Fabric of Love, Pain, Anger," *Washington*

Post, October 8, 1989, D3.

41. Zarembo, "AIDS at 25," A1.

42. Ibid.; Halberstam, *In a Queer Time and Space,* 2.

43. Fee and Fox, *AIDS: Making of a Chronic Disease,* 5.

44. David Groff, "Keeping Up with the Jones," *Poz,* September 2000, http://www.poz. com/articles/205_10157.shtml (accessed July 10, 2009).

45. Rebecca Minnich, "Loose Threads," *Poz,* June 2004, http://www.poz.com/articles/155_318.shtml (accessed July 10, 2009).

46. Zarembo, "AIDS at 25," A1.

47. Manny Fernandez, "Unfurling Their Love and Loss," *Washington Post,* June 26, 2004, B1.

48. Centers for Disease Control and Prevention, "HIV/AIDS in the United States," August 2008, http://www.cdc.gov/hiv/topics/resources/factsheets (accessed July 62009). As of December 4, 2010, the CDC lists 2006 as the "most recent year that data are available" (see Centers for Disease Control and Prevention, "Basic Statistics," 2008, http://www.cdc.gov/hiv/topics/surveillance/print/basic.htm, accessed December 4, 2010).

49. "Out of Control: AIDS in Black America," *ABC News,* August 24, 2006.

50. Ibid.; Zarembo, "AIDS at 25," A1.

51. Minnich, "Loose Threads"; Zarembo, "AIDS at 25," A1.

52. Jesse McKinley, "Fight Over Quilt Reflects Changing Times in Battle Against AIDS," *New York Times,* January 31, 2007, A16. This article inspired a lengthy debate on the "Forum" page of *Poz,* "Is the AIDS Quilt Obsolete?" See http://forums.poz.com/index.php?topic=8638.0.

53. McKinley, "Fight over Quilt," A16; Christensen, "A Rip in the Quilt," 28.

54. Christensen, "A Rip in the Quilt," 28.

55. Jia-Rui Chong, "AIDS at 25; 'You Don't Give Up Looking' for Lifeboats," *Los Angeles Times,* June 5, 2006, A9.

56. "Dropping Names," *Poz,* September 2004, http://www.poz.com/articles/158_423.shtml (accessed July 10, 2009).

57. Bowers's art installation is discussed in Sharon Mizota, "Politics Sewn to Art, Panel by Quilt-Like Panel," *Los Angeles Times,* June 9, 2007, E12; and in "The Weight of Relevance," Andrea Bowers and Susanne Vielmetter, *Los Angeles Projects,* 2007, http://www.vielmetter.com/index.php?site=artists&fromlink=&a_id=49&detail=exhibitions&artistname=ANDREA_BOWERS&e_id=138&xh_action=pressrelease (accessed July 2, 2009).

58. Roberts, "The AIDS Quilt Comes of Age," 9.

59. The youth programs and their successes are described on the NAMES Project Web site, http://www.aidsquilt.org/programs.htm (accessed July 1, 2009).

60. Zarembo, "AIDS at 25," A1.

61. Southern AIDS Living Quilt can be found at http://www.livingquilt.org/.

62. James Darsey, "From 'Gay Is Good' to the Scourge of AIDS: The Evolution of Gay Liberation Rhetoric, 1977–1990," *Communication Studies* 42 (1991): 43–66.

63. Heather Love, "Spoiled Identity: Stephen Gordon's Loneliness and the Difficulties of Queer History," *GLQ* 7 (2001): 496. She develops these themes in her book, *Feeling Backward: Loss and the Politics of Queer History* (Cambridge: Harvard University Press, 2007), 492, 494.

64. Ibid., 497.

65. Minnich, "Loose Threads."

66. Roberts, "The AIDS Quilt Comes of Age," A9.

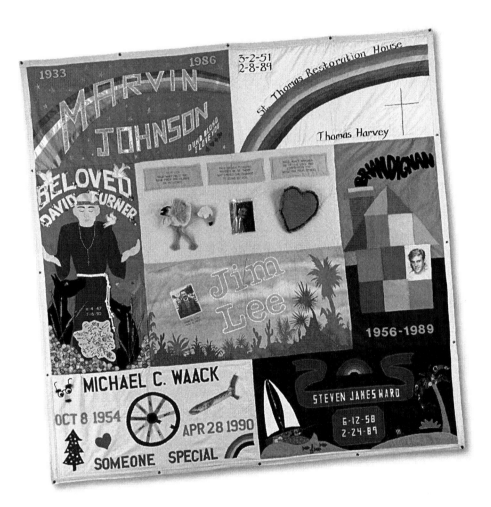

Experiencing the Quilt

Charles E. Morris III

As I close this volume I am taken back to my first encounter with the AIDS Quilt in Washington, D.C., in 1992. I was a young, closeted graduate student who along with my friend and peer Rick Pucci joined Carole Blair at the display, where Carole was conducting research for her project on U.S. commemorative culture. I couldn't have predicted the profound influence that personally seeing and touching those panels, the rush of manifold affective response, interactions with my friends and strangers, the bird's-eye view, inscribing the signature panel, the ACT UP flyer announcing a political funeral—all constitutive of my *experience* of the Quilt—would have on my coming out, my politics, my pedagogy, my scholarship.

In light of that memory I am saddened that on October 11, 2009, the National Equality March on Washington for LGBT Rights, orchestrated by a resurgent Cleve Jones, did not include a large-scale display of the AIDS Quilt. This is not 1987, of course, and as has been discussed in these pages there are many reasons for this absence, some more seemly than others, and we could certainly engage in a spirited and principled political and theoretical debate over the boon or bane of such a display. Whether understood as an ongoing political intervention, or archival exhibition, or embodied performance of cultural memory (all of these, in my judgment), the intimate and sublime event of the AIDS Quilt should be, must be, experienced.[1] And while certainly advocating the deeply powerful and significant ongoing local displays in schools and places of worship and community centers, I also believe that the Quilt should return en masse, if no more in full, to Washington, D.C., again and again, for multitudes to encounter together there.

The important and protracted debates about where and how the Quilt should go (or go at all) notwithstanding for this moment, I want to emphasize the paramount importance of experiencing it, of being proximate to those panels, of finding oneself intimately situated, indeed enveloped, in the environs and scene of its display, of participating in the performance of the Quilt. In that spirit I want to offer a few considerations especially for those scholars of rhetorical studies, though the issues raised here have wider applicability.

The first concerns materiality. For quite some time now, Carole Blair has encouraged rhetorical scholars to take seriously the differential experiences of the objects we analyze, and therefore "translate," and the critical difference "being there" can make:

> It is now common enough to acknowledge the positive, democratizing effects of the "mechanical reproduction" of artworks, but we must also remember the flattening effect of such reproduction—not just the literal two-dimensionalizing of a place and its inhabitant artworks, but also the metaphorical "flattening" of experience. And in doing so, we must pose the question of how we, as critics, make the object "real." How do we make it *matter* to our readers? The term "matter" has an important double edge here, as a noun that suggests substance and presence, but also as a verb that implies a rendering of significance.[2]

Elsewhere, with the same issues of reproduction and "experiential habitat" at stake, Blair asked, "What happens when the first of the Quilt's panels disintegrates? The NAMES Project will preserve all panels to the extent possible and reproduce them in photographs and into photo representations on its website; however, the literal feel of the panels will be lost, as will the rendered work of therapy for survivors that those panels contain."[3] Blair's question reminded me of Thomas Yingling's powerful observation on materiality, identity, and community within the context of AIDS:

> It is only in structures such as the quilt or, to a greater or lesser extent, in any demonstration or performance—in the making of artifacts about AIDS—that the disease can become meaningful in a way that allows those affected and infected by it to secure it as an experience and not merely as information. It allows as well an affirmation of identity not fated to succumb to the traps of affirmative, bourgeois culture in its determination to seal that identity and those meanings in a world of alienation and death. Only in such artifacts may the collective experience of AIDS be encountered, and only in encountering that collective knowledge may the gay and lesbian community continue to become visible to itself as something quite other than the site *par excellence* of social atrophy and alienation.[4]

In different registers—agent and audience, individual and collective, activist and academic—we see here the vital issue of how AIDS, past and present, gets materialized and mediated, enlivened and flattened, and how important experience and experiential habitat can be to making such materializations matter. If you have taken up AIDS and its history in the classroom, as I have for the past decade among those ever-increasingly "removed" from the epidemic, then this issue resonates as all the more pressing, material.[5]

Second, rhetorical critics and rhetorical theorists of social protest have yet to substantively engage affect—feelings and emotions—as it centrally figures in activist culture, biography, strategy, and performance. From the emotional dimensions of mobilization to the "shared and reciprocal emotions," "taste in tactics," "emotional common sense," and "affective public culture" that sustain and splinter activists personally and communally, to the individual and collective effervescence of tactical performance, to the burnout that often alters or ends activist commitment, *affect matters.*[6]

That much of the best scholarship on affect to date concerns AIDS activism, as well as GLBT people, also suggests both the need and a means by which to sharpen the queer turn in this field.

Moreover, in thinking again of Blair's notion of "being there," rhetorical critics and rhetorical theorists of social protest would do well to follow Phaedra Pezzullo's lead into the fray. This means to take seriously Pezzullo's advice, following Robert Asen, Dwight Conquergood, and others that we should engage and account for "actually existing" counterpublics and movements, engage and account for activist bodies, embodiment, interaction, interanimation, and cultural performance.[7] In doing so, we can better understand, indeed we critically manifest, what Pezzullo calls "presence":

> More than simply "showing up," being present as a mode of advocacy suggests that the materiality of a place promises the opportunity to shape perceptions, bodies, and lives with respect to the people and places hosting the experience. Being "present," like roll call in school, indicates the significance of someone literally coexisting with another in a particular space and time. Yet, a rhetorical appreciation of "presence" also can indicate when we *feel as if* someone, someplace, or something matters, whether or not she/he/it is physically present with us. Presence also refers, then, to the *structure of feeling* or one's *affective* experience when certain elements—and, perhaps, more important, relationships and communities—in space and time appear more immediate to us, such that we can imagine their "realness" or "feasibility" in palpable and significant ways.[8]

Following Pezzullo, or Joshua Gamson, Dana Cloud, Ann Cvetkovich, Deborah Gould, Patrick Johnson, and Jeffrey Bennett, among others, such "rhetorical appreciation" may require greater ethnographic commitment, a commitment to oral history, and our presence as participant observers.[9]

Finally, insofar as any present or future display of the Quilt would constitute memory of activism and activist memory, rhetorical scholars of social protest should further consider how the past materializes in the activist present, how activists experience and deploy, activate and are limited by memory and history. Rarely has social movement and public memory scholarship intersected in rhetorical studies.[10] However, the dynamic relationship between memory and activism makes such critical scrutiny crucial. Kristen Hoerl has demonstrated the extent to which various agents and institutions of mainstream culture distort and obliterate activist legacies and constrain the possibilities of activist countermemory.[11] Ann Cvetkovich revealed not only consequential differences between dominant and counter memories of the AIDS epidemic, but also the affective and strategic import of activist memory and amnesia for activists themselves across time and generation. As she observed, "Like the dead, memories of activism can also be kept alive as something that one has recourse to, even difficult memories."[12] The activist propulsion derived from memory is also made plain in Alexandra Juhasz's reflection on her AIDS video archive and experimental documentary *Video Remains*:

> The intrusion of present-day AIDS—suffered differently, represented less, lacking a movement aware of the awful and inspiring legacy of the past—enlivens my old tape and recommits to a contemporary conversation about AIDS, its representations, feelings, activism, and history. I conjured Jim from the AIDS activist video archive, both personal and institutional, private and public, and wondered what others might see in him, and whether we might be ready to revisit this past, not so much to heal as to think again together.[13]

Here the conjunction of memory and movement, a genealogy of activist performance, and queer archive activism all suggest the rich critical and political potential of the Quilt's pasts and presence. As Peter Hawkins concluded, "For in addition to its ongoing reproduction, the NAMES Project may well give rise to other symbols and strategies than its own, other responses to AIDS extended not only to the dead but to the living."[14]

My hope is that this volume in some meaningful way will provide inducement to experience the Quilt, and, like the Quilt itself, impel us to feel, and fathom, and fight AIDS with greater vigor and lasting commitment.

NOTES

1. In thinking about the importance of materiality, the experiential, in relation to the
   Quilt, a justificatory montage of emotional and theoretical fragments comes to mind.
   I think of the striking headline of an article in the *San Francisco Chronicle's* "AIDS
   at 25" series: "How to Respond to the Devastating Disease? *Live Theater . . .*" (my
   emphasis). Steven Winn, "How to Respond to the Devastating Disease? Live Theater—More Than Any Other Art—Has Asked the Most Profound Questions, *San
   Francisco Chronicle,* June 7, 2006, E1. Then there is this passage by David Román:
   "The book is dedicated to writing the history of various local interventions of AIDS
   activism and performance which need to circulate more widely, performances which
   official history has in many ways and for many reasons either neglected or forgot-
   ten. Such a practice is in part my own way of coping with loss and disappearance"
   (*Acts of Intervention: Performance, Gay Culture, and AIDS* [Bloomington: Indiana
   University Press, 1998], xiv). I recall the provocative title of Scott Dillard's memorial
   performance to his partner who died of AIDS, *Breathing Darrell* (Dillard, *"Breathing
   Darrell:* Solo Performance as a Contribution to a Useful Queer Mythology," *Text and
   Performance Quarterly* 20 [2000]: 74–83). And I contemplate articulations of queer
   archival activism. See Ann Cvetkovich, *An Archive of Feelings: Trauma, Sexuality,
   and Lesbian Public Cultures* (Durham, NC: Duke University Press, 2003); Judith
   Halberstam, *In a Queer Time and Place: Transgender Bodies, Subcultural Lives* (New
   York: New York University Press, 2005); Lucas Hilderbrand, "Retroactivism," *GLQ:
   A Journal of Lesbian and Gay Studies* 12 (2006): 303–317; Alexandra Juhasz, "Video
   Remains," *GLQ: A Journal of Lesbian and Gay Studies* 12 (2006): 319–328; Horacio
   N. Roque Ramírez, "A Living Archive of Desire: Teresita la Campesina and the Em-
   bodiment of Queer Latino Community Histories," in *Archive Stories: Facts, Fictions,
   and the Writing of History,* ed. Antoinette Burton (Durham, NC: Duke University
   Press, 2005), 111–135; Charles E. Morris III, "Archival Queer," *Rhetoric and Public
   Affairs* 9 (2006): 145–151; E. Patrick Johnson, *Sweet Tea: Black Gay Men of the South*
   (Chapel Hill: University of North Carolina Press, 2008); K. J. Rawson, "Accessing
   Transgender // Desiring Queer(er?) Archival Logics," *Archivaria* 68 (2009): 123–140.
   Finally, I think of Diana Taylor's distinction between archive and repertoire in *The
   Archive and the Repertoire: Performing Cultural Memory in the Americas* (Durham,
   NC: Duke University Press, 2003).

2. Carole Blair, "Reflections on Criticism and Bodies: Parables from Public Places,"
   Western Journal of Communication 65 (2001): 275.

3. Carole Blair, "Contemporary U.S. Memorial Sites as Exemplars of Rhetoric's Materiality," in *Rhetorical Bodies*, ed. Jack Selzer and Sharon Crowley (Madison: University of Wisconsin Press, 1999), 38. See also Jacqueline Lewis and Michael R. Fraser, "Patches of Grief and Rage: Visitor Responses to the NAMES Project AIDS Memorial Quilt," *Qualitative Sociology* 19 (1996): 433–451. I take the idea of "experiential habitat" from Carole Blair and Neil Michel, "Commemorating in the Theme Park Zone: Reading the Astronauts Memorial," in *At the Intersection: Cultural Studies and Rhetorical Studies*, ed. Thomas Rosteck (New York: Guilford Press, 1999), 59.

4. Thomas Yingling, "AIDS in America: Postmodern Governance, Identity, and Experience," in *Inside/Out: Lesbian Theories, Gay Theories*, ed. Diana Fuss (New York: Routledge, 1991), 307.

5. In her discussion of the "Activism's Afterlives," Cvetkovich quotes Kim Christensen, whose reflection on the memory of ACT UP should deepen for us the concern about the challenges of materializing the history of the epidemic: "[I taught a] gay and lesbian studies class for a friend of mine, about ACT UP, and these were 90 percent young, out, gay and lesbian people, and a good percent had never heard of ACT UP. Those who had had very bizarre notions about what we had done, and it was really depressing. It was like, 'Oh, my God, this was only ten years ago, and it's already gone from public memory.' Something has to happen here because they can't reinvent the wheel every single generation" (Cvetkovich, *An Archive of Feelings*, 227). For the first time in my own teaching career, students in the spring 2009 semester of my course covering the history of AIDS activism had never heard of ACT UP or the AIDS Quilt.

6. Deborah B. Gould, "Life during Wartime: Emotions and the Development of ACT UP," *Mobilization: An International Journal* 7 (2002): 177–200; Deborah B. Gould, *Moving Politics: Emotion and ACT UP's Fight Against AIDS* (Chicago: University of Chicago Press, 2009); Griff M. Tester, "Resources, Identity, and the Role of Threat: The Case of AIDS Mobilization, 1981–1986," *Research in Political Sociology* 13 (2004): 47–75; James M. Jasper, *The Art of Moral Protest: Culture, Biography, and Creativity in Social Movements* (Chicago: University of Chicago Press, 1999), chaps. 5, 8, 9, 10; Jeff Goodwin, James Jasper, and Francesca Polletta, eds., *Passionate Politics: Emotions and Social Movements* (Chicago: University of Chicago Press, 2001); Cvetkovich, *An Archive of Feelings*, 168–204; Eve Kosofsky Sedgwick, *Touching Feeling: Affect, Pedagogy, Performativity* (Durham, NC: Duke University Press, 2003); Sara Ahmed, *The Cultural Politics of Emotion* (New York: Routledge,

2004); Amin Ghaziani, *The Dividends of Dissent: How Conflict and Culture Work in Lesbian and Gay Marches on Washington* (Chicago: University of Chicago Press, 2008); Janet Staiger, Ann Cvetkovich, and Ann Reynolds, eds., *Political Emotions: New Agendas in Communication* (New York: Routledge, 2010). For a notable exception in the field, see Karma R. Chávez, "Spatializing Gender Performativity: Ecstasy and Possibilities for Livable Life in the Tragic Case of Victoria Arellano," *Women's Studies in Communication* 33 (2010): 1–15.

7. Phaedra C. Pezzullo, "Resisting 'National Breast Cancer Awareness Month': The Rhetoric of Counterpublics and Their Cultural Performances," in *Readings on the Rhetoric of Social Protest,* ed. Charles E. Morris III and Stephen Howard Browne (State College, PA: Strata, 2006), 269–272. See Robert Asen, "Seeking the 'Counter' in Counterpublics," *Communication Theory* 10 (2000): 424–446; Dwight Conquergood, "Rethinking Ethnography: Toward a Critical Cultural Politics," *Communication Monographs* 58 (1991): 191–193; Kirk W. Fuoss, *Striking Performances/Performing Strikes* (Jackson: University Press of Mississippi, 1997); Kevin Michael DeLuca, "Unruly Arguments: The Body Rhetoric of Earth First!, ACT UP, and Queer Nation," *Argumentation and Advocacy* 36 (1999): 9–21; Jeffrey Bennett and Isaac West, "'United We Stand, Divided We Fall': AIDS, Armorettes, and the Tactical Repertoires of Drag," *Southern Journal of Communication* 74 (2009): 300–313.

8. Phaedra C. Pezzullo, *Toxic Tourism: Rhetorics of Pollution, Travel, and Environmental Justice* (Tuscaloosa: University of Alabama Press, 2007), 9.

9. Joshua Gamson, "Silence, Death, and the Invisible Enemy: AIDS Activism and Social Movement 'Newness,'" *Social Problems* 36 (1989): 351–367; Dana L. Cloud, "The Null Persona: Race and the Rhetoric of Silence in the Uprising of '34," *Rhetoric and Public Affairs* 2 (1999): 177–209; Cvetkovich, *An Archive of Feelings*; Gould, *Moving Politics*; E. Patrick Johnson, *Appropriating Blackness: Performance and the Politics of Authenticity* (Durham, NC: Duke University Press, 2003); Jeffrey A. Bennett, *Banning Queer Blood: Rhetorics of Citizenship, Contagion, and Resistance* (Tuscaloosa: University of Alabama Press, 2009).

10. See Cindy Koenig Richards, "Inventing Sacagawea: Public Women and the Transformative Potential of Epideictic Rhetoric," *Western Journal of Communication* 73 (2009): 1–22; Charles J. G. Griffin, "Movement as Memory: Significant Form in *Eyes on the Prize*," *Communication Studies* 54 (2003): 196–210; Kyra Pearson, "Mapping Rhetorical Inventions in 'National' Feminist Histories: Second Wave Feminism and *Ain't I a Woman*," *Communication Studies* 50 (1999): 158–173; Stephen H. Browne, "Remembering Crispus Attucks: Race, Rhetoric, and the Politics of

Commemoration," *Quarterly Journal of Speech* 85 (1999): 169–187; Bonnie J. Dow, "Feminism, Miss America, and Media Mythology," *Rhetoric and Public Affairs* 6 (Spring 2003): 127–149.

11. Kristen Hoerl, "Mississippi's Social Transformation in Public Memories of the Trial Against Byron de la Beckwith for the Murder of Medgar Evers," *Western Journal of Communication* 72 (2008): 62–82; Kristen Hoerl, "Burning Mississippi into Memory? Cinematic Amnesia as a Resource for Remembering Civil Rights," *Critical Studies in Media Communication* 26 (2009): 54–79. See also my discussion of mnemonicide in Larry Kramer's queer countermemory of Abraham Lincoln. Charles E. Morris III, "My Old Kentucky Homo: Abraham Lincoln, Larry Kramer, and the Politics of Queer Memory," in my *Queering Public Address: Sexualities and American Historical Discourse* (Columbia: University of South Carolina Press, 2007), 93–120.

12. Cvetkovich, *An Archive of Feelings*, 235, chaps. 6, 7.

13. Juhasz, *Video Remains,* 320.

14. Peter S. Hawkins, "Naming Names: The Art of Memory and the NAMES Project AIDS Quilt," *Critical Inquiry* 19 (1993): 779.

Contributors

BRYANT KEITH ALEXANDER is professor of Performance, Pedagogy and Culture in the Department of Communication Studies at California State University Los Angeles. The former chair of the Department of Liberal Studies, he currently serves as the associate dean of the College of Arts and Letters. He is the author of *Performing Black Masculinity: Race, Culture and Queer Identity* and a coeditor with education scholars Gary L. Anderson and Bernardo Gallegos of *Performance Theories in Education: Power, Pedagogy and the Politics of Identity*. His essays appear in a wide variety of scholarly journals and book volumes.

ERIC AOKI is an award-winning teacher-scholar of Interpersonal, Co-Cultural, and Intercultural Communication. His publications include "Mexican American Ethnicity in Biola, CA: An Ethnographic Account of Hard Work, Family, and Religion," in *The Howard Journal of Communications,* and "The Absence: Living Everyday Life without Gay Male Friends," in the anthology *On the Meaning of Friendship between Gay Men*. Eric has also published, alongside exceptional colleagues Brian L. Ott and Greg Dickinson, in *Communication and Critical/Cultural Studies, Rhetoric and Public Affairs, Women's Studies in Communication,* and *Western Journal of Communication*.

JEFFREY A. BENNETT is assistant professor of Communication Studies at the University of Iowa. He is the author of *Banning Queer Blood: Rhetorics of Citizenship, Contagion, and Resistance*, which examines the federal donor deferral policies that prohibit men who have sex with men from giving blood. Jeff's work has also appeared in the *Quarterly Journal of Speech, Critical Studies in Media Communication, Communication and Critical/Cultural Studies, Text and Performance Quarterly,* and the *Journal of Homosexuality*. In 2009 Jeff was the recipient of the Karl R. Wallace Memorial Award from the National Communication Association.

CAROLE BLAIR is professor of Communication Studies at the University of North Carolina at Chapel Hill. Her research focuses on the rhetorical dimensions of public commemorative places and artworks of the twentieth-century United States. She has been a recipient of numerous research awards, and she is a Fellow of the Institute for Arts and Humanities at the University of North Carolina. She is coeditor of *Places of Public Memory: The Rhetoric of Memorials and Museums*.

DANIEL C. BROUWER is associate professor in the School of Human Communication at Arizona State University. His research explores theories and practices of publics, rhetorics, and cultural performances. He is a co-editor of two books, *Counterpublics and the State* and *Public Modalities: Rhetoric, Culture, Media, and the Shape of Public Life*, and the author of essays in *Rhetoric and Public Affairs, Critical Studies in Media Communication,* and *Argumentation and Advocacy*.

KEVIN MICHAEL DELUCA is associate professor in the Department of Communication at University of Utah. Author of the book *Image Politics: The New Rhetoric of Environmental Activism*, DeLuca explores humanity's relations to nature and how those relations are mediated and transformed by technological and ideological discourses. Having published essays on environmental politics, social movement practices, and visual rhetoric, DeLuca is now writing and doing documentary film work on environmental activism in China.

Greg Dickinson is associate professor and director of graduate studies in the Department of Communication Studies at Colorado State University. He has won the Gerald R. Miller Dissertation Award and, along with his coauthors, Brian L. Ott and Eric Aoki, the NCA Visual Communication Division Excellence in Scholarship Award. His essays have appeared in *Communication and Critical/Cultural Studies, Quarterly Journal of Speech, Rhetoric Society Quarterly, Southern Journal of Communication,* and *Western Journal of Communication.* He coedited *Places of Public Memory: The Rhetoric of Museums and Memorials.*

Christine Harold is assistant professor of communication at the University of Washington. Her work explores commercial rhetoric and consumer practices in an era of globalized capitalism. She is author of *OurSpace: Resisting the Corporate Control of Culture.* Harold serves on the editorial boards of *Quarterly Journal of Speech, Communication and Critical/Cultural Studies,* and *Western Journal of Communication.*

Cleve Jones is a former assistant to Harvey Milk and historical consultant on the film *Milk.* He is the founder of the AIDS Memorial Quilt and the author of *Stitching a Revolution: The Making of an Activist.* He planned the October 2009 National Equality March in Washington, D.C. Currently he is a labor activist working for Unite Here.

Neil Michel is vice president of creative and product development at Prosper Creative Media, where he directs projects in web, video, and web-based software. A founding partner of Axiom, a commercial art studio based in Davis, California, he received his master of arts degree from the University of California in 1993. He is a noted critic and photographer whose publication credits appear in numerous books, journals, newspapers and magazines, including *The New York Times, San Francisco Chronicle, Washington Post,* and *Landscape Architecture Magazine.*

CHARLES E. MORRIS III is associate professor in the Department of Communication at Boston College. He is editor of *Queering Public Address: Sexualities in American Historical Discourse* and coeditor of *Readings on the Rhetoric of Social Protest*. His queer history and criticism has regularly appeared in the *Quarterly Journal of Speech*, as well as *Rhetoric and Public Affairs, Communication and Critical/Cultural Studies*, and the *Southern Communication Journal*. He has received several awards from the National Communication Association, most recently the Randy Majors Memorial Award from the Caucus on LGBTQ Concerns, and his second Golden Monograph Award for article of the year.

BRIAN L. OTT teaches media studies at the University of Colorado Denver. He is an award-winning teacher and scholar whose work has appeared widely in national and international journals. He is the author of *The Small Screen: How Television Equips Us to Live in the Information Age* and *Critical Media Studies: An Introduction* (with Robert L. Mack), as well as a coeditor of *It's Not TV: HBO in the Post-Television Era* (with Marc Leverette and Cara Buckley) and *Places of Public Memory: The Rhetoric of Museums and Memorials* (with Greg Dickinson and Carole Blair). He currently serves as the editor in chief of the *Western Journal of Communication*.

KYRA PEARSON is associate professor of Communication Studies at Loyola Marymount University in Los Angeles. Her research explores the relationship between rhetoric, civic life, and social change. She is especially interested in the embodied rhetorics of feminism and queer politics, and the controversies these rhetorics incite. Her work appears in *Communication and Critical/Cultural Studies, Feminist Media Studies,* and *Text and Performance Quarterly,* among others. She is currently completing a book manuscript on the embodied rhetorics of U.S. feminism that explores the role of body politics in democratic public cultures.

ERIN J. RAND is assistant professor in the Department of Communication and Rhetorical Studies at Syracuse University. Her work theorizes resistance and rhetorical agency in activist and social movement discourses through contemporary rhetorical theory and criticism, as well as feminist and queer theories. She has published essays in journals such as the *Quarterly Journal of Speech, Communication and Critical/Cultural Studies,* and *Rhetoric and Public Affairs.*

KENNETH RUFO is a stay-at-home father and an independent media scholar living in the wild outskirts of Seattle, where he survives by harvesting books and hunting video game.

GUST A. YEP is professor of Communication Studies at San Francisco State University. His research focuses on communication at the intersections of culture, race, class, gender, sexuality, and nation. He is the author of more than sixty articles in various inter/disciplinary journals and anthologies and the author/editor of three books, including *Queer Theory and Communication.* In addition to serving as the editor of the National Communication Association Non-serial Publication Program (2005–2008), he is the recipient of several teaching, mentoring, research, and community service awards at the university, local community, regional, and national levels.